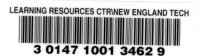

DATE DUE

Neonatal Jaundice

Monographs in Clinical Pediatrics

This series is one for all professionals concerned with child health and disease. It covers a number of clinically relevant topics, with each monograph dealing with a specific theme or disease entity. Volumes are oriented towards practical aspects of clinical pediatrics, but contain sufficient basic science to enable the reader to understand the logical basis of the subject under discussion. Common clinical problems are covered and controversies highlighted, providing authoritative guidance for the investigation and management of diseases seen in pediatric practice.

Series Editor

Philip Lanzkowsky, MD, FRCP, DCH, FAAP
Schneider Children's Hospital of Long Island Jewish Medical Center,
New Hyde Park, New York, USA

This book is part of a series. The publisher will accept continuation orders which may be cancelled at any time and which provide for automatic billing and shipping of each title in the series upon publication. Please write for details.

Neonatal Jaundice

Edited by

M. Jeffrey Maisels

Chairman, Department of Pediatrics
William Beaumont Hospital
Royal Oak, Michigan, USA

and

Jon F. Watchko

Chief, Division of Neonatology and Developmental Biology
University of Pittsburgh School of Medicine
Pittsburgh, Pennsylvania, USA

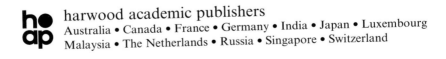
harwood academic publishers
Australia • Canada • France • Germany • India • Japan • Luxembourg
Malaysia • The Netherlands • Russia • Singapore • Switzerland

Amsteldijk 166
1st Floor
1079 LH Amsterdam
The Netherlands

British Library Cataloguing in Publication Data

Neonatal jaundice. – (Monographs in clinical pediatrics;
   v. 11)
   1. Jaundice, Neonatal   2. Jaundice, Neonatal – Diagnosis
   3. Jaundice, Neonatal – Treatment
   I. Maisels, M. Jeffrey   II. Watchko, Jon F.
   618.9'2'01

   ISBN: 90-5702-626-0
   ISSN: 1044-4882

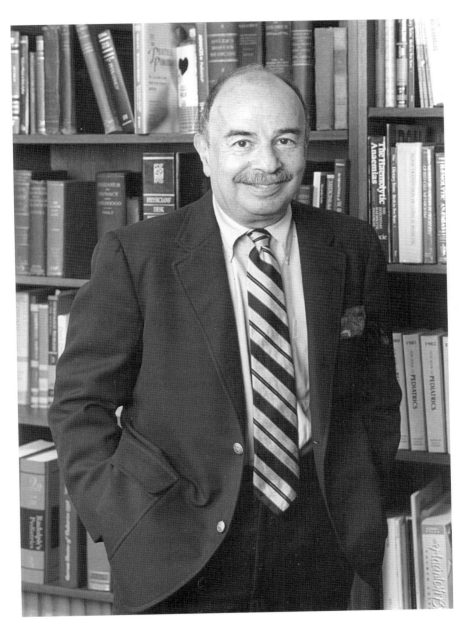

Frank A. Oski
1932–1996

Contents

Clinical Management

Preface

Although it is 150 years since Hervieux made neonatal jaundice the subject of his doctoral thesis, there is no indication that the problem has disappeared. If anything, the advent of short hospital stays following birth has both complicated and exacerbated the issue for the clinician and, in view of the many advances made over the last two decades, we felt that a volume was needed to bring together the relevant basic science and clinical information necessary for managing the jaundiced newborn. We are fortunate to have had the help of outstanding contributors, each of whom has made major contributors to the field and we have called on their considerable knowledge and experience to create a book that can serve as a reference for the investigator and the clinician.

We have come a long way in the last 20–30 years but not withstanding the enormous amount of clinical and basic research that has been devoted to this remarkably common problem, much is to be learned. For example, we have yet to fully understand the pathophysiology of bilirubin toxicity and we still have a long way to go before we are able to identify from the myriad of normal babies in our nurseries, which of them is likely to develop extreme hyperbilirubinemia and run the risk of developing kernicterus.

But there have been many exciting advances as well. An understanding of the pathways of heme catabolism and the potential for the inhibition of heme oxygenase production has produced a pharmacologic intervention that decreases bilirubin production, and the characterization of UDPGT gene has allowed us to identify the relevant mutations responsible for the inborn errors of bilirubin metabolism. The latter work has led to the recognition that Gilbert's disease, previously thought to be a condition that affects only those beyond their adolescent years, actually contributes to neonatal jaundice.

This mutation also interacts with other genetic defects such as G6PD deficiency and congenital spherocytosis to produce hyperbilirubinemia. Even more exciting is the potential for genetic therapy in the management of defects such as Crigler-Najjar syndrome. Unfortunately, space restrictions prevented us from dealing with the subject of cholestatic jaundice and the important topic of the laboratory measurement of bilirubin.

Finally we would like to dedicate this volume to the memory of Frank A. Oski, MD, a mentor, colleague and friend to both of us. Perhaps the foremost clinical scholar of pediatrics in our era, Frank had an abiding curiosity about the subject of neonatal jaundice, and challenged the pediatric community to think critically about the evaluation and management of these newborns. We are grateful for his vision, his provocative contributions to the debate and his lifetime of service to pediatrics and the newborn. We were privileged to have known and worked with him and will always remember his kind and gentle manner, his complete absence of pretension, his friendship and support, and his unyielding spirit of inquiry. We will not see his like again.

M. Jeffrey Maisels
Jon F. Watchko

Contributors

Mamdouha Ahdab-Barmada
The WHY-NMD Institute for the Study
  of Neuromuscular Disorders
Pittsburgh, Pennsylvania
USA

John M. Bowman
Department of Pediatrics and Child
  Health
Faculty of Medicine
University of Manitoba
Winnipeg, MN
Canada

Thor Willy Ruud Hansen
Section on Neonatology
Department of Pediatrics
Rikshospitalet, Oslo
Norway

M. Jeffrey Maisels
Department of Pediatrics
William Beaumont Hospital
Royal Oak, Michigan
USA

Steven M. Shapiro
Division of Child Neurology
Medical College of Virginia
Richmond, Virginia
USA

Timos Valaes
Department of Pediatrics
Tufts University School of Medicine
Boston, Massachusetts
USA

Jon F. Watchko
Division of Neonatology and
  Developmental Biology
Department of Pediatrics
University of Pittsburgh School of
  Medicine
Pittsburgh, Pennsylvania
USA

Metabolism

1 Fetal and Neonatal Bilirubin Metabolism

Thor Willy Ruud Hansen

Section on Neonatology, Department of Pediatrics, Rikshospitalet, Oslo, Norway

THE METABOLISM OF HEME AND BILIRUBIN IN THE FETUS

Bilirubin Formation and Conjugation in the Fetus

Bilirubin is formed in the organism through oxidation-reduction reactions as the end product of heme catabolism (Figure 1.1). Hemoglobin is the main source, but myoglobin, cytochrome, and catalase also contribute. Beginning in the yolk sac, production of erythrocytes is first observed in the fetus at 2–3 weeks of gestation. It enters the hepatic phase at about 6 weeks and the marrow phase at 20 weeks of gestation.[1] The mean life span of red cells in the newborn infant has been estimated to be between 45–90 days.[2] The life span of red cells in early fetal life has not been determined, but values in premature infants appear to be approximately 35–50 days.[2]

Heme oxygenase is found in several tissues, with significant levels in the liver, spleen, and erythropoietic tissue. In the fetus, hepatic microsomal heme oxygenase activity has been measured to be eight times higher than in adult liver.[3] Heme oxygenase activity is necessary for the conversion of heme to biliverdin, and therefore must be present by the time bilirubin appears in the human fetus at 14 weeks gestation as the IXβ isomer.[4] Two weeks later unconjugated bilirubin-IXα appears in bile. By 20 weeks of gestation IXα constitutes 6% of bilirubin in bile, IXβ 87%, IXγ 0.5%, and IXδ 6%.[5] By 38 weeks gestation bilirubin-IXα has replaced IXβ as the main isomer[4] (Table 1.1).

In umbilical vein blood samples obtained from non-immunized fetuses total bilirubin concentrations increased from a mean of $\approx$25 µmol/l (1.5 mg/dl) at 20 weeks of gestation to $\approx$30 µmol/l (1.8 mg/dl) near term.[6] The production rate of bilirubin at term has been calculated to about 8.5 mg/kg/day, which is more than double the rate in adults.[7]

Odell investigated the activity of glucuronyl transferase in liver from fetuses at 20–23 weeks gestational age and found this to be approximately 1/3 of adult values.[8]

Address for correspondence: Thor Willy Ruud Hansen, M.D., Ph.D., Section on Neonatology, Department of Pediatrics, Rikshospitalet, N-0027 Oslo, NORWAY, Phone: 011-47-22868942, Fax: 011-47-22422822, E-mail: t.w.r.hansen@klinmed.uio.no

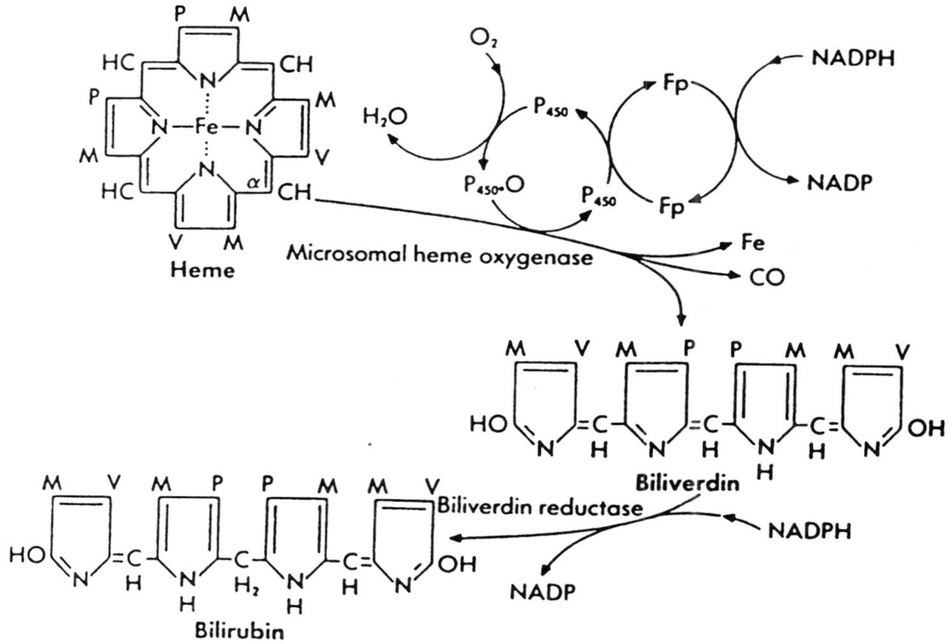

Figure 1.1. Formation of biliverdin and unconjugated bilirubin from heme, in a planar presentation. From Tenhunen *et al.*,[140] with permission.

Table 1.1. Time course of formation of bilirubin* isomers, conjugates, and glucuronosyl transferase activity in the human fetus and newborn.

Weeks of gestation	Bilirubin isomers	Bilirubin conjugates	Glucuronosyl transferase activity
14	IXβ appears		
16	IXα appears		0.1% of adult
20	IXβ predominant	IXα glycosyl conjugates appear	
22–23		Monoglucuronide appears	
30			
38–40	IXα predominant	IXα monoglucuronide predominant	1% of adult
Age 2–3 months			Adult levels
Adult		IXα diglucuronide predominant	

 * Data from references 4, 9–12.

Kawade and Onishi[9] found considerably lower activities, from 0.1% at 16–32 weeks increasing to ≈1% of adult values at term (Figure 1.2). Conjugated bile pigments have been found in the liver of fetuses with Rhesus incompatibility.[10] Bilirubin IXα glycosyl conjugates appear in human fetal bile at 20 weeks gestation, while monoglucuronide is first seen 2–3 weeks later.[4] From 30 weeks monoconjugates of bilirubin IXα are the predominant bilirubins in human fetal bile, but only at term is

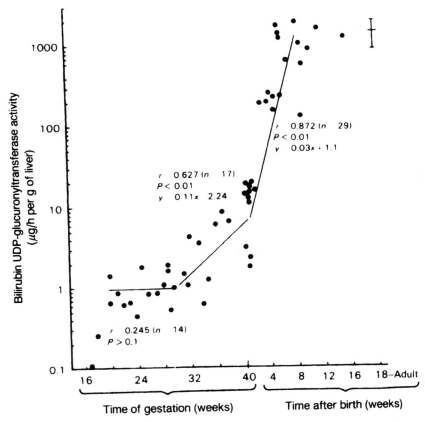

Figure 1.2. Developmental pattern of human hepatic uridine diphosphoglucuronosyl transferase (UDPGT) activity. Samples were obtained from fetal livers after elective abortion, at autopsy from premature and term infants surviving <7 days, and from liver biopsies of infants, children, and adults undergoing laparotomy. Each point represents a single patient, except patients 18 weeks and older, which are represented with the mean ± SD. From Kawade *et al.,*[9] with permission.

bilirubin-IXα monoglucuronide the major pigment present.[4,11] In adults bile contains an average 80% bilirubin-IX diglucuronide (Table 1.1) and 18% monoglucuronide.[12] Bilirubin metabolism must of necessity be different in the fetus compared to the situation after birth. Conjugation and excretion into bile is of limited use as long as bowel contents cannot be evacuated, although an amount of bilirubin equal to between 5–10 times daily production has been estimated to be present in meconium at birth.[13] Further, conversion of bilirubin into water-soluble isomers or conjugates would prevent the transfer of bilirubin across the placenta into the maternal circulation and thus limit excretion.

There appears to be marked species differences in fetal handling of bilirubin,[14] suggesting caution when extrapolating from animal data to the human situation. Thus, while fetal dog and sheep liver excrete about 50% of injected radiolabeled bilirubin as conjugates, fetal monkey liver excretes only about 5% of the dose, and very little as conjugates.[15–17] In rats monoconjugates appear in the intestines on fetal day 18, while diconjugates show up two days later.[18] On day 18, 80% of intestinal bilirubin is unconjugated, while from day 20 the conjugated pigment predominates. Thus, in this species there appears to be a rapid development of the conjugation mechanisms in the last few days of fetal life.

Ligandin, which is responsible for binding bilirubin in the hepatocytes, belongs to the glutathione S-transferases. The activity of glutathione S-transferase in fetal rat liver is <5% of adult values on day 16 of pregnancy and ~10% on day 20, using dinitrobenzene as substrate.[19] In fetal monkey liver ligandin is found in reduced amounts.[20] In human fetal livers basic monomers of glutathione S-transferase are present in the cytosol at 21 weeks gestation, while near-neutral isoenzymes do not appear until 30 weeks.[21]

Bilirubin Formation in Fetal Hemolytic Disease

Hemolysis may occur in the fetus in the presence of maternal red blood cell allo-immunization. In this situation the concentration of total bilirubin in serum may increase from ~25 μmol/l (1.5 mg/dl) at 20 weeks of gestation to ~70 μmol/l (4.1 mg/dl) at 32 weeks, and an inverse relationship is seen between total bilirubin and hemoglobin concentrations.[6] In fetuses who developed a hematocrit <30%, 82% had total serum bilirubin (TSB) concentrations that exceeded the 97.5 percentile. The increase in TSB was detectable weeks before anemia developed, and a TSB of >50 μmol/l (3 mg/dl) was associated with a high risk of severe antenatal anemia. Goodrum *et al.* examined the effect of repeated intrauterine transfusions in red cell alloimmunization and found a mean total serum bilirubin value of ~95 μmol/l (5.6 mg/dl, range 22–185 μmol/l [1.3–10.8 mg/dl]) at the time of the third transfusion, almost all of which was unconjugated.[22] This shows that in spite of the ability of bilirubin to pass the placenta, fetal hemolytic disease is associated with some degree of fetal hyperbilirubinemia. Although some of this bilirubin is conjugated and thus not able to cross the placenta, the major fraction is unconjugated.[22,23] One must therefore assume that the placenta has a finite capacity for transfer of bilirubin, and that this capacity is exceeded in fetal hemolytic disease.

BILIRUBIN METABOLISM AND THE MATERNAL-FETAL DYAD

Bilirubin Transfer and Metabolism in the Placenta

Unconjugated bilirubin in the mammalian fetus can be disposed of either by crossing the placenta into the maternal circulation, or by passing through the fetal liver and being excreted into the fetal bile. Placental membranes are essentially impermeable to polar compounds such as biliverdin and bilirubin conjugates, but nonpolar compounds such as unconjugated bilirubin can diffuse across.[24] The rhesus monkey placenta is structurally quite similar to that in humans, and is a major site of bilirubin excretion in the fetus. Bernstein *et al.* infused radiolabeled unconjugated bilirubin into rhesus monkey fetuses and found that more than 50% was transferred intact across the placenta and was eventually excreted in maternal bile, while only 3–6% was found in fetal bile.[25] Bashore *et al.* gave bilirubin IV to pregnant monkeys and found that it transferred rapidly to the fetus.[26] There was also a rapid transfer of bilirubin into and removal from the amniotic fluid. Rosenthal compared serum bilirubin in samples from umbilical artery and vein as well as from maternal serum.[27] The umbilical artery contained bilirubin in a concentration nearly twice that of umbilical vein, clearly showing that bilirubin is cleared quite efficiently from fetal blood when it passes through the placenta. The transplacental gradient of bilirubin from fetus to mother was ~10:1 in Rosenthal's study, while Monte *et al.* found a gradient of ~5:1.[28]

Bilirubin in the Amniotic Fluid

Bilirubin has been found in amniotic fluid from the 12th week of gestation, but gradually disappears as the volume of amniotic fluid increases, and under normal circumstances the amniotic fluid near term does not contain measurable bilirubin.[29] Studies in rhesus monkeys appear to show that bilirubin can enter the amniotic fluid from the maternal circulation.[26] Bilirubin was first found in the amniotic fluid in cases of Rhesus immunization.[30] The levels of amniotic fluid bilirubin were subsequently shown to correlate with the degree of fetal affection.[31] As amniotic fluid is primarily a fetal product, it is thought that bilirubin in this fluid most likely comes from the fetus itself. Fetal tracheal and pulmonary secretions containing bilirubin are possible sources.[32] The fetus swallows significant amounts of amniotic fluid, and it has been speculated that this ingested bilirubin may be absorbed across the intestinal mucosa and excreted by the mother.[33] This might explain why elevated levels of bilirubin may be seen in the amniotic fluid of fetuses with anencephaly or high intestinal obstructions, i.e. whose with compromised swallowing mechanisms.

Maternal Hyperbilirubinemia and the Fetus

Medical literature contains a few reports concerning infants who *in utero* have been exposed to significant maternal hyperbilirubinemia. Furhoff reported on the outcomes of 133 children born to 58 women with jaundice in pregnancy due to cholestasis or hepatitis.[34] None of these children appear to have suffered neurologic sequelae. However, the report does not mention maternal or infant serum bilirubin levels, and the follow-up was limited to an interview in which the mothers described their children as "healthy". It is likely that most of these mothers had mainly conjugated hyperbilirubinemia, where due to the water-soluble nature of the molecule little transfer to the fetus may have taken place. Because of the limited scope of the follow-up, developmental and/or neurologic problems may well have been missed. Similar limitations apply to a report on 49 cases of jaundice in pregnancy by Roszkowski and Pisarek-Miedzinska.[35]

Waffarn *et al.*[36] described an infant born at 37 weeks to a mother with end-stage liver disease who on the day before delivery had a TSB of ~500 µmol/l (29 mg/dl) with an unconjugated fraction of ~220 μmol/l (13 mg/dl). Cord venous TSB levels were ~320 μmol/l (19 mg/dl) and ~185 μmol/l (11 mg/dl) for total and unconjugated bilirubin respectively. The infant exhibited significant neurological symptoms in the first days of life, and needed several exchange transfusions. However, follow-up examinations into the second year of life showed normal neurological and developmental outcome. Patients with Crigler–Najjar syndrome have life-long, severe, unconjugated hyperbilirubinemia.[37,38] An infant born post-term to a mother with this disorder had a cord TSB of 410 μmol/l (24.0 mg/dl) of which 217 μmol/l (12.7 mg/dl) was unconjugated and received phototherapy for 24 h with good response in the newborn period.[39] The initial neurological evaluation was normal, but follow-up at 18 months revealed evolving quadriplegia. In light of the limited duration of a moderate unconjugated hyperbilirubinemia after birth, it seems possible that the sequelae in this child may have been related to prolonged exposure to hyperbilirubinemia *in utero*. In a similar case reported by Smith and Baker maternal hyperbilirubinemia reached a maximum of 150 μmol/l (8.8 mg/dl) in the third trimester, with an umbilical cord bilirubin of 130 μmol/l (7.6 mg/dl) at birth. Jaundice in the infant resolved without need for treatment and apparently without sequelae.[40]

In an experimental study Yeary performed bile duct ligation in pregnant heterozygous Gunn rats.[41] One group had daily IP injections of bilirubin from day 9 through 15 of pregnancy, the others served as controls. The unconjugated hyperbilirubinemia induced by bilirubin injections was associated with significant embryotoxicity, while conjugated hyperbilirubinemia due to bile duct ligation had no effect on fetal survival. This supports a body of other data suggesting that unconjugated bilirubin is toxic while water-soluble isomers are not.

BILIRUBIN METABOLISM IN THE NEONATE

Bilirubin Production

Degradation of heme from red cells, as well as from muscle myoglobin, and certain liver enzymes such as cytochromes and catalases results, through the intermediary step of biliverdin, in the production of bilirubin[42] (Figures 1.1 and 1.3). Carbon monoxide, which is a byproduct of this process, can be measured in exhaled breath and provides an estimate of bilirubin production.[7,43,44] Based on such measurements bilirubin production in the neonate has been estimated to be ~8.5 mg/kg/day, which is more than double the production rate in adults.[7] The breakdown of certain hepatic microsomal cytochromes does not yield CO,[45] so the above estimate may slightly understate the real production rate.

The first step in the breakdown of heme is catalyzed by heme oxygenase (Figure 1.1), an enzyme which is found in the reticuloendothelial system, but also in tissue macrophages and in gut mucosa.[46,47] The subsequent step, reduction at the central C-10 carbon of biliverdin $IX\alpha$ to bilirubin $IX\alpha$ takes place in the cytosol and is catalyzed by biliverdin reductase.[48] Both of these processes are dependent on NADPH. Bilirubin $IX\alpha$ in the serum of humans occurs almost exclusively at the

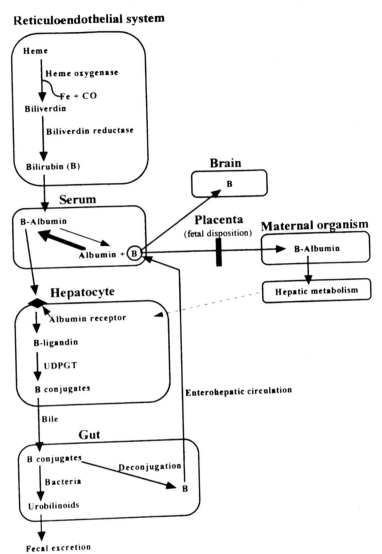

Figure 1.3. Schematic illustration of bilirubin metabolism in fetal and neonatal life. Bilirubin is formed in the reticuloendothelial system from heme through reactions catabolized by heme oxygenase and biliverdin reductase. In serum bilirubin is transported bound to albumin, but a minor fraction is unbound ("free") and can cross the blood–brain barrier or (in the fetus) the placental barrier. In the liver albumin is bound to a receptor on the surface of the hepatocyte. Bilirubin is transported into the cell and bound to ligandin. UDP-glucuronyl transferase (UDPGT) catabolizes the conversion of bilirubin to a water-soluble form through binding to one or two molecules of glucuronic acid, forming bilirubin conjugates. Excreted in the bile, these conjugates are subsequently transformed to urobilinoids through bacterial action. Conjugated bilirubin may also undergo de-conjugation and the unconjugated bilirubin can then be reabsorbed into the circulation (enterohepatic circulation). B, bilirubin; Fe, Iron; CO, carbon monoxide; UDPGT, uridine diphosphate glucuronyl transferase.

(4Z,15Z) isomer where the presence of intramolecular hydrogen bonds between the side groups (Z = zusammen) makes the molecule almost insoluble in water.[49] A schematic illustration of the pathways of bilirubin metabolism is given in Figure 1.3.

Transport and Protein Binding

Unconjugated bilirubin is transported in plasma bound to albumin with a binding affinity of $10^7-10^8 \, M^{-1}$ at the primary binding site.[50] However, there is also a secondary binding site on albumin where bilirubin is bound with lower affinity.[50–54] Because of the relatively high affinity of albumin for bilirubin, equilibrium concentrations of free or unbound bilirubin in plasma are only in the low nanomolar range even in the presence of significant hyperbilirubinemia.[50,55–57] However, once the molar concentration of bilirubin exceeds that of albumin the primary binding site becomes saturated and free bilirubin concentrations may increase significantly.[56] The binding of bilirubin to albumin increases with postnatal age,[58–60] but is reduced in sick infants[58,61] and in the presence of exogenous or endogenous binding competitors.[62–65]

In addition to albumin, bilirubin can also bind to other proteins (e.g., α-fetoprotein and ligandin),[67–69] as well as to lipoproteins,[70–71] and to erythrocytes.[72,73] Data suggest that lysine is involved in bilirubin binding both to albumin and ligandin, and possibly also to other proteins.[74–82] Indeed, recent findings suggest that binding to lysine may play a role in the mediation or modulation of bilirubin toxicity.[82]

Uptake, Conjugation, and Excretion of Bilirubin in Hepatocytes

When the bilirubin–albumin complex passes through the hepatic circulation and comes into contact with the hepatocytes, bilirubin, but not albumin, is transported into the cell. This process may be carrier mediated.[83] Newer data suggest that three different transport proteins may be implicated.[84–86] These transport systems appear to be dominant at different substrate concentrations and to have different driving forces. Binding of albumin to the hepatocyte surface was believed to be mediated by a receptor.[87] Newer data make that concept more controversial.[84–86] It has been suggested that the apparent receptor effect may derive from the presence of clusters of membrane proteins with high affinities for specific classes of ligands.[84] These protein clusters are thought to be located in the sinusoidal liver cell plasma membrane.

Within the hepatocyte ~60% of bilirubin is found in the cytosol and ~25% in microsomes.[88] The principal intracellular binding protein is ligandin, a glutathione S-transferase.[89–91] Uptake of bilirubin into hepatocytes seems to increase with increasing concentrations of ligandin.[83] Ligandin contains two binding sites for bilirubin, one with high ($Ka = 5 \times 10^7 \, M^{-1}$) and one with lower ($Ka = 3 \times 10^5 \, M^{-1}$) affinity.[92] The high affinity site is not identical to the binding site for catalytic activity, but binding to the low affinity site is associated with competitive inhibition of the enzymatic activity of ligandin.[92,93] As mentioned, lysine appears to be involved in the binding of bilirubin to ligandin. In monkeys ligandin concentrations in the liver are low at birth, but appear to reach adult values within 1–2 weeks.[94] The concentration of ligandin in hepatocytes can be increased by pharmacologic agents such as phenobarbital.[83]

Glucuronyl transferase (UDP glucuronate β-glucuronosyl transferase EC 2.4.1.17) catalyzes the binding first of one molecule of glucuronic acid to bilirubin, thus forming bilirubin monoglucuronide. This process takes place in the endoplasmic reticulum of the microsomes.[13] Conversion to diglucuronide is believed to occur at the cell membrane, thus possibly facilitating transfer of the diglucuronide from liver to bile.[95] Bilirubin-UDP-glucuronyl transferase in humans is a tetramer with molecular weight 209 kD.[96] Whereas the monomer can convert unconjugated bilirubin to the monoglucuronide, the tetramer appears to be required to convert the monogluc-uronide to the diglucuronide.[96] The importance of this process is that the essentially water-insoluble unconjugated bilirubin is converted to a water soluble form which can be excreted in the bile. Conjugation of bilirubin in the liver is controlled by a gene complex on chromosome 2, at 2q37.[97] Mutations and amino acid substitutions are responsible for genetic errors in bilirubin conjugation such as the Crigler–Najjar syndrome types 1 and 2, and Gilbert's disease (see Chapter 4).

The activity of glucuronyl transferase increases one hundred-fold after birth and reaches adult values by 4–8 weeks of age.[9] Premature birth accelerates the development of glucuronyl transferase activity in human liver.[9] The two isomeric mono-conjugates appear in serum during the first 1–2 days of life in both premature and term infants, followed by the diconjugate on the third day.[98] In the first days of life conjugated bilirubin constitutes <2% of total bile pigment in serum, well below the 3.6% documented in adults.[99] However, because of the higher total bilirubin concentration in neonates, the absolute concentrations of conjugates are 2- to 6-fold higher than in adults. Diconjugates constitute only 20% of the total conjugated fraction in contrast to a mean of 54% in adults.[99] In the hepatocyte both mono- and diconjugated bilirubin remain bound to ligandin.[91]

Administration of phenobarbital to the pregnant woman antenatally increases conjugation in the neonate.[100] For this reason phenobarbital has been used both ante-natally and postnatally for prevention and/or treatment of neonatal jaundice.[101–103] Increased glucuronyl transferase activity is also seen following administration of a thyroid analog,[104] dexamethasone,[105] and clofibrate.[106]

The organism can excrete heme directly in bile,[107] a phenomenon which is currently being exploited in the prevention and treatment of neonatal jaundice through the use of metal meso- and protoporphyrins,[108,109] inhibitors of heme oxygenase. However, direct excretion of heme in the bile would result in the loss of iron, whereas conversion of heme to biliverdin conserves this valuable resource for the body. Biliverdin can also be excreted in bile,[110] and although it makes sense for the fetus to reduce biliverdin to bilirubin which can cross the placenta, it is something of a biological puzzle why we continue after birth to produce and excrete potentially toxic bilirubin rather than stop the process at non-toxic biliverdin. Birds appear to lack biliverdin reductase in their reticuloendothelial system and thus excrete biliverdin rather than bilirubin.[48] The recent discovery that bilirubin is a free radical quencher could possibly be a piece in this puzzle.[111]

As mentioned above, the last step of the bilirubin conjugation process takes place at the cell membrane.[95] Excretion of conjugated bilirubin into bile then takes place against a concentration gradient, and thus necessarily must be an energy requiring process. In rabbits excretion of conjugated bilirubin into bile is enhanced by IV infusion of glucose.[112] Clearance of bilirubin from the hepatocyte is a saturable process, and after the first week of life appears to be the rate-limiting step in the excretion of bilirubin.[113,114] The excretory transport maximum can be increased by drugs that stimulate bile flow, such as e.g., barbiturates.[13]

In addition to the normal metabolic pathways for bilirubin disposition through the liver, alternate pathways may also exist. In Gunn rats treatment with dioxins results in the excretion of polar bilirubin metabolites in the liver, probably through induction of cytochrome P450-dependent oxygenases in the microsomal fraction.[115,116] Recent data suggest that both hemin, bilirubin, and biliverdin can activate the aryl hydrocarbon receptor which in turn activates hepatic CYP1A1 gene expression.[117] Thus, there is evidence that hemin, biliverdin, and bilirubin can induce an alternative pathway in bilirubin metabolism. The importance of such pathways in human infants is not currently known. However, a study of indole-3-carbinol, a constituent of cruciferous vegetables, is now underway in Crigler–Najjar type I patients.[86] When used enterally in Gunn rats and two patients with Crigler–Najjar syndrome, this compound resulted in a 60% decrease in serum unconjugated bilirubin levels.[86]

MECHANISMS OF PHYSIOLOGIC JAUNDICE

Almost every newborn infant will develop a serum unconjugated bilirubin $>30\,\mu mol/l$ (1.8 mg/dl) during the first week of life.[118–120] The incidence of significant neonatal jaundice varies between populations and geographic locations. Some of the reasons for these differences are known. For example significant neonatal jaundice occurs more frequently in populations with a high incidence of G6PD deficiency.[121–123] The incidence of neonatal jaundice is increased in populations living at high altitudes, presumably due to the increased red cell mass.[124,125] On the other hand, the reason for the increased incidence of newborn hyperbilirubinemia in certain regions of Greece compared to Greek infants born elsewhere is not fully known.[126]

Because of these differences, and because definitions of "significant jaundice" vary, precise numbers for the incidence of neonatal jaundice cannot be given. However, a few epidemiological studies will be cited to provide a frame of reference. In a study of 2416 well infants Maisels and Gifford found that 6.1% had serum bilirubin levels $>220\,\mu mol/l$ (12.9 mg/dl).[127] Moore *et al.* examined newborns at 3100 m altitude in Colorado and found that 32.7% had serum bilirubin levels $>205\,\mu mol/l$ (12 mg/dl).[124] Palmer and Drew reviewed 41,000 live births (including preterm and sick infants) and found that 10.7% of the infants had serum bilirubin values $>154\,\mu mol/l$ (9 mg/dl).[128] Thus it is clear that jaundice is a very common phenomenon in neonates and, due to the potential for neurotoxicity, a very frequent reason for clinical concern and investigation. The course of hyperbilirubinemia in neonates is affected significantly by both the method of feeding and the infant's race (see Chapter 3). In general, the bilirubin level peaks between the 3rd and 5th days of life and declines thereafter.

The term physiologic jaundice describes the occurrence of jaundice in newborns due to the normal occurrences of increased breakdown of red blood cells in the presence of a low capacity for uptake, conjugation and excretion of bilirubin in the liver, as well as reabsorption of bilirubin from the gut due to relatively low nutrient intake and thus reduced intestinal transit in the first days of life. However, one should note that the distinction between physiologic and pathologic jaundice in newborns is often not clear cut, and that each of the normally occurring mechanisms that produce hyperbilirubinemia may be exaggerated by both endogenous and exogenous factors. In the following the various steps in the metabolism of bilirubin in the neonate will be discussed briefly.

Increased Heme Catabolism

In order to provide sufficient oxygen carrying capacity the fetus utilizes a hemoglobin that is structurally different from the one formed in postnatal life, and also generates a higher hemoglobin concentration. After birth the infant no longer needs these mechanisms to provide a sufficient oxygen supply to its tissues. Production of adult hemoglobin starts and the high hemoglobin concentration is no longer needed. Catabolism of fetal erythrocytes results in a production of bilirubin which is at least twice that of adults on a per kilogram basis.[7] This aspect of bilirubin metabolism may become an important contributor to pathologic jaundice in the neonate. Thus, hemolysis may be increased above normal in various types of congenital hemolytic anemias, in immunological conditions such as maternal-fetal blood group incompatibilities, and due to drugs or toxins. Red cell survival may also be shortened by infections or bruising/hematomas. Splenic and hepatic heme oxygenase activities increase in response to hemolysis and fasting.[129] On the other hand heme oxygenase may be inhibited by a number of metal meso- and protoporphyrins, a phenomenon which is currently under investigation from a therapeutic perspective.[108,109,130]

Decreased Hepatic Uptake, Conjugation, and Excretion of Bilirubin

Bromosulfophthalein clearance data suggest that a deficiency in the uptake mechanism for bilirubin may exist in the immature organism.[131] No further details as far as the specifics of this phenomenon appear to be available. Estrogens stimulate the uptake of bromosulfophthalein and bilirubin in adult rats.[132,133] This could possibly explain why females normally have lower plasma bilirubin levels than males.[134] However, there appear to be no data in the literature that specifically address the influences of estrogen on these mechanisms in the newborn infant.

The neonate is deficient in ligandin, the hepatocellular binding protein for bilirubin. This may decrease the ability to retain bilirubin inside the hepatocyte and consequently may cause bilirubin to reflux into the circulation. The concentration of ligandin can be increased by drug therapy pre- or postnatally. There is no evidence that deficiency of ligandin beyond the physiological is implicated in pathological jaundice. It is generally accepted that the human neonate has a deficiency of UDP-glucuronyl transferase.[13] At birth UDPGT activities are $\sim$1% of adult values.[9] The activity increases in the first weeks of life and reaches adult values at 14 weeks of age. Conjugation appears to be the rate-limiting step in bilirubin metabolism in the first 3–4 days of life. In the next few days hepatic uptake and excretion are limiting, and during the rest of life excretion is the rate-limiting step.

Increased Enterohepatic Circulation

Fluid and nutrient intake is limited in the newborn until breast milk production is established. Thus there is a lack of a binding vehicle in the intestinal lumen to transport bilirubin conjugates through the gut. Deconjugation occurs in the gut lumen, probably through the action of a β-glucuronidase,[13] and unconjugated bilirubin may be reabsorbed through the intestinal mucosa (Figure 1.3). The infant is born with a sterile gut, and the intestinal microbial flora which normally contributes to further break-down of bilirubin is established during the first days and weeks of life. This phenomenon tends to make more bilirubin available for reabsorption from the gut. Meconium also contains a significant amount of bilirubin, estimated to be as much as 5 to 10 times the daily production.[13] Half of this is unconjugated and thus capable of being reabsorbed.

Enterohepatic circulation is enhanced by any condition associated with delayed or interrupted passage of intestinal contents. This is evident in intestinal atresias,[135] in infants kept off oral feeds for reasons of severe illness, and in infants receiving inadequate nutrition due to difficulties in establishing lactation ("lack-of-breast-milk jaundice"). It is also possible that increased enterohepatic circulation is involved in so called breast milk jaundice.[13] On the other hand, enterohepatic circulation is reduced following the successful establishment of enteral nutrition, by increasing the frequency of feeding,[136] by oral feeding of agar which tends to bind bilirubin in the gut,[137] and by oral administration of bilirubin oxidase.[138,139]

CONCLUSION

Bilirubin metabolism undergoes significant changes during fetal and neonatal life. This applies both to the isomers that predominate and to the processes involved in uptake into the hepatocyte, binding and conjugation inside the hepatocyte, and excretion into the bile. Several steps in the process that causes neonatal jaundice can be modulated both by endogenous (e.g., hormones) and exogenous (e.g., drugs) compounds. Drugs that increase the concentration of ligandin or the activity of bilirubin UDP-glucuronyl transferase are well documented, but appear not to be widely used. Drugs that limit bilirubin production by inhibiting heme oxygenase are undergoing trials, but their eventual place in the routine management of neonatal jaundice remains to be determined. Natural compounds that stimulate alternate pathways for hepatic bilirubin metabolism may provide a therapeutic option for patients with

Crigler–Najjar type I, but much work will be required to bring this beyond the experimental stage. Enterohepatic circulation contributes to neonatal jaundice, and is also amenable to therapeutic intervention by formula feeds or other bilirubin binding or degrading agents.

References

1. Sieff, C.A. and Nathan, D.G., The anatomy and physiology of hematopoiesis. In: Nathan, D.G. and Oski F.A., eds. Hematology of infancy and childhood. Philadelphia: WB Saunders Company, 1993, pp. 156–215.
2. Oski, F.A., The erythrocyte and its disorders. In: Nathan, D.G. and Oski, F.A., eds. Hematology of infancy and childhood. Philadelphia: WB Saunders Company, 1993, pp. 18–43.
3. Abraham, N.G., Lin, J.H., Mitrione, S.M., Schwartzman, M.L., Lever, R.D. and Shibahara, S. Expression of heme oxygenase gene in rat and human liver, *Biochem. Biophys. Res. Commun.* 1988; **150**: 717–722.
4. Blumenthal, S.G., Taggart, D.B., Rasmussen, R.D., Ikeda, R.M. and Ruebner, B.H., Conjugated and unconjugated bilirubins in humans and rhesus monkeys: structural identity of bilirubins from biles and meconiums of newborn humans and rhesus monkeys, *Biochem. J.* 1979; **179**: 537–547.
5. Yamaguchi, T. and Nakajima, H., Changes in the composition of bilirubin-IXα isomers during human prenatal development, *Eur. J. Biochem.* 1995; **233**: 467–472.
6. Weiner, C.P., Human fetal bilirubin levels and fetal hemolytic disease, *Am. J. Obstet. Gynecol.* 1992; **166**: 1449–1454.
7. Maisels, M.J., Pathak, A., Nelson, N.M., Nathan, D.G. and Smith, C.A., Endogenous production of carbon monoxide in normal and erythroblastotic newborn infants, *J. Clin. Invest.* 1971; **50**: 1–8.
8. Odell, G.B., Neonatal jaundice. In: Popper, H. Schaffner, F., eds. Progress in Liver Diseases, Volume 5. New York: Grune & Stratton, 1976, pp. 457–475.
9. Kawade, N. and Onishi, S., The prenatal and postnatal development of UDP-glucuronyl transferase activity towards bilirubin and the effect of premature birth on this activity in the human liver, *Biochem. J.* 1981; **196**: 257–260.
10. De Wolf-Peeters, C., Moens-Bullens, A.M., Van Assche, A. and Desmet, V., Conjugated bilirubin in foetal liver in erythroblastosis, *Lancet* 1969; **1**: 471.
11. Blumenthal, S.G., Stucker, T., Rasmussen, R.D., Ikeda, R.M., Ruebner, B.H., Bergstrom, D.E. and Hanson, F.W., Changes in bilirubins in human prenatal development, *Biochem. J.* 1980; **186**: 693–700.
12. Fevery, J.M., Van de Vijver, M., Michiels, R., De Groote, J. and Heirwegh, K.P.M., Comparison in different species of biliary bilirubin-IXα conjugates with the activities of hepatic and renal bilirubin-IXα uridine diphosphate glycosyltransferases, *Biochem. J.* 1977; **164**: 737–746.
13. Gourley, G.R. and Odell, G.B., Bilirubin metabolism in the fetus and neonate. In: Lebenthal, E., ed. Human gastrointestinal development. New York: Raven Press, 1989, pp. 581–621.
14. Fevery, J. and Heirwegh, K.P.M., Bilirubin metabolism. In: Javitt, N.B., ed. Liver and Biliary tract physiology. International Review of Physiology, Volume 21. Baltimore: University Park Press, 1980, pp. 171–220.
15. Alexander, D.P., Andrews, W.H.H., Britton, H.G. and Nixon, D.A., Bilirubin in the foetal sheep, *Biol. Neonate* 1970; **15**: 103–111.
16. Gartner, L.M., Lee, K., Vaisman, S., Lane, D. and Zarufu, I., Development of bilirubin in the newborn rhesus monkey, *J. Pediatr.* 1977; **90**: 513–531.
17. Lester, R., Jackson, B.T., Smallwood, R.A., Watkins, J.B., Klein, P.D., Smith, P.M. and Little, J.M., Fetal and neonatal function II, *Birth Defects* 1976; **12**: 307–314.
18. Muraca, M., Blanckaert, N., Rubaltelli, F.F. and Fevery, J., Unconjugated and conjugated bilirubin pigments during perinatal development. I. Studies on rat serum and intestine, *Biol. Neonate* 1986; **49**: 90–95.
19. Di Ilio, C., Del Boccio, G., Casalone, E., Aceto, A. and Sacchetta, P., Activities of enzymes associated with the metabolism of glutathione in fetal rat liver and placenta, *Biol. Neonate* 1986; **49**: 96–101.
20. Levi, A.J., Gatmaitan, Z. and Arias, I.M., Deficiency of hepatic organic anion-binding protein, impaired organic uptake by liver and "physiologic" jaundice in newborn monkeys, *N. Engl. J. Med.* 1970; **283**: 1136–1139.

21. Faulder, C.G., Hirrell, P.A., Hume, R. and Strange, R.C., Studies on the development of basic, neutral, and acidic isoenzymes of glutathione S-transferase in human liver, adrenal, kidney, and spleen, *Biochem. J.* 1987; **241**: 221–228.
22. Goodrum, L.A., Saade, G.R., Belfort, M.A., Carpenter, R.J. and Moise, K.J., The effect of intrauterine transfusion on fetal bilirubin in red cell alloimmunization, *Obstet. Gynecol.* 1997; **89**: 57–60.
23. Jansen, F.H., Heirwegh, K.P.M. and Devriendt, A., Foetal bilirubin conjugation, *Lancet* 1969; **1**: 702–704.
24. Schanker, L.S., Passage of drugs across body membranes, *Pharmacol. Rev.* 1962; **14**: 501–530.
25. Bernstein, R.B., Novy, M.J., Piasecki, G.J., Lester, R. and Jackson, B.T., Bilirubin metabolism in the fetus, *J. Clin. Invest.* 1969; **48**: 1678–1688.
26. Bashore., R.A., Smith, F. and Schenker, S., Placental transfer and disposition of bilirubin in the pregnant monkey, *Am. J. Obstet. Gynecol.* 1969; **103**: 950–958.
27. Rosenthal, P., Human placental bilirubin metabolism, *Pediatr. Res.* 1990; **27**: 223A.
28. Monte, M.J., Rodriguez-Bravo, T., Macias, R.I.R., Bravo, P., El-Mir, M.Y., Serrano, M.A., Lopez-Salva, A. and Marin, J.J.G., Relationship between bile acid transport gradients and transport across the fetal-facing plasma membrane of the human trophoblast, *Pediatr. Res.* 1995; **38**: 156–163.
29. Mandelbaum, B., LaCroix, G.C. and Robinson, A.R., Determination of fetal maturity by spectrophotometric analysis of amniotic fluid, *Obstet. Gynecol.* 1967; **29**: 471–474.
30. Bevis, D.C.A., The antenatal prediction of hemolytic disease of the newborn, *Lancet* 1952; **1**: 395–398.
31. Walker, A.H.C., Liquor amnii studies in the prediction of hemolytic disease of the newborn, *Br. Med. J.* 1957; **2**: 376.
32. Goodlin, R. and Lloyd, D., Fetal tracheal excretion of bilirubin, *Biol. Neonate* 1968; **12**: 1–12.
33. Brown, A.K., Perinatal aspects of bilirubin metabolism, *Obstet. Gynecol. Annu.* 1985; **4**: 191–212.
34. Furhoff, A.-K., Fate of children born to women with jaundice in pregnancy, *Arch. Gynäk.* 1974; **217**: 165–172.
35. Roszkowski, I. and Pisarek-Miedzinska, D., Jaundice in pregnancy. II. Clinical course of pregnancy and delivery and condition of neonate, *Am. J. Obstet. Gynecol.* 1968; **101**: 500–503.
36. Waffarn, F., Carlisle, S., Pena, I., Hodgman, J.E., Bonham, D., Fetal exposure to maternal hyperbilirubinemia, *Am. J. Dis. Child.* 1982; **136**: 416–417.
37. Crigler, J.F.J. and Najjar, V.A., Congenital familial nonhemolytic jaundice with kernicterus, *Pediatrics* 1952; **10**: 169–180.
38. Rosenthal, I.M., Zimmerman, H.J. and Hardy, N., Congenital nonhemolytic jaundice with disease of the central nervous system, *Pediatrics* 1956; **18**: 378–386.
39. Taylor, W.G., Walkinshaw, S.A., Farquharson, R.G., Fisken, R.A. and Gilmore, I.T., Pregnancy in Crigler–Najjar syndrome, Case report, *Br. J. Obstet. Gynaecol.* 1991; **98**: 1290–1291.
40. Smith, J.F. Jr. and Baker, J.M., Crigler–Najjar disease in pregnancy, *Obstet. Gynecol.* 1994; **84**: 670–672.
41. Yeary, R.A., Embryotoxicity of bilirubin, *Am. J. Obstet. Gynecol.* 1977; **127**: 497–498.
42. Ostrow, J.D., Jandl, J.H. and Schmid, R., The formation of bilirubin from hemoglobin *in vivo*, *J. Clin. Invest.* 1962; **41**: 1628–1637.
43. Coburn, R.F., Endogenous carbon monoxide production, *N. Engl. J. Med.* 1970; **282**: 207–209.
44. Bartoletti, A.L., Stevenson, D.K., Ostrander, C.R. and Johnson, J.D., Pulmonary excretion of carbon monoxide in the human infant as an index of bilirubin production. I. Effects of gestational and postnatal age and some common neonatal abnormalities, *J. Pediatr.* 1979; **94**: 952–955.
45. Bissell, D.M. and Guzelian, P.S., Degradation of endogenous hepatic heme by pathways not yielding carbon monoxide, *J. Clin. Invest.* 1980; **65**: 1135–1140.
46. Tenhunen, R., Marver, H.S. and Schmid, R., Microsomal heme oxygenase. Characterization of the enzyme, *J. Biol. Chem.* 1969; **244**: 6388–6394.
47. Raffin, S.B., Woo, C.H., Roost, K.T., Price, D.C. and Schmid, R., Intestinal absorption of hemoglobin iron-heme cleavage by mucosal heme oxygenase, *J. Clin. Invest.* 1974; **54**: 1344–1352.
48. Colleran, E. and O'Carra, P., Enzymology and comparative physiology of biliverdin reduction. In: Berk, P.D. and Berlin, N.R., eds. International symposium on chemistry and physiology of bile pigments. Washington, D.C.: US Government Printing Office, 1977; 69.
49. Brodersen, R., Physical chemistry of bilirubin: binding to macromolecules and membranes. In: Heirwegh, K.P.M. and Brown, S.B., eds. Bilirubin. Chemistry. Boca Raton: CRC press, Inc., 1982, pp. 75–123.

50. Brodersen, R., Binding of bilirubin to albumin, *Crit. Rev. Clin. Lab. Sci.* 1980; **11**: 305–399.
51. Brodersen, R., Bilirubin. Solubility and interaction with albumin and phospholipids, *J. Biol. Chem.* 1979; **254**: 2364–2369.
52. Jacobsen, J. and Brodersen, R., Albumin–bilirubin binding mechanism, *J. Biol. Chem.* 1983; **258**: 613–626.
53. Hrkal, Z. and Klementova, S. Bilirubin and haeme binding to human serum albumin studied by spectroscopy methods, *Int. J. Biochem.* 1984; **16**: 799–804.
54. Brodersen, R., Knudsen, A. and Pedersen, A.O., Cobinding of bilirubin and sulfonamide and of two bilirubin molecules to human serum albumin: A site model, *Arch. Biochem. Biophys.* 1987; **252**: 561–569.
55. Meisel, P., Jährig, D., Bleyer, H. and Jährig, K., Indikationen zur Blutaustauschtransfusionen bei Neugeborenen mit Hyperbilirubinämie, *Kinderarztl Prax* 1981; **49**: 449–459.
56. Jacobsen, J. and Wennberg, R.P., Determination of unbound bilirubin in the serum of newborns. *Clin. Chem.* 1974; **20**: 783–789.
57. Cashore, W.J., Free bilirubin concentrations and bilirubin-binding affinity in term and preterm infants, *J. Pediatr.* 1980; **96**: 521–527.
58. Robertson, A.F., Karp, W.B., Bunyapen, C., Catterton, W.Z. and Davis, H.C., Clinical and chemical correlates of the bilirubin-binding capacity in newborns, *Am. J. Dis. Child.* 1981; **135**: 525–528.
59. Kapitulnik, J., Horner-Mibashan, R., Blondheim, S.H., Kaufmann, N.A. and Russell, A., Increase in bilirubin-binding affinity of serum with age of infant, *J. Pediatr.* 1975; **86**: 442–445.
60. Ebbesen, F. and Nyboe, J., Postnatal changes in the ability of plasma albumin to bind bilirubin, *Acta. Paediatr. Scand.* 1983; **72**: 665–670.
61. Ebbesen, F., Foged, N., and Brodersen, R., Reduced albumin binding of MADDS – a measure of bilirubin binding in sick children, *Acta. Paediatr. Scand.* 1986; **75**: 550–504.
62. Brodersen, R., Prevention of kernicterus, based on recent progress in bilirubin chemistry, *Acta. Paediatr. Scand.* 1977; **66**: 625–634.
63. Bratlid, D., Pharmacologic aspects of neonatal hyperbilirubinemia, *Birth Defects: Original Article Series* 1976; **12**: 184–189.
64. Odell, G.B., Cukier, J.O., Seungdamrong, S. and Odell, J.L., The displacement of bilirubin from albumin, *Birth Defects: Original Article Series* 1976; **12**: 192–200.
65. Blanc, W.A., and Johnson, L., Studies on kernicterus. Relationship with sulfonamide intoxication, report on kernicterus in rats with glucuronyl transferase deficiency, and review of pathogenesis, *J. Neuropathol. Exp. Neurol.* 1959; **18**: 165–189.
66. Cormode, E.J., Lyster, D.M. and Israels, S., Analbuminemia in a neonate, *J. Pediatr.* 1975; **86**: 862–867.
67. Blauer, G., Complexes of bilirubin with proteins, *Biochim. Biophys. Acta.* 1986; **884**: 602–604.
68. Aoyagi, Y., Ikenaka, T. and Ischida, F., α-Fetoprotein as a carrier protein in plasma and its bilirubin-binding ability, *Cancer Res.* 1979; **39**: 571–574.
69. Jagt, D.L.V. and Garcia, K.B., Immunochemical comparisons of proteins that bind heme and bilirubin: Human serum albumin, (alfa)-fetoprotein and glutathione S-transferases from liver, placenta and erythrocyte, *Comp. Biochem. Physiol.* 1987; **87B**: 527–531.
70. Takahashi, M., Sugiyama, K., Shumiya, S. and Nagase, S., Penetration of bilirubin into the brain in albumin-deficient and jaundiced rats and Nagase analbuminemic rats, *J. Biochem.* 1984; **96**: 1705–1712.
71. Suzuki, N., Yamaguchi, T. and Nakajima, H., Role of high-density lipoprotein in transport of circulating bilirubin in rats, *J. Biol. Chem.* 1988; **263**: 5037–5043.
72. Bratlid, D., Bilirubin binding by human erythrocytes, *Scand. J. Clin. Lab. Invest.* 1972; **29**: 91–97.
73. Bratlid, D., The effect of pH on bilirubin binding by human erythrocytes, *Scand. J. Clin. Lab. Invest.* 1972; **29**: 453–459.
74. Jacobsen, C., Lysine residue 240 of human serum albumin is involved in high-affinity binding of bilirubin, *Biochem. J.* 1978; **171**: 453–459.
75. Jacobsen, C., Chemical modification of the high-affinity bilirubin-binding site of human serum albumin. *Eur. J. Biochem.* 1972; **27**: 513–519.
76. Mir, M.M., Fazili, K.M. and Abul Qasim, M., Chemical modification of buried lysine residues of bovine serum albumin and its influence on protein conformation and bilirubin binding, *Biochim. Biophys. Acta.* 1992; **1119**: 261–267.
77. Lo Bello, M., Pastore, A., Petruzelli, R., Parker, M.W., Wilce, M.C.J., Federici, G. and Ricci, G., Conformational states of human placental glutathione transferase as probed by limited proteolysis, *Biochem. Biophys. Res. Comm.* 1993; **194**: 804–810.

78. Xia, C., Meyer, D.J., Chen, H., Reinemer, P., Huber, R. and Ketterer, B., Chemical modification of GSH transferase P1-1 confirms the presence of Arg-13, Lys-44 and one carboxylate group in the GSH binding domain of the active site, *Biochem. J.* 1993; **293**: 357–362.
79. Gurba P.E. and Zand, R., Bilirubin binding to myelin basic protein, histones and its inhibition *in vitro* of cerebellar protein synthesis, *Biochem. Biophys. Res. Comm.* 1974; **58**: 1142–1147.
80. Zhu, X.X., Brown, G.R. and St-Pierre, L.E., Adsorption of bilirubin with polypeptide-coated resins, *Biomater Artif Cells Artif Organs* 1990; **18**: 75–93.
81. Chandy, T. and Sharma, C.P., Polylysine-immobilized chitosan beads as adsorbents for bilirubin, *Artif Organs* 1992; **16**: 568–576.
82. Hansen, T.W.R., Mathiesen, S.B.W. and Walaas, S.I. Modulation of the effect of bilirubin on protein phosphorylation by lysine-containing peptides, *Pediatr. Res.* 1997; **42**: 615–617.
83. Wolkoff, A.W., Goresky, C.A., Sellin, J., Gatmaitan, Z. and Arias, I., Role of ligandin in transfer of bilirubin from plasma to liver, *Am. J. Physiol.* 1979; **236**: E638–648.
84. Berk, P.D., Potter, B.J. and Stremmel, W., Role of plasma membrane ligand-binding proteins in the hepatocellular uptake of albumin-bound organic anions. *Hepatology* 1987; **7**: 165–176.
85. Tiribelli, C. and Ostrow, J.D., New concepts in bilirubin chemistry, transport and metabolism: Report of the International Bilirubin Workshop, April 6–8, 1989, Trieste, Italy. *Hepatology* 1990; **11**: 303–313.
86. Tiribelli, C. and Ostrow, J.D., New concepts in bilirubin chemistry, transport and metabolism: Report of the Second International Bilirubin Workshop, April 9–11, 1992, Trieste, Italy, *Hepatology* 1993; **17**: 715–736.
87. Weisiger, R., Gollan, J. and Ockner, R., Receptor for albumin on the liver cell surface may mediate uptake of fatty acids and other albumin-bound substances, *Science* 1981; **211**: 1048–1050.
88. Bernstein, L.H., Ezzer, J.B., Gartner, L. and Arias, I.M., Hepatic intracellular distribution of tritium-labeled unconjugated and conjugated bilirubin in normal and Gunn rats, *J. Clin. Invest.* 1966; **45**: 1194–1201.
89. Litwack, G., Ketterer, B. and Arias, I.M., Ligandin: a hepatic protein which binds steroids, bilirubin, carcinogens and a number of exogenous organic anions, *Nature* 1971; **234**: 466–467.
90. Ketley, J.N., Habig, W.H. and Jakoby, W.B., Rat liver glutathione S-transferase: a family of binding proteins, *Fed. Proc.* 1975; **34**: 504.
91. Wolkoff, A.W., Ketley, J.N. and Waggoner, J.G., Hepatic accumulation and intracellular binding of conjugated bilirubin, *J. Clin. Invest.* 1978; **61**: 142–149.
92. Bhargava, M.M., Listowsky, I. and Arias, I.M., Ligandin. Bilirubin binding and glutathione-S-transferase activity are independent processes, *J. Biol. Chem.* 1978; **253**: 4112–4115.
93. Sugiyama, Y., Stolz, A., Sugimoto, M. and Kaplowitz, N., Evidence for a common high affinity binding site on glutathione- S-transferase B for lithocholic acid and bilirubin, *J. Lipid Res.* 1984; **25**: 1177–1183.
94. Levi, A.J., Gatmaitan, Z. and Arias, I.M., Deficiency of hepatic organic anion-binding protein, impaired organic anion uptake by liver and "physiologic" jaundice in newborn monkeys, *N. Engl. J. Med.* 1970; **283**: 1136–1139.
95. Jansen, P.L.M., Chowdhury, J.R., Fischberg, E.B. and Arias, I.M., Enzymatic conversion of bilirubin monoglucuronide to diglucuronide by rat liver plasma membranes, *J. Biol. Chem.* 1977; **252**: 2710–2716.
96. Peters, W.H.M., Jansen, P.L.M. and Nauta, H., The molecular weights of UDP-glucuronyl transferase determined with radiation-inactivation analysis: a molecular model of bilirubin UDP-glucuronyl transferase, *J. Biol. Chem.* 1984; **259**: 11701–11705.
97. Van Es, H.H., Bout, A., Liu, J., Anderson, L., Duncan, A.M., Bosma, P., Elferink, O.R., Jansen, P.L., Chowdhury, J.R. and Schurr, E., Assignment of the human UDP glucuronosyltransferase gene (UGT1A1) to chromosome region 2q37, *Cytogenet. Cell. Genet.* 1993; **63**: 114–116.
98. Rosenthal, P., Blanckaert, N., Kabra, P.M. and Thaler, M.M., Formation of bilirubin conjugates in human newborns, *Pediatr. Res.* 1986; **20**: 947–950.
99. Muraca, M., Rubaltelli, F.F., Blanckaert, N. and Fevery, J., Unconjugated and conjugated bilirubin pigments during perinatal development. II. Studies on serum of healthy newborns and of neonates with erythroblastosis fetalis, *Biol. Neonate* 1990; **57**: 1–9.
100. Rayburn, W., Donn, S., Piehl, E. and Compton, A. Antenatal phenobarbital and bilirubin metabolism in the very low birth weight infant, *Am. J. Obstet. Gynecol.* 1988; **159**: 1491–1493.
101. Epstein, M.F., Leviton, A., Kuban, K.C., Pagano, M., Meltzer, C., Skoutelli, H.N., Brown, E.R. and Sullivan, K.F., Bilirubin, intraventricular hemorrhage and phenobarbital in very low birth weight babies, *Pediatrics* 1988; **82**: 350–354.

102. Valaes, T., Petmezaki, S. and Doxiadis, S.A., Effect on neonatal hyperbilirubinemia of phenobarbital during pregnancy or after birth: practical value of the treatment in a population with high risk of unexplained severe neonatal jaundice, *Birth Defects: Original Article Series* 1970; **6**: 46–54.
103. Margies, D. and Jährig, K., Der Platz der Phototherapie bei der Prophylaxe und Behandlung des Icterus neonatorum, *Kinderarztl Prax.* 1975; **43**: 19–28.
104. Neufeld, N.D., Corbo, L., Brunnerman, S. and Melmed, S., Stimulation of neonatal hepatic UDP-glucuronyl transferase activity with prenatal thyroid analog therapy, *Pediatr. Res.* 1985; **19**: 178A.
105. Leaky, J.E.A., Althaus, Z.R., Bailey, J.R. and Slikker, W.J., Dexamethasone increases UDP-glucuronyl transferase activity towards bilirubin, oestradiol and testosterone in foetal liver from rhesus monkey during late gestation, *Biochem. J.* 1985; **225**: 183–188.
106. Lindebaum, A., Hernandorena, X., Vial, M. *et al.*, Traitement curatif de l'ictere du nouveau-ne a terme par le clofibrate, *Arch. Fr. Pediatr.* 1981; **38**: 867–873.
107. Hintz, S.R., Kwong, L.K., Vreman, H.J. and Stevenson, D.K., Recovery of exogenous heme as carbon monoxide and biliary heme in adult rats after tin protoporphyrin treatment, *J. Pediatr. Gastroenterol. Nutr.* 1987; **6**: 302–306.
108. Drummond, G.S. and Kappas, A., Prevention of neonatal hyperbilirubinemia by tin protoporphyrin IX, a potent competitive inhibitor of heme oxidation, *Proc. Natl. Acad. Sci. USA* 1981; **78**: 6466–6470.
109. Kappas, A., Drummond, G.S., Manola, T., Petmezaki, S. and Valaes, T., Sn-Protoporphyrin use in the management of hyperbilirubinemia in term newborns with direct Coombs-Positive ABO incompatibility, *Pediatrics* 1988; **81**: 485–497.
110. Royer, M., Rodriguez Garay, E. and Argerich, T., Action of biliverdin on biliary elimination of bilirubin and biliverdin in the rat, *Acta. Physiol. Latinoam.* 1962; **12**: 84–95.
111. Stocker, R., Yamamoto, Y., McDonagh, A.F., Glazer, A.N. and Ames, B.N., Bilirubin is an antioxidant of possible physiological importance, *Science* 1987; **235**: 1043–1046.
112. Munoz, M.E., González, J. and Esteller, A., Effect of glucose administration on bilirubin excretion in the rabbit, *Experientia* 1987; **43**: 166–168.
113. Arias, I.M., Johnson, L. and Wolfson, S., Biliary excretion of injected conjugated and unconjugated bilirubin by normal and Gunn rats, *Am. J. Physiol.* 1961; **200**: 1091–1094.
114. Natschka, J.C. and Odell, G.B., The influence of albumin on the distribution and excretion of bilirubin in jaundiced rats, *Pediatrics* 1966; **37**: 51–61.
115. Kapitulnik, J. and Ostrow, J.D., Stimulation of bilirubin catabolism in jaundiced Gunn rats by an inducer of microsomal mixed-function monooxygenases, *Proc. Natl. Acad. Sci. USA* 1977; **75**: 682–685.
116. De Matteis, F., Dawson, S.J., Boobis, A.R. and Comoglio, A., Inducible bilirubin-degrading system of rat liver microsomes: Role of cytochrome P450IA1, *Molec. Pharmacol.*, 1991; **40**: 686–691.
117. Sinal, C.J. and Bend, J.R., Aryl hydrocarbon receptor-dependent induction of CYP1A1 by bilirubin in mouse hepatoma HEPA 1C1C7 cells, *Molec. Pharmacol.* 1997; **52**: 590–599.
118. Linn, S., Schoenbaum, S.C., Monson, R.R., Rosner, B., Stubblefield, P.G. and Ryan, K.J. Epidemiology of neonatal hyperbilirubinemia, *Pediatrics* 1985; **75**: 770–774.
119. Clarkson, J.E., Cowan, J.O. and Herbison, G.P., Jaundice in full term healthy neonates – a population study, *Aust. Paediatr. J.* 1984; **20**: 303–308.
120. Maisels, M.J., Gifford, K., Antle, C.E. and Leib, G.R., Jaundice in healthy newborn infant: A new approach to an old problem, *Pediatrics* 1988; **81**: 505–511.
121. Tan, K.L., Glucose-6-phosphate dehydrogenase status and neonatal jaundice, *Arch. Dis. Child.* 1981; **56**: 874–877.
122. Gibbs, W.N., Gray, R. and Lowry, M., Glucose-6-phosphate dehydrogenase deficiency and neonatal jaundice in Jamaica, *Br. J. Haematol.* 1979; **43**: 263–274.
123. Roux, P., Karabus, C.D. and Hartley, P.S., The effect of glucose-6-phosphate dehydrogenase deficiency on the severity of neonatal jaundice in Cape Town, *S. Afr. Med. J.* 1982; **61**: 781–782.
124. Moore, L.G., Newberry, M.A., Freeby, G.M. and Crnic, L.S., Increased incidence of neonatal hyperbilirubinemia at 3100m in Colorado, *Am. J. Dis. Child.* 1984; **138**: 157–161.
125. Cohen, R.S., Brown, M.S. and Stevenson, D.K., Effect of altitude on neonatal bilirubin production, *Pediatr. Res.* 1987; **21**: 357A.
126. Drew, J.H. and Kitchen, W.H., Jaundice in infants of Greek parentage: The unknown factor may be environmental, *J. Pediatr.* 1976; **89**: 248–252.
127. Maisels, J.M. and Gifford, K., Normal serum bilirubin levels in the newborn and the effect of breast-feeding, *Pediatrics* 1986; **78**: 837–843.

128. Palmer, D.C. and Drew, J.H., Jaundice: a 10 year review of 41,000 live born infants, *Aust. Paediatr. J.* 1983; **19**: 86–89.
129. Whitington, P.F. and Gartner, L.M., Disorders of bilirubin metabolism. In: Nathan, D.G. and Oski, F.A., eds. Hematology of infancy and childhood. Philadelphia: WB Saunders Company; 1993, pp. 74–114.
130. Kappas, A., Drummond, G.S., Henschke, C. and Valaes, T., Direct comparison of Sn-mesoporphyrin, and inhibitor of bilirubin production, and phototherapy in controlling hyperbilirubinemia in term and near-term newborns, *Pediatrics* 1995; **95**: 468–474.
131. Obrinsky, W., Denley, M.L. and Brauer, R.W., Sulfobromophthalein sodium excretion test as a measure of liver function in premature infants, *Pediatrics* 1952; **9**: 421–438.
132. Orzes, N., Bellentani, S., Aldin, R., Simoni, P., Ferretti, I., Lunazzi, G.C., Sottocasa, G.L. and Tiribelli, C., Sex differences in the hepatic uptake of sulfobromophthalein in the rat, *Clin. Sci.* 1985; **69**: 587–593.
133. Persico, M., Bellentani, S., Marchegiano, P., Orzes, N., Lunazzi, G.C., Sottocasa, G.L. and Tiribelli, C., Sex steroids modulation of the hepatic uptake of organic anions in rat. *J. Hepatol.* 1988; **6**: 343–349.
134. O'Kell, R.T. and Elliott, J.R., Development of normal values for use in multitest biochemical screening of sera, *Clin. Chem.* 1970; **163**: 161–165.
135. Bogg, T.R. Jr. and Bishop, H., Neonatal hyperbilirubinemia associated with high obstruction of the small bowel, *J. Pediatr.* 1965; **66**: 349–356.
136. DeCarvalho, M., Klaus, M.H. and Merkatz, R.B., Frequency of breast-feeding and serum bilirubin concentration, *Am. J. Dis. Child.* 1982; **136**: 737–738.
137. Odell, G.B., Gutcher, G.R., Whitington, P.F. and Yang, G., Enteral administration of agar as an effective adjunct to phototherapy in neonatal jaundice, *Pediatr. Res.* 1983; **17**: 810–814.
138. Johnson, L.H., Gourley, G., Kreamer, W. and Dalin, C., Bilirubin oxidase was non-toxic, decreased stool bilirubin products and retained activity in stools during 22 days of feeding to four children with Crigler Najjar syndrome aged 3 to 7 years, *Pediatr. Res.* 1996; **39**: 219A.
139. Johnson, L.H., Bhutani, V.K., Abbasi, S., Gerdes, J.S., Kraemer, W., Dalin, C. and Gourley, G., Bilirubin oxidase in addition to intensive phototherapy to eliminate or delay need for exchange, *Pediatr. Res.* 1997; **41**: 156A.
140. Tenhunen, R., Marver, H.S. and Schmid, R., The enzymatic conversion of hemoglobin to bilirubin, *Trans. Assoc. Am. Physicians* 1969; **82**: 363–371.

Fetal Therapy

2 The Management of Alloimmune Fetal Hemolytic Disease

J.M. Bowman

Department of Pediatrics and Child Health, Faculty of Medicine, University of Manitoba, Winnipeg, MB, Canada

INTRODUCTION

Hemolytic disease of the newborn (HDN) was first reported in 1609 by a French midwife in a set of twins. One was hydropic and stillborn; the other became severely jaundiced and died. The cause of hemolytic disease was elucidated by Levine in 1941[1] following the discovery of the Rh blood group system by Landsteiner and Weiner in 1940.[2] After a hydropic stillbirth, a woman had a severe reaction following transfusion with her husband's blood. She was found to be Rh(D) negative with a powerful antibody against her husband's Rh positive red cells and the red cells of a panel of Rh positive Caucasians.[1] In the early 1940's, when perinatal mortality in Canada was more than 40 per thousand births, 10% of these deaths were due to HDN.

OTHER ANTIBODIES CAUSING HDN

Although the Rh antibody (anti-D) was, and still is, the most common cause of severe HDN, as Rh immunization has decreased due to Rh prevention programs, other alloimmune antibodies have become relatively more important as a cause. Anti-c, Kell, and Fy^a may cause severe HDN, as less commonly do anti-C and anti-E. Other antibodies are rare causes of significant HDN.[3] In the 34 year period ending October 31, 1996, the only alloantibodies other than anti-D encountered by our center, that required intensive investigation and treatment of the fetus or the baby, were anti-c, Kell, Fy^a, Jk^a, -C, $-C^W$, -E, -k, $-Kp^a$, and -S.

Address for correspondence: J.M. Bowman, M.D., Rh Laboratory, Women's Hospital, Health Sciences Centre, 735 Notre Dame Avenue WINNIPEG, Manitoba R3E OL8, Canada

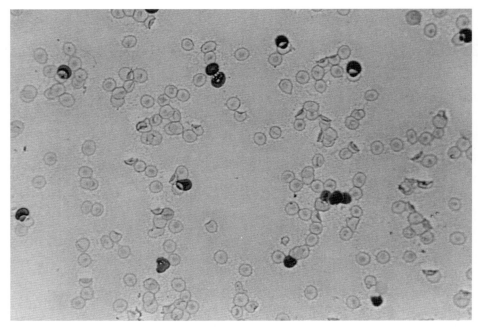

Figure 2.1. Acid elution technique of Kleihauer. Fetal red blood cells (RBC) stain with eosin (appear dark). Adult RBC do not stain (appear as ghosts). This maternal blood smear contained 9% fetal RBC, representing a transplacental hemorrhage of about 400 ml of blood. From Bowman, J.M., Hemolytic disease of the newborn. In: Conn, R.B., ed. *Current Diagnosis* **5**. Philadelphia: WB Saunders Company, 1977.

ETIOLOGY OF ALLOIMMUNIZATION

In 1954 Dr. Bruce Chown, the founder of the Rh Laboratory in Winnipeg, published his findings demonstrating that the cause of Rh immunization was the transfer of fetal Rh(D) positive red cells into the maternal circulation[4] (Figure 2.1). Kleihauer Betke measurements indicated that 75% of women have such hemorrhages.[5] More sensitive (molecular) detection measures indicate that such hemorrhages are universal.

The likelihood of Rh immunization is 16% if the Rh positive fetus is ABO compatible with its mother; 1.5 to 2% if ABO incompatible; 4 to 5% following induced abortion; 2% following spontaneous abortion. Invasive procedures such as amniocentesis, chorionic villus sampling, and fetal blood sampling all increase the risk of fetomaternal hemorrhage and, therefore, alloimmunization.

DEGREES OF SEVERITY OF Rh(D) HDN

About one half of affected newborn infants are so mildly affected that they require no treatment. Approximately one quarter will be born near term, in good condition, but, without treatment, will become extremely jaundiced and either die of kernicterus

(90%) or will be left severely damaged with neurosensory deafness, spastic choreo-athetosis, and some degree of intellectual retardation (10%).[6] The remaining one quarter are so severely affected that they develop hydrops *in utero*, about one half before 34 weeks' gestation, occasionally as early as 17 to 18 weeks' gestation; the other half between 34 weeks and term.[6] In the early 1940's before there were any treatment measures, the perinatal mortality rate from Rh(D) HDN was 50%.

EXCHANGE TRANSFUSION

The first major advance in the treatment of Rh(D) HDN occurred in 1945 when Wallerstein introduced exchange transfusion.[7] A successful treatment was now available for the infant born near term in good condition but otherwise doomed to die of kernicterus. With the advent of exchange transfusion perinatal mortality from Rh(D) HDN fell to 25%.

EARLY DELIVERY IN SEVERE HDN

Although exchange transfusion was very successful, there remained the problem of the fetus doomed to become hydropic *in utero*. Chown hypothesized that such a fetus might survive if delivered following induction at 32 to 34 weeks' gestation (prior to the development of hydrops) and treated with prompt exchange transfusion. He was proven brilliantly correct.[8] By 1961, the perinatal mortality from hemolytic disease in Manitoba had dropped to 16%. The major problem with early delivery was the risk of prematurity and death from hyaline membrane disease and our lack of ability to predict accurately the severity of hemolytic disease *in utero*.

PREDICTIVE MEASURES

Antibody Titre and Past History of Hemolytic Disease

Before 1961, antibody titres and a history of HDN in previous pregnancies were the only measures available to predict the severity of hemolytic disease before delivery. Although both of these measures determine the need for further and potentially more invasive measures, by themselves, they are only 62% accurate in predicting the severity of HDN.[6]

In Vitro Cell Mediated Maternal Functional Assays

Attempts have been made to improve the prediction of severity of hemolytic disease by measuring the binding (avidity) of the antibody for the antigen on the red cell membrane and its ability to lyse affected red cells. A review of these various assays indicates that the chemiluminescence assay of Hadley[9] may be the most accurate and does not use radio isotopes. Nevertheless, none of the tests are completely accurate and occasionally may be misleading. Because their only function may be to reduce, moderately, the number of invasive investigative procedures, cell mediated maternal functional assays are not used widely.

Fetal D Antigen Determination

A major advance has been the ability to determine the fetal Rh(D) (and also Kell and PLA1) status by PCR technology, when the father is heterozygous for the offending antigen.[10–12] The use of amniotic fluid fetal cellular elements for this purpose is now well established. In the very near future, routine fetal antigen typing will be possible using fetal nucleated erythroid progenitors found during early pregnancy in maternal blood[10–12] and, ultimately, such determinations will be made by PCR testing of fetal DNA in maternal plasma and serum.[11,12]

Amniotic Fluid Spectrophotometry

This definitive investigative procedure, described by Bevis, was first used in the management of Rh sensitized pregnancies by Liley in 1961.[13] Measurement of deviation from linearity at 450 nm (the Δ O.D. 450), the wavelength at which bilirubin absorbs light, was an important advance in determining the severity of hemolytic disease (Figure 2.2). Although, the Δ O.D. 450 is more accurate in predicting severity in the third trimester than in mid to late second trimester, the use of serial

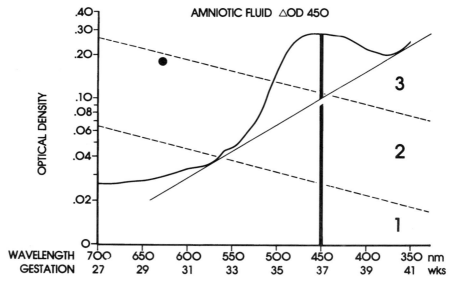

Figure 2.2. Amniotic fluid spectrophotometric reading, Liley method. In this example the Δ O.D. 450 is 0.200 and falls high in zone II at 29½ weeks' gestation, indicating severe Rh erythroblastosis. Curved line indicates analysis of O.D. on patient's liquor; full straight line indicates O.D. baseline. From Bowman, J.M., Haemolytic disease of the newborn (erythroblastosis fetalis). In: Roberton, N.R.C., ed. Textbook of Neonatology, Edinburgh: Churchill Livingstone, 1986.

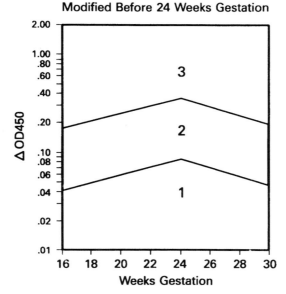

Figure 2.3. Modification of Liley's Δ O.D. 450 zone boundaries before 24 weeks' gestation. Zone boundary angle of inclination before 24 weeks gestation is the same as the zone boundary angle of declination after 24 weeks gestation. From Bowman, J.M., Pollock, J.M., Manning, F.A. *et al.*, Maternal Kell blood group alloimmunization, *Obstet. Gynecol.* 1992; **79**: 239–244.

measurements and the alteration of the zone boundaries by extending them upward rather than downward before 24 weeks' gestation[14] (Figure 2.3), has improved the accuracy of prediction of HDN in the second trimester. In serial measurements, the last Δ O.D. 450 falling into the 75 to 85% level of zone II or a single Δ O.D. 450 falling into zone III (at one time a reason for intrauterine [intraperitoneal] transfusion), is now an indication for fetal blood sampling. The prevalence of fetomaternal trans-placental hemorrhage due to placental trauma at the time of amniocentesis, initially 10%, has been reduced to 2.5% in the ultrasound era. Indeed, if ultrasound indicates that the placenta cannot be avoided by the amniocentesis needle, amniocentesis is not undertaken. With the introduction of amniotic fluid spectrophotometry, by 1964, perinatal mortality from Rh disease in Manitoba was reduced to 13%.

Amniocentesis is indicated whenever there is a maternal serum Rh antibody titer of 16 or greater, or a history of prior hemolytic disease severe enough to require intrauterine transfusion, early delivery or exchange transfusion, or which resulted in fetal or neonatal death.

Perinatal Ultrasonography

The development of ultrasound (US) techniques in the late 1970's, marked another advance in the management of maternal blood group alloimmunization.[15] With US

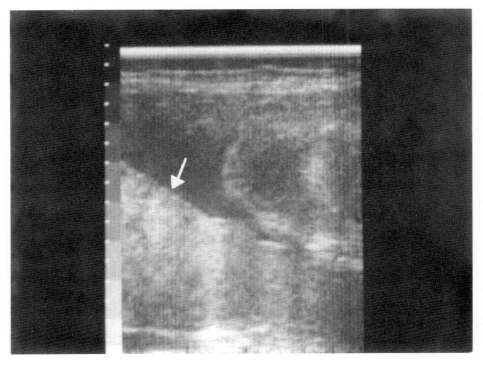

Figure 2.4. Sonogram of fetus with hydrops fetalis. Placenta is enormously thickened and edematous (arrow). Fetal abdomen, which is grossly distended with ascitic fluid, can be seen to the right of the arrow. From Bowman, J.M., Maternal blood group immunization. In, Creasy, R.K. and Resnik, R. eds. Maternal-Fetal Medicine: Principles and Practice. 2nd ed. Philadelphia: WB Saunders, 1989.

one can make the diagnosis of hydrops (ascites, edema, pleural and pericardial effusions) with great accuracy (Figure 2.4), but unfortunately one may not be able to make the diagnosis of impending hydrops. US is of value in assessing fetal well being in decreasing the incidence of placental trauma at amniocentesis and in directing the needle at both intraperitoneal (IPT) and intravascular fetal transfusions (IVT). After IPT, US confirms that blood is present in the peritoneal cavity and serial examinations monitor its absorption. At IVT, US observation of turbulence within the umbilical vessel as the blood is injected, confirms that it is being injected into the fetal circulation. After fetal transfusions, US biophysical profile scoring provides an ongoing assessment of fetal condition.

Percutaneous Umbilical Blood Sampling

With the introduction of sophisticated ultrasound equipment and the availability of perinatologists skilled in its use, percutaneous umbilical blood sampling (PUBS) became feasible in the mid 1980's[16] (Figure 2.5). PUBS allows the measurement of all blood parameters which can be measured after birth and PUBS is the most accurate

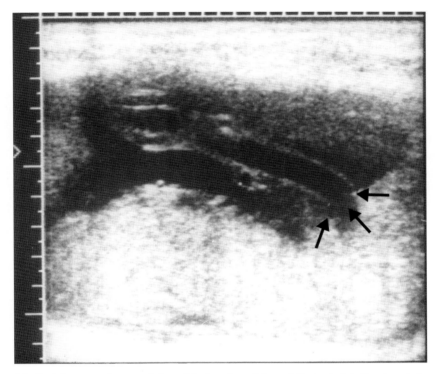

Figure 2.5. Real time scan ultrasound view of the insertion of the umbilical vein into the placenta (arrows), the placenta is posterior. The wall of the umbilical vein is sonar lucent. From Bowman, J.M., Maternal blood group immunization. In: Creasy, R.K. and Resnik, R. eds. Maternal-Fetal Medicine: Principles and Practice. 2nd ed. Philadelphia: WB Saunders, 1989.

means of determining the severity of HDN in the absence of hydrops. When serial spectrophotometric measurements of amniotic fluid demonstrate a Δ O.D. falling into the 75–85% level of zone II or a single Δ O.D. falling into zone III, PUBS is indicated. The procedure is relatively benign, carrying a fetal mortality of less than 1%. Since it carries with it a great hazard of fetomaternal transplacental hemorrhage, it should be carried out only when serial amniotic fluid Δ O.D. 450 readings indicate a fetus at risk, or when an anterior placenta precludes amniocentesis, and the maternal history and/or maternal antibody titre indicate a fetus at risk. Fetal blood sampling may be possible as early as 17 to 18 weeks' gestation; it usually is feasible by 20 to 21 weeks.

PREVENTION OF MATERNAL Rh ALLOIMMUNIZATION

The ability to prevent Rh immunization has been a major milestone in the management of this condition. Unless the father of the child is known to be Rh D-negative, Rh immune globulin (Rhogam, WinRho) is given to Rh D-negative women at 28 weeks gestation and following the birth of an Rh D-positive infant.[17] Rh immune globulin must also be given after abortion or threatened abortion, and after amniocentesis or chorionic-villus sampling or any other invasive intrauterine procedure. The dose used in the US is 300 µg, but in many other countries is 100–125 µg. If the Kleihauer–Betke test determines that there is a transplacental hemorrhage of more than 30 ml of fetal blood (which occurs in 1 in 400 pregnancies), the dose of Rh_0 (D) immune globulin must be at least 10 µg/ml of fetal blood in the maternal circulation. The use of Rh immunoglobulin in this way has reduced the likelihood of natural Rh alloimmunization by 96%. It is not known exactly how Rh_0 (D) immune globulin works. Its action does not appear to be due simply to clearance of Rh D-positive fetal red cells or to binding of the antibody to antigenic sites on the red cell membrane.

MANAGEMENT OF MATERNAL ALLOIMMUNIZATION

Antibody Suppression

Attempts to depress Rh antibody progression with Rh hapten, Rh positive RBC stroma, and administration of promethazine hydrochloride have not been of benefit; neither has administration of Rh Immune Globulin once Rh immunization has begun, no matter how weak the antibody.

A moderately beneficial effect can be achieved by intensive plasma exchange (removal of 10 to 15 L of plasma per week, and partial replacement of the removed plasma with 5% albumin and intravenous immune globulin [IVIG]),[18] or the administration of IVIG 1 gram per kilogram body weight weekly.[19] In the author's experience, the only value of either procedure is to postpone the need for PUBS and IVT until a gestation is reached at which these procedures are feasible. Institution of either plasmapheresis or IVIG therapy, does not obviate the need for carrying out amniocentesis and/or fetal blood sampling at the usual gestation, (18 to 20 weeks).

Intrauterine Fetal Transfusion (IUT)

Intraperitoneal fetal transfusion (IPT)

In 1961, induced premature delivery could not be carried out before 32 weeks' gestation because of the prohibitive mortality from prematurity and severe HDN. Eight percent of fetuses will become hydropic before 32 weeks' gestation. The introduction of IPT by Liley in 1963[20] dramatically changed the outlook for these most severely affected fetuses. Fetal diaphragmatic movements are required for absorption of RBC to occur.

Under ultrasound guidance a Tuohy needle is introduced into the fetal peritoneal cavity. An epidural catheter is then threaded down the needle. The needle is withdrawn and 1 to 1.5 ml of radiopaque medium are injected. An x-ray confirms proper placement of the catheter by showing contrast free in the peritoneal cavity, under the diaphragm and outside of fetal bowel (semilunes), or diffusing into ascitic fluid, indicating the presence of fetal ascites and hydrops fetalis.

Anti-CMV negative and irradiated packed RBC, less than four days old, group 0, Rh (D) negative, Kell negative, crossmatch compatible with the mother's serum, are then injected in 10 ml aliquots to a volume calculated by the formula: (gestation [wk] − 20) ×10 ml. Salvage rates after IPT were 30% in the first two years but increased to 76% in the ultrasound era. Most IPT survivors are normal both physically and intellectually.

IPT has its problems. It is of no value for the moribund, non breathing fetus. If the placenta must be traversed by the Tuohy needle, the mortality per procedure is 7%. After multiple IPT spontaneous labor occurs in 70% of patients, fortunately usually after 30 weeks of gestation. Finally, the decision to carry out IPT is dependent upon amniotic fluid Δ O.D. 450 readings (serial fluids in which the last reading is in the upper 85% of Liley's zone II or a single fluid reading is in zone III). Amniotic fluid readings, particularly in the second trimester, have a 5 to 10% inaccuracy rate.

Direct intravascular fetal transfusion (IVT)

With the introduction of PUBS, it became possible to follow the sampling procedure with direct IVT,[21] (Figure 2.5). Under ultrasound guidance, a needle is introduced into an umbilical blood vessel, a fetal blood sample is obtained and the hemoglobin measured immediately. When a rapid alkaline denaturation test confirms that the blood sample is fetal, additional measurement of all fetal blood parameters are done. These include: hemoglobin, hematocrit, ABO, Rh, and other pertinent blood groups, direct antiglobulin tests, reticulocyte count, platelet count, serum proteins, and erythropoietin levels.

If the hemoglobin level is less than 110 g/l, IVT is indicated. Injection of 0.5 ml of saline prior to the transfusion produces turbulence in the fetal vessel and confirms that the needle tip is positioned properly in the vessel. If fetal movements are likely to displace the needle, the fetus is paralyzed with intravenous pancuronium.

The transfusion is carried out in 10 ml aliquots, to a volume of 50 ml per estimated kg body weight, or until it is calculated that the total circulating hemoglobin and hematocrit are in the range of 190 to 200 g/l and 55 to 60% respectively. We have encountered no hyperviscosity or developmental problems with transfusions up to that level. The perinatal ultrasonographer monitors turbulence in the blood vessel, which confirms that the transfusion is into the fetal vessel. The ultrasonographer also assesses fetal condition. If turbulence disappears, the procedure is discontinued immediately; the needle is repositioned and evidence that the tip is properly placed is again obtained before the transfusion is begun again. If, from observation of fetal heart rate, fetal doppler heart rate pattern, and cardiac ventricular volume, there is evidence of hypervolemia producing cardiac stress, a relatively rare event, the procedure is stopped before the full volume is administered.

In Manitoba, from January 2, 1964 to September 30, 1997, 518 fetuses have had 1583 IUT (IPT and IVT) (Table 2.1). The overall survival rate with IUT is 71%. IVT has many advantages over IPT and is the preferred procedure.[22] It is the only hope

Table 2.1. Intrauterine transfusion survival – Winnipeg 1964–97.

Total intrauterine transfusions (intraperitoneal and intravascular)	1583
Total Fetuses	518
Total Survivors	363 (70%)

Table 2.2. Intrauterine transfusion in the ultrasound era – Winnipeg.

	Intraperitoneal transfusion n =204 July 80–Oct 86		Intravenous transfusion n =705 May 86–Sept 97	
	Total	% Alive	Total	% Alive
Fetuses	75	76	164	88
Non Hydrops	45	87	113	96
Hydrops	30	60	51	71
Non Moribund	22	82	31	37
Moribund	8	0	20	60

for the moribund, non breathing, hydropic fetus. Elevation of circulating hemoglobin levels is immediate. The risk of IVT is less than 0.8% versus 3.5% per procedure with IPT. IVT survival rates in Winnipeg are superior to IPT survival rates in every category (Table 2.2). The overall IVT survival rate is 88%.

CONCLUSION

The use of these approaches to investigate and treat alloimmune hemolytic disease in the fetus has reduced the perinatal mortality per affected pregnancy in Manitoba from 50% in the 1940's, to 1.5% in the 1990's.

References

1. Levine, P., Katzin, E.M. and Burnham, L., Isoimmunization in pregnancy: Its possible bearing on the etiology of erythroblastosis fetalis, *JAMA* 1941; **116**: 825–827.
2. Landsteiner, K. and Weiner, A.S., An agglutinable factor in human blood recognized by immune sera for rhesus blood, *Proc. Soc. Exp. Biol. Med.* 1940; **43**: 223.
3. Bowman, J.M., Treatment Options for the fetus with alloimmune hemolytic disease, *Transf. Med. Rev.* 1990; **IV**: 191–207.
4. Chown, B., Anemia from bleeding of the fetus into the mother's circulation, *Lancet* 1954; **1**: 1213–1215.
5. Bowman, J.M., Pollock, J.M. and Penston, L.E., Feto maternal transplacental hemorrhage during pregnancy and after delivery, *Vox. Sang.* 1986; **51**: 117–121.
6. Bowman, J.M. and Pollock, J.M., Amniotic fluid spectrophotometry and early delivery in the management of erythroblastosis fetalis, *Pediatrics* 1965; **35**: 815–835.

7. Wallerstein, H., Treatment of severe erythroblastosis by simultaneous removal and replacement of blood of the newborn, *Science* 1946; **103**: 583–585.
8. Chown, B. and Bowman, W.D., The place of early delivery in the prevention of foetal death from erythroblastosis, *Pediatr. Clin. North Am.* 1958; May: 279–288.
9. Hadley, A.G., *In vitro* assays to predict the severity of hemolytic disease of the newborn, *Transf. Med. Rev.* 1995; **IX**: 302–313.
10. Hyland, C.A., Wolter, L.C. and Saul, A., Identification and analysis of Rh Genes: Application of PCR and RFLP typing tests, *Transf. Med. Rev.* 1995; **IX**: 289–301.
11. Lo, Y.M.D., Corbetta, N., Chamberlain, P.F. *et al.*, Presence of fetal DNA in maternal plasma and serum, *Lancet* 1997; **350**: 485–487.
12. Lo, Y.M.D., Hjelm, N.M., Fidler, C. *et al.*, Prenatal diagnosis of fetal RhD status by molecular analysis of maternal plamsa, *New Eng. J. Med.* 1998; **339**: 1734–1738.
13. Liley, A.W., Liquor amnii analysis in management of pregnancy complicated by rhesus immunization, *Am. J. Obstet. Gynecol.* 1961; **82**: 1359–1371.
14. Bowman, J.M., Pollock J.M., Manning F.A. *et al.*, Maternal Kell blood group alloimmunization, *Obstet. Gynecol.* 1992; **79**: 239–244.
15. Chitkara, U., Wilkins, I., Lynch, L. *et al.*, The role of sonography in assessing severity of fetal anemia in Rh- and Kell-isoimmunized pregnancies, *Obstet. Gynecol.* 1988; **71**: 393–395.
16. Daffos, F., Capella-Pavlovsky, M. and Forestier, F., Fetal blood sampling during pregnancy with use of a needle guided by ultrasound: A study of 606 consecutive cases, *Am. J. Obstet. Gynecol.* 1985; **153**: 655–660.
17. Bowman, J.M., RhD hemolytic disease of the newborn, *New Eng. J. Med.* 1998; **339**: 1775–1777.
18. Graham-Pole, J., Barr, W. and Willoughby, M.L.N., Continuous flow plasmapheresis in management of severe Rhesus disease, *Br. Med. J.* 1977; **1**: 1185–1188.
19. Margulies, M., Voto, L.S., Mathet, E. and Margulies, M., High-dose intravenous IgG for the treatment of severe Rhesus alloimmunization, *Vox Sang* 1991; **61**: 181–189.
20. Liley, A.W., Intrauterine transfusion of fetus in hemolytic disease, *Br. Med. J.* 1963; **2**: 1107–1109.
21. Berkowitz, R.L., Chikara, U., Goldberg, J.D. *et al.*, Intrauterine intravascular transfusions for severe red blood cell isoimmunization: Ultrasound guided percutaneous approach, *Am. J. Obstet. Gynecol.* 1986; **155**: 574–581.
22. Harman, C.R., Bowman, J.M., Manning, F.A. *et al.*, Intrauterine transfusion – Intraperitoneal versus intravascular approach: A case-control comparision, *Am. J. Obstet. Gynecol. 1990;* **162**: 1053–1059.

Epidemiology and Causes of Indirect Hyperbilirubinemia

3 Epidemiology of Neonatal Jaundice

M. Jeffrey Maisels

Department of Pediatrics, William Beaumont Hospital, Royal Oak, Michigan, USA

There is a wide range of factors that affect neonatal bilirubin levels and these are listed in Table 3.1. Some of these factors have been identified only in large epidemiologic studies,[1] and their clinical relevance is questionable, but there are some that have been shown repeatedly to have an important influence on serum bilirubin levels and these are identified in the table.

GENETIC, ETHNIC AND FAMILIAR INFLUENCES

East Asian[2–4] and native American[5,6] infants have mean maximal serum bilirubin levels that are significantly higher than Caucasian infants. The reasons for this are not clear but recent studies provide intriguing information regarding the East Asian population. One of the mutations of the bilirubin diphosphate-glucuronosyl-transferase (UGT1A1) gene is a missense mutation (Gly71Arg) associated with Gilbert's syndrome.[7] Akaba *et al.* have reported that this mutation is prevalent in the Japanese, Korean and Chinese populations[8] and two studies have found that it occurs more commonly in Japanese newborns who receive phototherapy.[9,10] Thus it appears to be an important contributor to the high incidence of hyperbilirubinemia in Japanese newborns. Increased bilirubin production has also been found in these infants[6,11] so that the combined effect of increased production and poor clearance could explain why they have higher bilirubin levels than infants of other racial groups.

Black infants in the US and in Britain have lower bilirubin levels than white infants.[1,3,4,12,13] This occurs in spite of the fact that a polymorphism in the promoter of the UGT1A1 gene (the TA7 promoter genotype), which both causes Gilbert's syndrome[7] and is associated in Caucasian newborns with higher bilirubin levels,[14] is more common in black newborns.[15] Thus, other factors must play a role in lowering the bilirubin in these infants.

Address for correspondence: M. Jeffrey Maisels, M.D., 3535 W. 13 Mile Road, Royal Oak, MI 48073, Phone: (248) 551-0412, Fax: (248) 551-5998, E-mail: jmaisels@beaumont.edu

Table 3.1. Epidemiology of neonatal jaundice.

Associated factors	Effect on neonatal serum bilirubin levels		
	Increase	*Decrease*	*No effect*
Race	East Asian Native American Greek	African American[a]	

Genetic or familial	Previous sibling with jaundice[a]
	Variant promoter or mutation of
	   UGT1A1 gene associated
	   with Gilbert's syndrome		

Maternal	Older mothers Diabetes[a] Hypertension Oral contraceptive use at time of conception First-trimester bleeding Decreased plasma zinc level	Smoking	
Drugs administered to mother	Oxytocin[a] Diazepam Epidural anesthesia Promethazine	Phenobarbital Meperidine Reserpine Aspirin Chloral hydrate Heroin Phenytoin Antipyrine Alcohol	Beta-adrenergic agents
Labor and delivery	Premature rupture of membranes Forceps delivery Vacuum extraction Breech delivery		Fetal distress Low Apgar scores
Infant	Low birth weight Decreasing gestation[a] Male gender[a] Delayed cord clamping Elevated cord blood bilirubin level Delayed meconium passage Breast-feeding[a] Caloric deprivation[a] Larger weight loss after birth[a] Low serum zinc and magnesium		
Drugs administered to infant	Chloral hydrate Pancuronium		
Other	Altitude Short hospital stay after birth[a]		

[a] Most common clinically important factors.
From Maisels.[1]

Neonatal jaundice runs in families.[16–18] In a study of 3,301 infants, Khoury *et al.* found that if a previous sibling had a TSB level >12mg/dl (205 µmol/l), the risk of a similar TSB in a subsequent sibling was 3.1 times higher than in controls. When the TSB in the previous sibling was >15 mg/dl (257 µmol/l) the risk in subsequent siblings was 12.5 times greater than controls.[17] Others have also identified a significant correlation between the peak bilirubin levels of siblings.[18]

MATERNAL FACTORS

Smoking

Most studies suggest that infants of mothers who smoke during pregnancy have lower serum bilirubin levels than infants of nonsmokers[3,19–21], although some studies have not found this.[16,22] These data are confounded by the fact that women who smoke are much less likely to breast-feed[19] and the likelihood of breast-feeding is inversely related to the number of cigarettes smoked per day.[23]

Diabetes

Infants of insulin dependent diabetic mothers (IDM) who are large for their gestational age or have an elevated birth weight–length ratio have higher bilirubin levels than controls.[24–26] This is most likely related to an increase in bilirubin production – the rate of carbon monoxide production (and excretion) is directly related to the degree of macrosomia in these infants.[27] They have high erythropoietin levels and increased erythropoiesis[28] and as many as 24% of macrosomic IDM's are polycythemic.[25] Thus, ineffective erythropoiesis and polycythemia are probably responsible for their increased bilirubin production. In addition, diabetic mothers have 3 times more beta-glucuronidase in their breast milk than nondiabetic mothers.[25] This enzyme enhances the enterohepatic reabsorption of bilirubin. (See below)

Other Maternal Factors

Some investigators have found that primiparous mothers are more likely to have jaundiced infants,[16,29] but others have not found this.[3,30] A significant association between jaundice and increasing maternal age has been described; infants of teenage mothers had the lowest risk for hyperbilirubinemia.[16]

EVENTS DURING LABOR AND DELIVERY

Induction of Labor by Oxytocin

Multiple studies and several controlled trials have shown an association between the use of oxytocin to induce or augment labor and an increased incidence of neonatal hyperbilirubinemia, although the mechanism for this is unclear.[19,31]

Anesthesia and Analgesia

Epidural anesthesia, specifically bupivacaine, has been associated with neonatal jaundice in several studies.[12,16,32,33] These anesthetic agents readily cross the placenta and produce measurable blood levels in the newborn.[34]

Tocolysis

Tocolytic agents have not been associated with higher TSB levels or an increase in bilirubin production,[35,36] nor has any effect of nifedipine, ritodrine or terbutaline been found on carboxyhemoglobin levels or the need for phototherapy.[37,38]

Other Drugs

The administration of narcotic agents, barbiturates, aspirin, chloral hydrate, reserpine and phenytoin sodium are associated with lower bilirubin concentrations.[39] In the case of aspirin, this is possibly the result of the displacement of bilirubin from its binding to albumin (see Chapter 1). The use of diazepam increased TSB levels, but by less than 1 mg/dl (17 µmol/l).[39] Antipyrine administered to mothers before delivery decreases TSB levels and infants of heroin addicted mothers have lower bilirubin levels.[40] Phenobarbital, if given in sufficient doses to the mother significantly lowers TSB levels during the first week (see Chapter 13).

Route of Delivery

Vaginal delivery has been associated with higher neonatal TSB levels than Cesarean section birth,[41] although this was not confirmed in a controlled trial involving low birth weight infants.[42] When compared with forceps delivery, the use of vacuum extraction did not increase the number of infants who required phototherapy, although more clinical jaundice was seen with vacuum extraction.[43,44] Recent studies suggest an increased risk of severe hyperbilirubinemia following instrumented vaginal deliveries.[45]

Placental Transfusion and Hyperviscosity

Although a high hematocrit is often considered a risk factor for neonatal jaundice, controlled trials of intervention for hyperviscosity (using partial exchange transfusions in symptomatic infants) showed no differences in the incidence of hyperbilirubinemia in the treated and control groups.[46–48] Controlled trials on the effects of placental transfusion have also produced conflicting results.[31] In one study infants were held 30 cm below the introitus. If cord clamping was delayed, mean bilirubin levels at age 72 hours were 7.7 mg/dl (132 µmol/l) compared with 3.2 mg/dl (55 µmol/l) in the early clamped group.[48]

Cord Blood Bilirubin Levels

There is a strong association between TSB levels in cord blood and the risk of hyper-bilirubinemia in infants with and without hemolytic disease.[49–53]

NEONATAL FACTORS

Birth Weight and Gestation

Low birth weight and decreasing gestational age are strongly correlated with an increased risk for hyperbilirubinemia.[3,12,16,19,33,54,55] In a well baby population, we found that infants of 35–36 weeks gestation, were 13 times more likely (than those $\geq$40 weeks gestation) to be readmitted to hospital for phototherapy and those between 36 $\frac{1}{7}$ and 38 weeks, 7 times more likely to require phototherapy.[55]

Although cared for in well-baby nurseries, infants of 35–38 weeks gestation are much more likely to nurse ineffectively, receive fewer calories, and have a greater weight loss than their truly term counterparts. When combined with less effective hepatic clearance (because of prematurity), it is not surprising that they become more jaundiced.

Gender

Male infants consistently have higher bilirubin levels than females.[3,12,16,19]

Calories and Protein Intake

Decreased caloric intake is associated with an increase in TSB levels[56,57] and a significant association exists between hyperbilirubinemia and weight loss in the first few days after birth.[16,19,29,30,33] The primary mechanism associated with low caloric intake appears to be an increase in the enterohepatic circulation.[58] Infants fed with parenteral nutrition solutions are much more likely to develop conjugated hyperbilirubin-emia.[59,60] A higher protein intake (3.6 gm/kg/day vs. 2.3 gm/kg/day) was associated with higher peak direct serum bilirubin levels and early onset of cholestatic jaundice.[61]

Type of Diet

Gourley and colleagues have evaluated the effect of diet on fecal output and neonatal jaundice in infants fed human milk or infant formulas.[62,63] Infants who consumed a casein-hydrolysate formula (Nutramigen) had significantly lower bilirubin levels from days 6–16 than those fed standard whey predominant formulas. The reason for this is not known, but may be related to the fact that Nutramigen contains a beta-glucuronidase inhibitor. This will reduce hydrolysis of bilirubin glucuronides and less unconjugated bilirubin will be available for intestinal absorption.[62] (See below) The cumulative stool output of the infants fed casein-hydrolysate was lower than that of infants fed other formulas, suggesting that factors other than stool output and its effect on the enterohepatic circulation must explain these observations.[62]

BREAST-FEEDING AND JAUNDICE

Multiple studies over the last 25 years have found a strong association between breast-feeding and an increased incidence of neonatal hyperbilirubinemia (Figure 3.1).[31,64–67] Although some studies have not found this,[68] a pooled analysis of 12 studies in over 8,000 newborns showed that breast-fed infants were 3 times more likely to develop TSB levels of 12 mg/dl (205 μmol) or higher and 6 times more likely to develop levels of 15 mg/dl (257 μmol) or higher than formula fed infants.[67] In studies of infants readmitted to hospital in the first 2 weeks of life because of severe hyperbilirubinemia, 90% or more were fully or partially breast-fed.[54,55,69,70] Some mothers nurse their infants very effectively, starting soon after delivery and these infants are less likely to develop breast feeding associated jaundice.[71,72]

Jaundice associated with breast-feeding in the first 2–4 days of age has been called "the breast-feeding jaundice syndrome" or "breast-feeding associated jaundice" and that which appears later (at 4–7 days of age) has been called the "breast milk jaundice syndrome".[73] There is considerable overlap between these two entities and evidence to support 2 distinct syndromes is meager. In addition to having higher bilirubin levels in the first 3–5 days (Figure 3.1),[66] as a group, breast-fed infants have serum bilirubin levels that are higher than formula fed infants for at least 3–6 weeks.[64,65,74] These are the same infants who have high bilirubin levels in the first week of life and it is

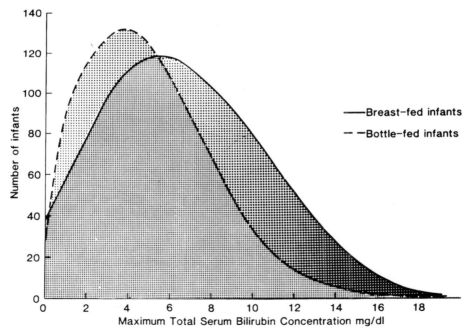

Figure 3.1. Distribution of maximum serum bilirubin concentrations in Caucasian infants who weigh >2500 gm. From Maisels *et al.*[66]

hard to believe that those who are still jaundiced at age 2–3 weeks represent a distinct group. Prolonged indirect hyperbilirubinemia (beyond 2–3 weeks) occurs in 20–30% of all breast-feeding infants[75] and in some infants may persist for up to three months. A recent study showed that 27% of breast fed infants who had TSB levels of more than 5.8 mg/dl (100 µmol/l) at age 28 days had the Gilbert's syndrome genotype.[76]

Pathogenesis of Jaundice Associated with Breast Feeding

The factors that play a role in the pathophysiology of jaundice associated with breast-feeding are listed in Table 3.2 and have recently been reviewed in detail.[73,77] Although most studies suggest that the primary contributors to breast-feeding jaundice are a decreased caloric intake and an increase in the enterohepatic circulation, some studies have suggested the role of inhibitory substances in breast milk and these are listed in Table 3.2. The roles of a progestational steroid, 3-alpha-20-beta-pregnanediol as well as free fatty acids have also been examined, but the data regarding the contribution of these substances to the jaundice associated with breast-feeding are conflicting.[73,77]

The management of hyperbilirubinemia associated with breast feeding is discussed in Chapter 10.

Intestinal reabsorption of bilirubin

Intestinal reabsorption of bilirubin (the enterohepatic circulation) appears to be the most important mechanism responsible for the jaundice associated with breast feeding. Breast fed infants receive fewer calories in the days after birth than do those fed formula, and caloric deprivation is strongly associated with an increase in the enterohepatic circulation of bilirubin.[58,78] Additional support for the important role of caloric deprivation and enterohepatic circulation is provided by the finding that increasing the frequency of breast feeding significantly reduced the risk of hyperbilirubinemia.[71,72,79] In the first few days, breast-fed infants also pass less stool by

Table 3.2. Factors that play a role in the pathophysiology of jaundice associated with breast feeding.

Decreased bilirubin clearance by the liver
  Genetic – Gilbert's syndrome genotype

Inhibitory substances in breast milk
  Pregnanediol
  Lipase – free fatty acids
  Unknown inhibitors

Increased intestinal reabsorption of bilirubin
  Decreased caloric intake
  Delayed meconium passage
  Decreased formation of urobilin
  Beta-glucuronidase
  Bile acid abnormalities

weight and their stools contain less bilirubin than those of formula fed infants.[77,80] The stools of breast-fed infants weigh less and their cumulative stool output is lower than in formula fed infants.[62] In breast-fed infants, an increase in the quantity of stool excreted in the first 21 days was associated with a decrease in serum bilirubin levels.[62] Infants fed human milk passed stool significantly less frequently than infants fed casein predominant formulas,[62] while those fed casein hydrolysate formulas passed less stool, cumulatively, than those given whey-predominant or casein-predominant formulas.[62] Alonso and colleagues[75] collected milk from unselected, normal mothers and serum from their infants at 16.3 ± 2.4 days. They labeled bilirubin with ^{14}C and studied its absorption when administered into the duodenum of adult rats. When bilirubin was administered with a bicarbonate buffer, $25.29 \pm 4\%$ was absorbed. Absorption was $4.67 \pm 2.4\%$ when given with Similac formula and $7.7 \pm 2.9\%$ when given with fresh human milk. There was a positive correlation between the percentage of bilirubin absorbed when administered with human milk and the serum bilirubin level in the rat being fed that milk. These data provide additional evidence that enhanced intestinal absorption of bilirubin contributes to the jaundice associated with breast-feeding. The fact that breast fed infants have higher TSB levels than formula fed infants for as long as 6 weeks, when the nursing infants are thriving and are not calorically deprived indicates that if this is the result of an increase in enterohepatic circulation, it cannot be caused by caloric deprivation.

Urobilin formation

In adults, bilirubin in the gut is rapidly reduced by the action of colonic bacteria to urobilin. At birth, the fetal gut is sterile and although there is an increase in the bacterial content of the gut after delivery, the neonatal intestinal flora do not convert conjugated bilirubin to urobilin. This leaves bilirubin in the bowel and allows it to be deconjugated and thus available for reabsorption. Formula-fed infants excrete urobilin in their stools earlier than breast-fed infants[81] perhaps due to the effect of formula feeding on the intestinal flora. Thus, the effect of breast milk on intestinal flora, by slowing the formation of urobilin, further enhances the possibility of intestinal reabsorption of bilirubin.

Beta-glucuronidase formation

Beta-glucuronidase is an enzyme that cleaves the ester-linkage of bilirubin-glucuronide, producing unconjugated bilirubin which can then be reabsorbed through the gut. Significant concentrations of beta-glucuronidase are found in the neonatal intestine and its activity is also higher in human milk than in infant formulas. Gourley and colleagues found a correlation between neonatal serum bilirubin levels and beta-glucuronidase activity in the first stool passed after birth.[82] They also found a positive relation between serum bilirubin levels and breast milk beta-glucuronidase activity in the first 3–4 days after birth,[83] but others have not been able to confirm these findings.[75,84–86]

Meconium passage

Because the enterohepatic circulation of bilirubin is an important contributor to neonatal hyperbilirubinemia, increasing the rate of bilirubin evacuation from the bowel should decrease the incidence of neonatal jaundice. Two randomized studies have shown that the early passage of meconium (stimulated by a rectal thermometer or a suppository) reduced peak serum bilirubin levels by about 1 mg/dl (17 µmol) when compared with control groups.[87,88]

PHENOLIC DETERGENTS

The use of phenolic detergents to disinfect incubators and other nursery surfaces has been associated with an epidemic of neonatal hyperbilirubinemia in 2 hospitals.[89,90] These detergents should not be used in the nursery.

ALTITUDE

Infants born at 3100 meters above sea level are four times more likely to have TSB levels above 12 mg/dl (205 µmol/l) than those born at sea level.[91] Both short and long-term exposure to high altitudes increases bilirubin levels in adults. The possible mechanisms for these observations include an increase in bilirubin load due to high hematocrits,[92] impaired conjugation,[93] and impaired excretion of bilirubin.[94]

DRUGS ADMINISTERED TO THE INFANT

Large doses of synthetic vitamin K analogs have been associated with significant hyperbilirubinemia, but the standard dose (1 mg) of IM vitamin K1 has no effect on neonatal bilirubin levels. The use of pancuronium[95] and chloral hydrate in the neonate[96,97] have been associated with an increased risk for hyperbilirubinemia. Chloral hydrate is metabolized to trichloroacetic acid and the toxic trichloroethanol, both of which accumulate in the tissues of compromised infants. The administration of chloral hydrate is associated with both indirect and direct hyperbilirubinemia[96] and this drug should be used with caution in newborns and particularly low-birth-weight, ventilator-dependent infants.

GLUCOSE-6-PHOSPHATE DEHYDROGENASE DEFICIENCY

Although G6PD deficiency affects millions of people around the world, most American pediatricians do not think about this enzyme deficiency as a likely cause for hyperbilirubinemia. This problem is particularly relevant in infants discharged early because the increase in bilirubin in G6PD-deficient infants may occur later than in other types of hemolytic disease. Recent evidence suggests that although some infants with G6PD deficiency have an increase in bilirubin production, in others, abnormal bilirubin conjugation appears to be the main reason for their hyperbilirubinemia.[98] (See Chapters 4 and 5)

References

1. Maisels, M.J., Neonatal jaundice, In: Avery G.B., Fletcher, M.A. and MacDonald, M.G., eds Neonatology: pathophysiology and management of the newborn. J.B. Lippincott Co., 5th ed. Philadelphia, 1999; 765–820.
2. Horiguchi, T. and Bauer C., Ethnic differences in neonatal jaundice: Comparison of Japanese and Caucasian newborn infants, *Am. J. Obstet. Gynecol.* 1975; **121**: 71–74.
3. Linn, S., Schoenbaum, S.C., Monson, R.R. *et.al.*, Epidemiology of neonatal hyperbilirubinemia, *Pediatrics* 1985; **75**: 770–774.
4. Newman, T.B., Easterling, M.J., Goldman, E.S. and Stevenson, D.K., Laboratory evaluation of jaundiced newborns: Frequency, cost and yield., *Am. J. Dis. Child.* 1990; **144**: 364–368.
5. Saland, J., McNamara, H. and Cohen, M.I., Navajo jaundice: Variant of neonatal hyperbilirubinemia associated with breast feeding, *J. Pediatr.* 1974; **85**: 271–275.
6. Johnson, J.D., Angelus, P., Aldrich, M. and Skipper, B.J., Exagerated jaundice in Navajo neonates: the role of bilirubin production, *Am. J. Dis. Child.* 1986; **140**: 889–890.
7. Bosma, P.J., Roy-Chowdhury, J., Bakker, C. *et al.*, The genetic basis of the reduced expression of bilirubin UDP-glucuronosyl transferase 1 in Gilbert's syndrome, *N. Engl. J. Med.* 1995; **333**: 1171–1175.
8. Doyle, P.E., Eidelman A.I., Lee K-S. *et al.*, Exchange transfusion and hypernatremia: Possible role in intracranial hemorrhage in very-low birthweight infants, *J. Pediatr.* 1978; **92**: 848.
9. Akaba, K., Toshiyuki, K., Sasaki, A., Tanabe S., Wakabayashi, T., Hiroi, M. *et al.*, Neonatal hyperbilirubinemia and a common mutation of the bilirubin uridine diphosphate-glucuronosyl-transferase gene in Japanese, *J. Hum. Genet.* 1998; **44**: 22–25.
10. Maruo, Y., Nishizawa, K., Sato H., Doida, Y. and Shimada, M., Association of Neonatal Hyperbilirubinemia with bilirubin UDP-glucuronosyltransferase polymorphism, *Pediatrics* 1999; **103**: 1224–1227.
11. Chen S.H., Endogenous formation of carbon monoxide in Chinese newborn with hyperbilirubinemia, *J. Formosan Med. Assoc.* 1981; **80**: 68–77.
12. Friedman, L., Lewis, P.J., Clifton, P. and Bulpitt, C.J., Factors influencing the incidence of neonatal jaundice, *Br. Med. J.* 1978; **1**: 1235–1237.
13. Hardy, J.B., Drage, J.S. and Jackson, E.C., The First Year of Life: The Collaborative Perinatal Project of the National Institutes of Neurological and Communicative Disorders and Stroke. Baltimore, MD: Johns Hopkins University Press, 1979.
14. Bancroft, J.D., Kreamer, B. and Gourley, G.R., Gilbert's syndrome accelerates development of neonatal jaundice, *J. Pediatr.* 1998; **132**: 656–660.
15. Beutler, E., Gelbart, T. and Demina, A., Racial variability in the UDP-glucuronosyltransferase 1 (UGT1A1) promoter: A balanced polymorphism for regulation of bilirubin metabolism? *Proc. Natl. Acad. Sci.* 1998; **95**: 8170–8174.
16. Gale, R., Seidman, D.S., Dollberg, S. and Stevenson, D.K., Epidemiology of neonatal jaundice in the Jerusulem population, *J. Pediatr. Gastro. Nutr.* 1990; **10**: 82–86.
17. Khoury, M.J., Calle, E.E. and Joesoef, R.M., Recurrence risk of neonatal hyperbilirubinemia in siblings, *Am. J. Dis. Child.* 1988; **142**: 1065–1069.
18. Nielsen, H, Haase, P, Blaabjerg, J, Stryhn, H. and Hilden, J., Risk factors and sib correlation in physiological neonatal jaundice, *Acta. Paediatr. Scand.* 1987; **76**: 504–511.
19. Maisels, M.J., Gifford, K.L., Antle, C.E. *et al.*, Jaundice in the healthy newborn infant: A new approach to an old problem, *Pediatrics* 1988; **81**: 505–511.
20. Diwan, V.K., Vaughan, T.L. and Yang, C.Y., Maternal smoking in relation to the incidence of early neonatal jaundice, *Gynecol. Obstet. Invest.* 1989; **27**: 22–25.
21. Hardy, J.B. and Mellits, E.D., Does maternal smoking during pregnancy have a long-term effect on the child? *Lancet* 1972; **2**: 1332–1336.
22. Knudsen, A. Maternal smoking and the bilirubin concentration in the first three days of life, *Eur. J. Obstet. Gynecol. Reprod. Biol.* 1991; **25**: 37–41.
23. Jones, J.B., The smoking disease, *Br. Med. J.* 1971; **1**: 228.

24. Peevy, K.J., Landaw, S.A. and Gross, S.J., Hyperbilirubinemia in infants of diabetic mothers, *Pediatrics* 1980; **66**: 417–419.
25. Berk, M.A., Mimouni, F., Miodovnik, M., Hertzberg, V. and Valuck, J., Macrosomia in infants of insulin-dependent diabetic mothers, *Pediatrics* 1989; **83**: 1029–1034.
26. Jährig, D., Jährig, K., Striet, S. *et al.*, Neonatal jaundice in infants of diabetic mothers, *Acta. Paediatr. Scand.* 1989; **360**: 101–107.
27. Stevenson, D.K., Ostrander, C.R., Cohen, R.S. *et al.*, Pulmonary excretion of carbon monoxide in the human infant as an index of bilirubin production. II. Evidence for the possible effect of maternal prenatal glucose metabolism on postnatal bilirubin production in a mixed population of infants, *Eur. J. Pediatr.* 1981; **137**: 255–259.
28. Widness, J.A., Susa, J.B., Garcia, J.F. *et al.*, Increased erythropoiesis and elevated erythropoietin in infants born to diabetic mothers and in hyperinsulinemic rhesus fetuses, *J. Clin. Invest.* 1981; **67**: 637–642.
29. Tudehope, D., Bayley, G., Monro, D. and Townsend, S., Breast feeding practices and severe hyperbiliurinaemia, *J. Paediatr. Child Health* 1991; **27**: 240–244.
30. Osborn, L.M., Reiff, M.I. and Bolus, R., Jaundice in the full term neonate, *Pediatrics* 1984; **73**: 520–526.
31. Maisels, M.J., Neonatal Jaundice. In: Sinclair J.C. and Bracken M.B., eds., Effective care of the newborn infant. Oxford: Oxford University Press, 1992; 507–561.
32. Sims, D.G. and Neligan, G.A., Factors affecting the increasing incidence of severe non-haemolytic neonatal jaundice, *Br. J. Obstet. Gynaecol.* 1975; **82**: 863–867.
33. Wood, B., Culley, P., Roginski, C., Powell, J. and Waterhouse, J., Factors affecting neonatal jaundice, *Arch. Dis. Child.* 1979; **54**: 111–115.
34. Pedersen, H., Morishima, H.O. and Finster, M., Uptake and effects of local anesthetics in mother and fetus, *Int. Anesthesiol. Clin.* 1978; **16**: 73–89.
35. Hancock, D.J., Setzer, E.S. and Beydown, S.N., Physiologic and biochemical effects of ritodrine therapy on the mother and perinate, *Am. J. Perinatol.* 1985; **2**: 1–6.
36. Hopper, A.O., Cohen, R.S., Ostrander, C.R., Brackman, F.S., Uekand, K. and Stevenson D.K., Maternal adrenergic tocolysis and neonatal bilirubin production, *Am. J. Dis. Child.* 1983; **137**: 58–60.
37. Caritis, S.N., Toig, G., Heddinger, L.A. and Ashmead, G., A double-blind study comparing ritodrine and terbutaline in the treatment of preterm labor, *Am. J. Obstet. Gynecol.* 1984; **150**: 7–14.
38. Ferguson, J.E., II, Schutz, T.E. and Stevenson, D.K., Neonatal bilirubin production after preterm labor tocolysis with nifedipine, *Dev. Pharmacol. Ther.* 1989; **12**: 113–117.
39. Drew, J.H. and Kitchen, W.H., The effect of maternally administered drugs on bilirubin concentrations in the newborn infant, *J. Pediatr.* 1976; **89**: 657–661.
40. Nathenson, G., Cohen, M.I., Litt, I.F. and McNamara, H., The effect of maternal heroin addition on neonatal jaundice, *J. Pediatr.* 1972; **81**: 899–903.
41. Yamauchi, Y. and Yamanouchi, I., Difference in TcB readings between full term newborn infants born vaginally and by cesarean section, *Acta. Paediatr. Scand.* 1989; **79**: 824–828.
42. Wallace, R.L., Schifrin, B.S. and Paul, R.H., The delivery route for very-low-birth-weight infants. A preliminary report of a randomized, prospective study, *J. Reprod. Med.* 1984; **29**: 736–740.
43. Dell, D.L., Sightler, S.E. and Plauche, W.C., Soft cup vacuum extraction: A comparison of outlet delivery, *Obstet. Gynecol.* 1985; **66**: 624–628.
44. Vacca, A., Grant, A., Wyatt, G. and Chalmers, I., Portsmouth operative delivery trial: A comparison of vacuum extraction and forceps delivery, *Brit. J. Obstet. Gynaecol.* 1983; **90**: 1107–1112.
45. Bhutani, V.K., Johnson, L.H., Sivieri, E. *et al.*, Clinical risk assessment of Coombs positive ABO isoimmunization for excessive neonatal hyperbilirubinemia, *Pediatr. Res.* 1999; **45**: 237A.
46. Black, V.D., Lubchenco, L.O., Koops, B.L., Poland, R.L. and Powell, D.P., Neonatal hyperviscosity: Randomized study of effect of partial plasma exchange transfusion on long-term outcome, *Pediatrics.* 1985; **75**: 1048–1053.
47. Goldberg, K., Wirth, F.H., Hathaway, W.E., Guggenheim, M.A., Murphy, J.R., Braithwaite, W.R., *et al.*, Neonatal hyperviscosity II. Effect of partial plasma exchange transfusion, *Pediatrics* 1982; **69**: 419–425.
48. Saigal, S., O'Neill, A., Surainder, Y., Chua, L.B. and Usher, R., Placental transfusion and hyperbilirubinemia in the premature, *Pediatrics* 1972; **49**: 406–419.
49. Davidson, L.T., Merritt, K.K. and Weech, A.A., Hyperbilirubinemia in the newborn, *Am. J. Dis. Child.* 1941; **61**: 958–980.
50. Saigal, S., Lunyk, O., Bennett, K.J. and Patterson, M.C., Serum bilirubin levels in breast- and formula-fed infants in the first 5 days of life, *Can. Med. Assoc. J.* 1982; **127**: 985–989.

51. Knudsen, A., Prediction of the development of neonatal jaundice by increased umbilical cord blood bilirubin, *Acta. Pediatr. Scand.* 1989; **78**: 217–221.
52. Rosenfeld, J., Umbilical cord bilirubin levels as a predictor of subsequent hyperbilirubinemia, *J. Fam. Pract.* 1986; **23**: 556–558.
53. Risemberg, H.M., Mazzi, E., MacDonald, M.G. *et al.*, Correlation of cord bilirubin levels with hyperbilirubinemia in ABO incompatibility, *Arch. Dis. Child.* 1977; **52**: 219–222.
54. Soskolne, E.L., Schumacher, R., Fyock, C. *et al.,* The effect of early discharge and other factors on readmission rates of newborns, *Arch. Pediatr. Adolesc. Med.* 1996; **150**: 373–379.
55. Maisels, M.J. and Kring, E.A., Length of stay, jaundice and hospital readmission, *Pediatrics* 1998; **101**: 995–998.
56. Barrett, P.V.D., Hyperbilirubinemia of fasting, *JAMA* 1971; **217**: 1349–1353.
57. Felsher, B.F., Rickard, D. and Redeker, A.G., The reciprocal relation between caloric intake and the degree of hyperbilirubinemia in Gilbert's syndrome, *N. Engl. J. Med.* 1970; **283**: 170–172.
58. Fevery, J., Fasting hyperbilirubinemia: Unraveling the mechanism involved, *Gastroenterology* 1997; **113**: 1707–1313.
59. Glass, E.J., Hume, R., Lang, M.A. and Forfar, J.O., Parenteral nutrition compared with transpyloric feeding, *Arch. Dis. Child.* 1984; **59**: 131–135.
60. Yu, V.Y.H., James, E., Hendry, P. and MacMahon, R.A., Total parenteral nutrition in very low birth weight infants: A controlled trial, *Arch. Dis. Child.* 1979; **54**: 653–661.
61. Vileisis, R.A., Inwood, R.J. and Hunt, C.E., Prospective controlled study of parenteral nutrition – associated cholestatic jaundice: Effect of protein intake, *J. Pediatr.* 1980; **96**: 893–897.
62. Gourley, G.R., Kreamer, B. and Arend, R., The effect of diet on feces and jaundice during the first three weeks of life, *Gastroenterology* 1992; **103**: 660.
63. Gourley, G.R., Kreamer, B., Cohnen, M, *et al.* Neonatal jaundice and diet, *Arch. Pediatr. Adolesc. Med.* 1999; **153**: 184–188.
64. Kivlahan, C. and James, E.J.P., The natural history of neonatal jaundice, *Pediatrics* 1984; **74**: 364–370.
65. Maisels, M.J. and D'Archangelo, M.R., Breast feeding and jaundice in the first six weeks of life (abstr), *Pediatr. Res.* 1983; **17**: 324A.
66. Maisels, M.J., Gifford, K., Antle, C.E. *et al.*, Normal serum bilirubin levels in the newborn and the effect of breast feeding, *Pediatrics* 1986; **78**: 837–843.
67. Schneider, A.P., Breast milk jaundice in the newborn. A real entity. *JAMA* 1986; **255**: 3270–3274.
68. Rubaltelli, F.F., Unconjugated and conjugated bilirubin pigments during perinatal development. IV. The influence of breast-feeding on neonatal hyperbilirubinemia, *Biol. Neonate.* 1993; **64**: 104–109.
69. Seidman, D.S., Stevenson, D.K., Ergaz, Z. and Gale, R., Hospital readmission due to neonatal hyperbilirubinemia, *Pediatrics* 1995; **96**: 727–729.
70. Maisels, M.J. and Kring, E., Risk of sepsis in newborns with severe hyperbilirubinemia, *Pediatrics* 1992; **90**: 741–743.
71. De Carvalho, M., Klaus, M.H. and Merkatz, R.B., Frequency of breastfeeding and serum bilirubin concentration, *Am. J. Dis. Child.* 1982; **136**: 737–738.
72. Yamauchi, Y. and Yamanouchi, I., Breast-feeding frequency during the first 24 hours after birth in full-term neonates, *Pediatrics* 1990; **86**: 171–175.
73. Auerbach, K.G., and Gartner, L.M., Breast feeding and human milk: Their association with jaundice in the neonate, *Clin. Perinatol.* 1987; **14**: 89–107.
74. Hall, R.T., Braun, W.J., Callenbach, J.C. *et al.*, Hyperbilirubinemia in breast-vs-formula-fed infants in the first six weeks of life: Relationship to weight gain, *Am. J. Perinatol.* 1983; **1**: 47–51.
75. Alonso, E.M., Whitington, P.F., Whitington, S.H., Rivard, W.A. and Given G. Enterohepatic circulation of non-conjugated bilirubin in rats fed with human milk, *J. Pediatr.* 1991; **118**: 425–430.
76. Monaghan, G., McLellan, A., McGeehan, A. *et al.*, Gilbert's syndrome is a contributory factor in prolonged unconjugated hyperbilirubinemia of the newborn, *J. Pediatr.* 1999; **134**: 441–446.
77. Gourley, G.R., Pathophysiology of breast-milk jaundice. In: Polin, R.A. and Fox W.W., eds. Fetal and Neonatal Physiology. 2nd ed. Philadelphia: W.B. Saunders, Co., 1998; 1499.
78. Gärtner, U., Goeser, T. and Wolkoff, A.W., Effect of fasting on the uptake of bilirubin and sulfobromophthalein by the isolated perfused rat liver, *Gastroenterology* 1997; **113**: 1707–1713.
79. Varimo, P., Similä, S., Wendt, L. and Kolvisto, M., Frequency of breast feeding and hyperbilirubinemia, *Clin. Pediatr.* 1986; **25**: 112.
80. De Carvalho, M., Robertson, S. and Klaus, M., Fecal bilirubin excretion and serum bilirubin concentration in breast-fed and bottle-fed infants, *J. Pediatr.* 1985; **107**: 786–790.
81. Yoshioka, H., Development and differences of intestinal flora in the neonatal period in breast-fed and bottle-fed infants, *Pediatrics* 1983; **72**: 317–321.

82. Gourley, G.R., Kremer, B. and Arend, R., Neonatal serum bilirubin levels correlate with beta glucuronidase activity in the first stool of life, *Hepatology* 1989; **10**: 728.
83. Gourley, G.R. and Arend, R.A., Beta-glucuronidase and hyperbilirubinemia in breast-fed and formula-fed babies, *Lancet* 1986; **1**: 644–646.
84. Wilson, D.C., Afrasiabi, M. and Reid, M.M., Breast-milk beta-glucuronidase and exaggerated jaundice in the early neonatal period, *Biol. Neonate*. 1992; **61**: 232–234.
85. Ince, Z., Coban, A., Peker, I. and Can, G., Breast milk beta-glucuronidase and prolonged jaundice in the neonate, *Acta. Paediatr*. 1995; **84**: 237–239.
86. LaTorre, A., Targioni, G. and Rubaltelli, F.F., Beta-glucuronidase and hyperbilirubinemia in breast-fed babies, *Biol. Neonate*. 1999; **75**: 82–84.
87. Cottrell, B.H., and Anderson, G.C., Rectal or axillary temperature measurement: Effect on plasma bilirubin and intestinal transit of meconium, *J. Pediatr. Gastroenterol. Nutr*. 1984; 3: 734–739.
88. Weisman, L.E., Merenstein, G.B., Digirol, M., Collins, J., Frank, G. and Hudgins, C., The effect of early meconium evacuation on early-onset hyperbilirubinemia, *Am. J. Dis. Child*. 1983; **137**: 666–668.
89. Daum, F., Cohen, M.I. and McNamara, H., Experimental toxicologic studies on a phenol detergent associated with neonatal hyperbilirubinemia, *J. Pediatr*. 1976; **89**: 853–853.
90. Wysowski, D.K., Flynt, J.W., Goldfield, M. *et al.*, Epidemic neonatal hyperbilirubinemia and use of a phenolic disinfectant detergent, *Pediatrics* 1978; **61**: 165–165.
91. Moore, L.G., Newberry, M.A., Freeby, G.M. and Crnic, L.S., Increased incidence of neonatal hyperbilirubinemia at 3,100 m in Colorado, *Am. J. Dis. Child*. 1984; **138**: 157–161.
92. Atland, P.D. and Parker, M.G., Bilirubinemia and intravascular hemolysis during acclimatization to high altitude, *Int. J. Biometeorol*. 1977; **21**: 165–170.
93. Berendsohn, S., Hepatic function at high altitudes, *Arch. Intern. Med*. 1962; **109**: 256–264.
94. Barron, E.S.G., Bilirubinemia, *Medicine* 1931; **10**: 114–115.
95. Freeman, J., Lesko, S., Mitchell A.A., Epstein, M.F. and Shapiro, S., Hyperbilirubinemia following exposure to pancuronium bromide in newborns, *Dev. Pharmacol. Ther*. 1990; **14**: 209–215.
96. Lambert, G.H., Muraskas, J., Anderson, C.L. and Myers, T.F., Direct hyperbilirubinemia associated with chloral hydrate administration in the newborn, *Pediatrics* 1990; **86**: 277–281.
97. Reimche, L.D., Sankaran, K., Hindmarsh, K.W., Kasian, G.F., Gorecki, D.K.J. and Tan, L., Chloral hydrate sedation in neonates and infants – clinical and pharmacologic considerations, *Dev. Pharmacol. Ther*. 1989; **12**: 57–64.
98. Kaplan, M. and Hammerman, C., Severe Neonatal Hyperbilirubinemia: A potential complication of glucose-6-phosphate dehydrogenase deficiency, *Clin. Perinatol*. 1998; **25**: 575–590.

4 Indirect Hyperbilirubinemia in the Neonate

Jon F. Watchko

Division of Neonatology and Developmental Biology, Department of Pediatrics, University of Pittsburgh School of Medicine, Pittsburgh, Pennsylvania, USA

Almost two-thirds of human newborns develop clinically evident indirect hyper-bilirubinemia in the first few days of life. This hyperbilirubinemia reflects an inter-play of developmentally modulated changes in bilirubin production and metabolism characterized by an increased bilirubin load on hepatocytes and decreased hepatic bilirubin clearance (Table 4.1). The increased bilirubin load is the result of i) the newborns large red cell mass combined with a reduced red cell lifespan and ii) the enterohepatic circulation of bilirubin. Decreased neonatal hepatic bilirubin clearance results primarily from a limited capacity for hepatic bilirubin conjugation. Both an increased bilirubin load and a decreased clearance probably contribute to the jaun-dice in any given infant; quantifying their individual contribution, however, is usually not possible in the clinical arena. In a small fraction of neonates, marked indirect hyperbilirubinemia develops that may pose a neurotoxic risk to the infant. In these cases, an additional superimposed process may exaggerate the hyperbilirubinemia. This chapter will review the causes of indirect hyperbilirubinemia and highlight the factors that may enhance its development.

INCREASED BILIRUBIN LOAD – HEMOLYTIC DISEASE

The reduced erythrocyte life span of normal newborn red cells (70–90 days as opposed to 120 days in the adult)[1,2] contributes to an enhanced level of bilirubin production and hepatic bilirubin load in neonates. Each gram of hemoglobin yields 35 mg of bilirubin[3] and the amount of bilirubin produced in the first three days of life as a result of a red cell life span of 70 days approximates 72 mg for the average term newborn.[1] It follows that an increase in red cell mass, i.e., polycythemia and factors known to accelerate red cell turn over, i.e., hemolytic disorders, are clinically important conditions that enhance the risk for developing hyperbilirubinemia in infants. Of these, hemolysis is the most potent contributor to the genesis of marked hyperbilirubinemia. The causes of hemolysis in the neonatal period are numerous but can be broadly grouped into three major categories: i) heritable defects in red

Table 4.1. Causes of indirect hyperbilirubinemia in newborn infants.

Increased production or bilirubin load on the liver
  Hemolytic disease
    Immune mediated
      Rh alloimmunization
      ABO and other blood group incompatibilities
    Heritable
      Red cell membrane defects
        spherocytosis[a], elliptocytosis, stomatocytosis, pyknocytosis
      Red cell enzyme deficiencies
        Glucose-6-phosphate dehydrogenase deficiency[a]
        pyruvate kinase deficiency and other erythrocyte enzyme deficiencies
      Hemoglobinopathies
        Alpha thalassemia, beta-γ-thalassemia
  Other causes of increased production
    Sepsis[a,b]
    Disseminated intravascular coagulation
    Extravasation of blood (hematomas, pulmonary, cerebral or other occult hemorrhage)
    Polycythemia
    Macrosomic infants of diabetic mothers
  Increased enterohepatic circulation of bilirubin
    Breast-milk jaundice
    Pyloric stenosis[a]
    Small or large bowel obstruction or ileus
Decreased clearance
    Prematurity
    Glucose-6-phosphate dehydrogenase deficiency
  Inborn errors of metabolism
    Crigler–Najjar syndrome, Types 1 and 2
    Gilbert's syndrome
    Tyrosinemia[b]
    Hypermethioninemia[b]
  Metabolic
    Hypothyroidism
    Hypopituitarism[b]

---

[a] Decreased clearance also part of the pathogenesis of indirect hyperbilirubinemia.
[b] Evaluation of direct-reacting bilirubin also occurs.

cell metabolism, membrane structure, or hemoglobin; ii) acquired disorders; and iii) immune mediated mechanisms (Table 4.1).

Heritable Causes of Hemolysis – Red Cell Membrane Defects

Of the many red cell membrane defects that lead to hemolysis only hereditary spherocytosis, elliptocytosis, stomatocytosis and infantile pyknocytosis may manifest themselves in the newborn period.[4–6] Establishing a diagnosis of these disorders is often difficult in neonates because newborns normally exhibit a marked variation in red cell membrane size and shape.[4,7,8] In premature infants, the high frequency of red cell dysmorphology in hematologically normal neonates is even more prevalent and can include target cells and acanthocytes.[7] Spherocytes, however, are not often seen on red cell smears of hematologically normal newborns and this morphologic abnormality, when prominent, may yield a diagnosis of hereditary spherocytosis in the immediate neonatal period. Given that approximately 75% of families affected with hereditary spherocytosis manifest an autosomal dominant phenotype, a positive family history can often be elicited and provide further support for this diagnosis. A recent observation shows that the presence of jaundice severe enough to require phototherapy in newborns with hereditary spherocytosis is strongly related to an interaction with the Gilbert's syndrome allele[9] a phenomenon also seen in infants with G6PD deficiency (see section on G6PD deficiency below). The diagnosis of hereditary spherocytosis can be confirmed using the incubated osmotic fragility test which is a reliable diagnostic tool in newborns when coupled with fetal red cell controls. One must rule out symptomatic ABO hemolytic disease by performing a direct Coombs test as infants so affected may also manifest prominent microspherocytosis.[10] Moreover, hereditary spherocytosis and symptomatic ABO hemolytic disease can occur in the same infant and result in severe anemia and hyperbilirubinemia.[11]

Hereditary elliptocytosis and stomatocytosis are rare but reported causes of hemolysis in the newborn period.[4] Infantile pyknocytosis, a transient red cell membrane abnormality manifesting itself during the first few months of life, is more common. The pyknocyte, an irregularly contracted red cell with multiple spines, can normally be observed in newborns, particularly premature infants where up to ~5% of red cells may manifest this morphologic variant.[6] In newborns affected with infantile pyknocytosis, up to 50% of red cells exhibit the morphologic abnormality and this degree of pyknocytosis is associated with jaundice, anemia and a reticulocytosis. Infantile pyknocytosis can cause hyperbilirubinemia that is severe enough to require control by exchange transfusion.[6] Red cells transfused into affected infants become pyknocytic and have a shortened life span suggesting that an extracorpuscular factor mediates the morphologic alteration.[6,12,13] Whatever the precise mechanism(s) underlying infantile pyknocytosis may be, this disorder tends to resolve after several months of life. Pyknocytosis may also occur in several other conditions including G6PD deficiency, vitamin E deficiency and herditary elliptocytosis and these conditions must be excluded before a diagnosis of infantile pyknocytosis is made. Although some investigators suggest that infantile pyknocytosis is rarely seen today, this author has seen three cases in the past two years.

Heritable Causes of Hemolysis – Red Cell Enzyme Deficiencies

The two most common red cell enzyme defects that may lead to hyperbilirubinemia in the neonatal period are glucose-6-phosphate dehydrogenase (G6PD)[14-17]and pyruvate kinase deficiency.[18] G6PD deficiency is a sex-linked disorder that may be associated with hemolysis in newborns following exposure to an appropriate trigger, usually an oxidative challenge. The most frequently reported hemolytic agent in G6PD deficient neonates is naphthalene, a common component in moth-balls.[15] Severe hemolysis and marked hyperbilirubinemia may occur in this context and result in kernicterus.[19,20] Another important hemolytic triggers in G6PD deficient newborns is infection.[14,15,17]

In most cases of marked hyperbilirubinemia in G6PD deficient neonates, how-ever, there is no overt evidence of hemolysis, i.e., anemia and reticulocytosis.[21,22] This observation has prompted some to conclude that in the majority of cases, hyper-bilirubinemia in G6PD deficiency is of hepatic origin.[14] These investigators speculate that G6PD deficiency in the liver results in impaired bilirubin clearance.[14] There is some evidence to support this view.[23,24] Others counter that hemolysis in G6PD deficiency is a self-limited postnatal phenomenon and the anemia is likely to be masked by other factors that modulate hemoglobin concentration in the immediate newborn period.[15] From their standpoint it is not necessary to invoke impaired hepatic clearance in the genesis of marked hyperbilirubinemia in G6PD deficient neonates.[15]

A recent study sheds some light on this controversy demonstrating that i) a molecular marker for Gilbert's syndrome [a congenital defect in bilirubin conjugating capacity – see below] was observed in ∼53% of G6PD deficient newborns, and ii) the combination of G6PD deficiency with Gilbert's syndrome significantly increased the risk of hyperbilirubinemia ($\geq$15 mg/dl [257 μmol/l]), as compared with G6PD defi-ciency alone (Table 4.2).[25] These investigators conclude that the presence of the Gilbert syndrome is an important factor in the pathogenesis of G6PD deficiency associated newborn jaundice.[25] Regardless of the mechanism(s) underlying jaundice in G6PD deficient newborns, it is clear that marked hyperbilirubinemia may develop in such infants and lead to neurotoxicity.[14–16] For a more detailed discussion of neonatal hyperbilirubinemia in G6PD deficiency see Chapter 5.

Pyruvate kinase deficiency is an autosomal recessive disorder that is less prevalent than G6PD deficiency and in contrast to G6PD deficiency typically presents with jaundice, anemia, and reticulocytosis.[18,26] Such jaundice may be severe; in one series a full third of affected infants required exchange transfusion to control their hyper-bilirubinemia[27] and kernicterus in the context of pyruvate kinase deficiency has been described.[28] The diagnosis of pyruvate kinase deficiency is often difficult as the enzymatic abnormality is frequently not simply a quantitative defect, but in many

Table 4.2. Incidence of hyperbilirubinemia ($\geq$15 mg/dl) as a func-tion of G6PD and Gilbert genotype.

G6PD	Incidence of Gilbert genotype			
	6/6	*6/7*	*7/7*	*Total*
$-/-$	6/62	18/57	6/12	30/131
	(9.7%)	(31.6%)	(50%)	(22.9%)
$+/+$	10/101	7/105	5/34	22/240
	(9.9%)	(6.7%)	(14.7%)	(9.2%)
P value	NS	$P < 0.0001$	$P = 0.02$	$p = 0.0005$

6/6, homozygous normal UDPGT genotype; 6/7, heterozygous variant UDPGT genotype; 7/7, homozygous Gilbert UDPGT genotype. *P* values are for G6PD$-/-$ (G6PD deficienct genotype) vs. G6PD$+/+$ (G6PD sufficient genotype). Reproduced with per-mission from *Proc. Natl. Acad. Sci. USA* 1997; **94**: 12128–12132.

cases involves abnormal enzyme kinetics or an unstable enzyme that decreases in activity as the red cell ages. The diagnosis of pyrutvate kinase deficiency should be considered whenever persistent jaundice and a picture of nonspherocytic, Coombs negative hemolytic anemia is observed.

Heritable Causes of Hemolysis – Hemoglobinopathies

Defects in hemoglobin structure or synthesis are rare disorders that infrequently manifest themselves in the neonatal period. Of these, the alpha-thalassemia syndromes are the most likely to be clinically apparent in newborns. Each human diploid cell contains four copies of the alpha-globin gene and thus, four alpha thalassemia syndromes have been described reflecting the presence of defects in 1, 2, 3, or 4 alpha-globin genes. Silent carriers have one abnormal alpha globin chain and are asymptomatic. Alpha thalassemia trait is associated with two alpha thalassemia mutations and in neonates is not associated with hemolysis. Alpha thalassemia trait, however, is common in Black populations and can be detected by a low mean corpuscular volume of $< 95 \, u^3$ [normal infants 100 to 120 u^3].[29] Hemoglobin H disease results from the presence of three thalassemia mutations and can cause hemolysis and anemia in neonates.[30] Homozygous alpha thalassemia (total absence of alpha chain synthesis) results in profound hemolysis, anemia, hydrops fetalis and almost always stillbirth or death in the immediate neonatal period.

The pure beta thalassemias do not manifest themselves in the newborn period and the gamma thalassemias are i) incompatible with life (homozygous form), ii) associated with transient mild to moderate neonatal anemia if one or two genes are involved that resolves when beta chain synthesis begins, or iii) in combination with impaired beta chain synthesis, associated with severe hemolytic anemia and marked hyperbilirubinemia.[31]

Acquired Causes of Hemolysis

Acquired causes of hemolysis comprise a miscellaneous group of disorders which include among others the i) microangiopathic hemolysis associated with disseminated intravascular coagulation or hemangiomas and ii) infection (bacterial sepsis or congenital infections).[26] The mechanism(s) underlying the hemolytic process in the latter is not fully understood.

Immune-mediated Hemolytic Disease

Immune mediated hemolysis encompasses the fetomaternal incompatibilities of the Rhesus (Rh), ABO (major), and minor blood group systems. Historically Rh incompatibility has been viewed as the most clinically important immune mediated hemolytic disorder. The incidence of isoimmunization to the Rh D antigen, however, has declined since the introduction of $Rh_0(D)$ immune globulin in 1968 and is now estimated at $\sim$1 case per 1,000 live births.[32] Most instances of Rh isoimmunization are due to the Rh D antigen.[33] The severity of hemolysis varies in the context of Rh isoimmunization but almost half of Rh positive infants born to Rh sensitized mothers will evince moderate or severe disease. Affected infants develop significant hyperbilirubinemia that frequently requires exchange transfusion, in addition to intensive phototherapy, to control. Isoimmunization secondary to minor blood group antigens, e.g., Kell, Duffy, and Kidd, can also lead to significant hemolysis *in utero* and postnatal hyperbilirubinemia, although these antigens are far less potent in inducing antibodies than Rh D. The incidence of clinically significant sensitization to the minor blood group antigens as determined by meta-analysis approximates 1:330 pregnancies.[34]

Hemolytic disease related to ABO incompatibility is generally limited to mothers who are blood group O and infants of blood group A or B.[35,36] Although this association exists in ∼15% of pregnancies, only a small fraction of infants born in this context will develop significant hyperbilirubinemia.[35,36] Defining which infants will become so affected is difficult to predict using laboratory screening tests. Indeed, a recent investigation demonstrated that of type A or B infants born to mothers who are blood group O, only one-third had a positive direct Coombs test, and of those with a positive direct Coombs test, only ∼15% had peak serum bilirubin levels ≥12.8 mg/dl.[36] Thus, evidence of symptomatic ABO hemolytic disease was found in only 4% of such incompatible mother–infant pairs and was not strongly predicted by the Coombs test. Similarly, group A or B infants born to respectively incompatible group B or A mothers are not likely to manifest symptomatic ABO hemolytic disease or have a positive direct Coombs test (<1%).[36] Infants born of ABO incompatible mother–infant pairs who have a negative direct Coombs test as a group appear to be at no greater risk for developing hyperbilirubinemia than their ABO compatible counterparts, regardless of the indirect Coombs test status.[36]

Despite the difficulty in predicting its development, symptomatic ABO hemolytic disease does occur and in individual instances may develop even in the absence of a positive direct Coombs test.[35,37] The latter may reflect a paucity of A and B antigens on newborn red cells and/or the absorption of serum antibody by A and B antigen epitopes throughout the body tissues and fluids.[35] The diagnosis of symptomatic ABO hemolytic disease should be considered in infants who develop marked jaundice in the context of ABO incompatibility that is generally accompanied by a positive direct Coombs test and prominent microspherocytosis on red cell smear.[35]

The hyperbilirubinemia seen with symptomatic ABO hemolytic disease is often detected within the first 12 to 24 hours of life ("icterus praecox"[38]) and usually is readily controlled with intensive phototherapy.[35] Few affected infants ever develop hyperbilirubinemia to levels requiring exchange transfusion.[39] Routine screening of all ABO-incompatible cord blood has been recommended in the past[40] and is common practice in many nurseries.[41] The current literature[36,41,42] however, suggests that such routine screening is probably not warranted given the low yield and cost, consistent with the tenor of recent recommendations of the American Association of Blood Banks.[43] A blood type and Coombs test is indicated, however, in the evaluation of any newborn with early and/or clinically significant jaundice.

INCREASED BILIRUBIN LOAD – ENTEROHEPATIC CIRCULATION

Once bilirubin conjugates reach the intestine they are either reduced by bacteria to urobilinogens and excreted in the feces, or they are deconjugated to glucuronic acid and unconjugated bilirubin by bacterial and tissue beta-glucuronidase (an enzyme also present in human milk).[44] The cleavage of glucuronic acid from bilirubin conjugates and the resultant intestinal absorption of unconjugated bilirubin is termed the enterohepatic circulation of bilirubin. In the fetus intestinal beta-glucuronidase activity can be detected as early as 12 weeks of gestation. The teleologic speculation is that fetal intestinal beta-glucuronidase activity facilitates intestinal bilirubin absorption *in utero*, thus enhancing bilirubin clearance by the placenta.[45] The enterohepatic circulation of bilirubin is exaggerated in the neonatal period, in part because the newborn intestinal tract is not yet colonized with bacteria that convert conjugated bilirubin to urobilinogen, and because intestinal beta-glucuronidase activity is high.[44] Studies in newborn humans and primates suggest that the enterohepatic circulation of bilirubin contributes significantly to neonatal jaundice,[46,47] accounting for up to 50% of the hepatic bilirubin load in neonates.[47] Moreover, recent evidence demonstrates that fasting hyperbilirubinemia is largely due to intestinal reabsorption of unconjugated bilirubin[48,49] and suggests that enterohepatic circulation of bilirubin may play a role in the marked jaundice associated with inadequate lactation and poor enteral intake in some neonates. Although various methods to limit the enterohepatic circulation of bilirubin have been studied (e.g., agar[47]), none are in clinical use.

INCREASED BILIRUBIN LOAD – EXTRAVASCULAR BLOOD

Internal hemorrhage, ecchymoses, and other extravascular blood collections will enhance the bilirubin load on the liver. Extravascular red cells have a markedly shortened life span and their heme fraction is quickly catabolized to bilirubin by tissue macrophages that contain heme oxygenase and biliverdin reductase.[45] Thus, cephalohematomas, subdural hemorrhage, massive adrenal hemorrhage, and marked bruising can be associated with increased serum bilirubin levels, typically manifest 48–72 hours following the extravasation of blood. This temporal pattern is consistent with the evolution of ecchymoses and bilirubin formation *in situ*[45] and also accounts for why extravascular blood can cause prolonged indirect hyperbilirubinemia. An unusual but dramatic example of how extravascular blood can contribute to the genesis of hyperbilirubinemia is found in reports of marked jaundice associated with the delayed absorption of intraperitoneal blood in infants who received fetal intraperitoneal red cell transfusions.[50,51] In one such case 13 exchange transfusions were necessary to control the hyperbilirubinemia that resolved only when ~87 cc of packed red cell were evacuated from the intraperitoneal cavity.[50] In this instance, the intraperitoneal blood had a hematocrit of 60% and the potential to contribute up to ~600 mg of bilirubin to the infant's bilirubin load over time. Although other causes of extravasation generally are not associated with such a volume of sequestered blood and resultant bilirubin load, they can nevertheless contribute to the development of jaundice.

DECREASED HEPATIC CLEARANCE OF BILIRUBIN – CONJUGATION

Once bilirubin enters the hepatocyte it is conjugated with glucuronic acid to form
the polar, water-soluble, and readily excretable bilirubin mono and diglucuronides.
The formation of these derivatives is catalyzed by hepatic bilirubin uridine diphosphate glucuronyl transferase (UDPGT), an enzyme that arises from the UDPGT1
gene complex whose transcription unit UDPGT1A1 encodes the physiologically
important UDPGT that conjugates bilirubin.[52–54] In addition to the A1 exon, the
UDPGT1 gene locus contains twelve variable exons (A2–A13) that encode other
UDPGT isoforms and an exon 2–5 cluster that is common to all (i.e., constant
domain) UDPGT isoforms (Figure 4.1).

Bilirubin UDPGT expression in humans is modulated in a developmental manner
such that its activity is 0.1% of adult levels at 17 to 30 weeks gestation, increasing to
1% of adult values between 30 and 40 weeks gestation, and reaching adult levels by 14
weeks of postnatal life.[55,56] A graded upregulation of hepatic bilirubin UDPGT over
the first few days of life is noted following birth regardless of the newborns gestational age. This developmentally determined pattern of hepatic bilirubin UDPGT
activity in conjunction with an increased bilirubin load accounts in large part for the
genesis of physiologic neonatal hyperbilirubinemia.

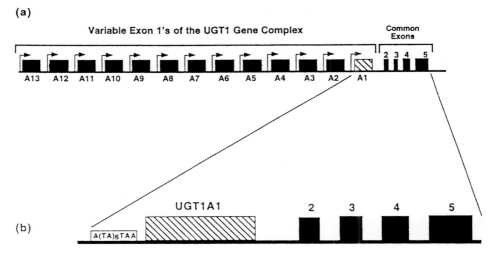

Figure 4.1. Schematic of the UDPGT1 gene. Panel (a) represents the entire gene complex including the
variable exons A1–A13 and constant domain, exons 2, 3, 4, and 5. Bilirubin UDPGT is defined by the
UDPGT1A1 locus and common exons 2–5 as shown in panel (b). The normal UDPGT1A1 TATA box
promoter sequence is also shown in panel (b) Genetic mutations in exon A1 and exons 2–5, as well as a
variant promoter sequence, have been identified as causes for the indirect hyperbilirubinemia syndromes.
Reprinted from *Clinica. Chimica. Acta.*, Volume 166, Clarke, D.J., Moghrabi, N., Monaghan, G., Cassidy,
A., Boxer, M., Hume, R. and Burchell, B., Genetic defects of the UDP-glucuronosyltransferase-1 (UGT1)
gene that cause familial non-haemolytic unconjugated hyperbilirubinemias, pp. 63–74, 1997, with permission from Elsevier Science.

Table 4.3. Inborn errors of hepatic bilirubin UDP glucoronosyltransferase expression.

Characteristic	Crigler–Najjar Type I	Crigler–Najjar Type II (Arias syndrome)	Gilbert's
Inheritance	AR	AR or AD	AD or AR
UDPGT1 Activity	Absent	<10%	50%
Genetics	Nonsense or stop mutation	Missense mutation	Variant promoter
Hyperbilirubinemia	>20 mg/dl	5–15 mg/dl*	3–5 mg/dl
Kernicterus	High Risk	Low Risk*	No apparent risk

*in some cases of Arias syndrome marked hyperbilirubinemia can occur which may place the infant at high risk for kernicterus. AR, autosomal recessive; AD, autosomal dominant.

In addition to the developmentally modulated postnatal transitions in hepatic bilirubin UDPGT activity, there are congenital inborn errors of bilirubin UDPGT expression, commonly referred to as the indirect hyperbilirubinemia syndromes.[57] These include the Crigler–Najjar type I and II (Arias) syndromes, and Gilbert's syndrome (Table 4.3). Crigler and Najjar first described a clinical syndrome of severe chronic nonhemolytic unconjugated hyperbilirubinemia in 1952.[58] Affected infants have complete absence of bilirubin UDPGT activity and are at significant risk for hyperbilirubinemic encephalopathy and its neurodevelopmental sequelae. Although inherited in an autosomal recessive pattern, the type I syndrome has marked genetic heterogeneity.[59] Currently, more than thirty different genetic mutations have been identified in Crigler–Najjar type I syndrome and defects common to both the UDPGT1A1 exon and those comprising the constant domain (exons 2–5)[54,60–62] underlie most cases, although there are exceptions to this rule.[54] Such gene defects are typically nonsense or "stop" mutations in nature.

Phototherapy is the mainstay of treatment for infants and children with Crigler–Najjar type I syndrome with useful potential adjuncts being tin-mesoporphyrin and oral calcium phosphate. Liver transplantation is currently the only definitive therapeutic intervention for this disorder,[63] although human hepatocyte transplantation to enhance hepatic UDPGT1 activity[64–66] holds promise as an alternative approach that could obviate the need for liver transplantation in patients with Crigler–Najjar type I syndrome. The ulitmate treatment for this inborn error of bilirubin UDPGT1 expression will reside in the development of an effective gene therapy strategy.[66] Gene therapy trials for Crigler–Najjar type I syndrome using chimeric oligonucleotides (DNA and RNA) that theoretically correct point mutations by initiating the cell's DNA mismatch machinery hold promise and are scheduled to begin soon.

In contrast, the Arias syndrome, typified by more moderate levels of indirect hyperbilirubinemi as well as low but detectable hepatic bilirubin UDPGT activity, appears in the majority of cases to be mediated by a missense mutations in the UDPGT1A gene alone.[54,67] In some cases, marked hyperbilirubinemia occurs in Arias syndrome making it difficult to distinguish this entity from Crigler–Najjar syndrome. These rare but important clinical syndromes must be included in the differential diagnosis of prolonged marked indirect hyperbilirubinemia.

Gilbert syndrome, originally described at the turn of the century,[68] is characterized by mild, chronic or recurrent unconjugated hyperbilirubinemia in the absence of liver disease or overt hemolysis.[69] Hepatic bilirubin UDPGT activity is reduced at least 50% in affected subjects and more than 95% of their total serum bilirubin is unconjugated.[69] Typically, the indirect hyperbilirubinemia associated with Gilbert's syndrome is seen during fasting associated with an intercurrent illness. Interestingly, in about half of patients there is also an unexplained, shortened red cell life span and increased bilirubin production.[70]

Gilbert's syndrome is common, affecting ~6% of the population[69] and a genetic basis for this disorder has recently been defined.[71] The start site on the UDPGT1 gene where transcription of message (messenger RNA) begins, i.e., the promoter element is abnormal. More specifically, the variant promoter for the gene encoding UDPGT1 contains a two base-pair addition (TA) in the TATAA promoter element giving rise to 7 (A[TA]$_7$TAA) rather than the more usual 6 (A[TA]$_6$TAA) repeats in affected subjects. This extra TA repeat (A[TA]$_7$TAA) impairs proper message transcription and accounts for a reduced UDPGT activity [Figure 4.1].[71] Indeed, as the repeat number increases, UDPGT1 activity decreases. Subjects with Gilbert's syndrome are homozygous for the (A[TA]$_7$TAA) variant promoter providing a unique genetic marker for this disorder. The expanded A[TA]$_7$TAA promoter motif is expressed in the heterozygous form in 40% of the population.[71]

Although Gilbert's syndrome is most commonly diagnosed in young adulthood, investigators have long speculated that this disorder might contribute to indirect hyperbilirubinemia in the newborn period.[45,57,72] Identification of a molecular marker for Gilbert's syndrome has provided investigators with an important tool to study the role of Gilbert's syndrome in the pathogenesis of neonatal jaundice.[71] Gourley and colleagues were the first to confirm an association between Gilbert's syndrome, as indexed by the variant promoter marker, and neonatal jaundice.[73–75] Their recently published study demonstrates that newborn infants with the A[TA]$_7$TAA polymorphism in the promoter region of UDPGT1 have an accelerated increase in neonatal hyperbilirubinemia and decreased fecal excretion of bilirubin mono and diglucuronides.[73–75] Roy-Chowdhury and co-workers in an analogous study have demonstrated that the presence of the A[TA]$_7$TAA variant UDPGT1 promoter in neonates is associated with higher postnatal serum bilirubin levels than those observed in newborns without the A[TA]$_7$TAA polymorphism (Figure 4.2).[76] As discussed above, the combination of the Gilbert's genotype and G6PD deficiency markedly increases a newborn's risk for hyperbilirubinemia.[25] Studies in adults confirm that the Gilbert's genotype in combination with G6PD deficiency,[77] and co-inherited Gilbert's and beta-thalassemia[78] result in accentuated hyperbilirubinemia in this age group as well. A more recent report also demonstrates that the A[TA]$_7$TAA variant UDPGT1 promoter is significantly more prevalent in breast-fed infants who develop prolonged neonatal hyperbilirubinemia.[79] Thus, the Gilbert genotype may contribute to the duration of neonatal jaundice as well. These newborn studies taken together demonstrate that Gilbert's syndrome is a factor contributing to the risk for neonatal jaundice. The role of Gilbert's syndrome in the genesis of extreme hyperbilirubinemia remains unclear although i) the low direct bilirubin

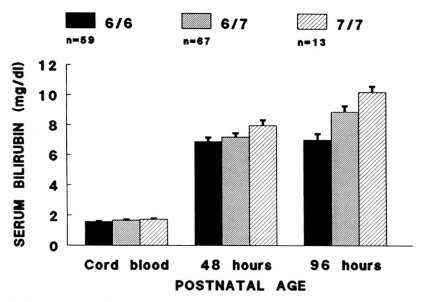

Figure 4.2. Newborn serum bilirubin levels as a function of postnatal age and presence of Gilbert promoter abnormality. Solid bars are homozygous normal UDPGT genotype [6/6]; fine hatched bars are heterozygous variant UDPGT genotype [6/7]; and coarse hatched bars are homozygous variant UDPGT genotype [7/7]. Values are means ± SEM. Adapted from *Hepatology* 1997; **26**: 370A, and reproduced with permission from Hepatology.

fractions, and ii) evidence of poor feeding and prominent weight loss (i.e., a state resembling fasting) reported in several of the published cases of extreme neonatal hyperbilirubinemia[80] suggest that Gilbert's syndrome might contribute to some cases of marked jaundice. This hypothesis is worthy of testing in future studies of the genetic determinants of neonatal hyperbilirubinemia.

Of related interest with respect to bilirubin metabolism and UDPGT1 promoter variation, is the report by Beutler and colleagues detailing the UDPGT1 promoter genotypes in persons of Asian, African, and Caucasian ancestry.[81] Population studies have demonstrated that Asian infants have a higher and African-American infants a lower incidence of hyperbilirubnemia as compared with their Caucasian counterparts.[82,83] Beutler and co-workers therefore speculated that the prevalence of the A[TA]$_7$TAA variant UDPGT1 promoter would be highest in Asian subjects, intermediate in Caucasians, and lowest in African-Americans. Contrary to this expectation, the A[TA]$_7$TAA variant was most common observed among African-Americans and least common among subjects of Asian origin.[81] Thus, although there is a relationship between UDPGT1 promoter repeat number and UDPGT1 activity (and jaundice) within a racial group, this correlation does not appear to hold across ethinic groups. These data underscore the multifactorial nature of jaundice.

Table 4.4. Differential diagnosis of prolonged indirect hyperbilirubinemia in newborns.

Breast milk jaundice
Hypothyroidism
Hemolytic disorders
Crigler–Najjar syndrome
Pyloric stenosis
Sequestered blood collections

From Maisels, M.S., 1994.[75]

MISCELLANEOUS CAUSES OF INDRECT HYPERBILIRUBINEMIA

There are several other conditions that predispose infants to indirect hyperbilirubinemia. The most common of these is breast milk feeding, a topic discussed in detail in Chapter 3. Other less common but important associated conditions include hypothryroidism, hypopituitarism, the Lucey-Driscoll syndrome, galactosemia, tyrosinosis, congenital dyserythropoietic anemia type I, and hypermethioninemia.[84] Several conditions can lead to prolonged indirect hyperbilirubinemia, the differential diagnosis of which is listed in Table 4.4.[84]

SUMMARY

Indirect hyperbilirubinemia is the most common clinical condition in neonates requiring evaluation or intervention, and is in large part accounted for by developmentally determined postnatal changes in bilirubin production and metabolism. Enhanced bilirubin production secondary to hemolytic disorders, an increased hepatic bilirubin load as a result of the enterohepatic bilirubin circulation, and the impaired hepatic bilirubin clearance associated with limited neonatal UDPGT activity, can singularly or in combination significantly increase serum indirect hyperbilirubinemia. An improved understanding of the genetic determinants of indirect hyperbilirubinemia, such as the recent report on G6PD deficiency and Gilbert syndrome,[25] provides important insights into the pathogenesis of newborn jaundice that will ultimately be translated into more rationale clinical management.

References

1. Pearson, H., Life-span of the fetal red blood cell, *J. Pediatr.* 1967; **70**: 166–171.
2. Vest, M.F., and Grieder, H.R., Erythrocyte survival in the newborn infant, as measured by chromium[51] and its relation to the postnatal serum bilirubin level, *J. Pediatr.* 1961; **59**: 194–199.
3. Crosby, W.H., The metabolism of hemoglobin and bile pigment in hemolytic disease, *Am. J. Med.* 1955; **18**: 112–122.
4. Oski, F.A., The erythrocyte and its disorders. In: Nathan, D.G. and Oski, F.A., eds. Hematology of Infancy and Childhood. Philadelphia: W.B. Saunders; 1993, pp. 18–43.
5. Caprari, P., Maiorana, A., Marzetti, G., Tarzia, A., Luciania, A. and Salvati, A.M., Severe neonatal hemolytic jaundice associated with pyknocytosis and alterations of red cell skeletal proteins, *Prenat. Neonat. Med.* 1997; **2**: 140–145.

6. Tuffy, P., Brown, A.K. and Zuelzer, W.W., Infantile pyknocytosis: common erythrocyte abnormality of the first trimester, *Am. J. Dis. Child.* 1959; **98**: 227–241.
7. Stockman, J.A., Physical properties of the neonatal red blood cell. In: Stockman, J.A. and Pochedly, C., eds. Developmental and Neonatal Hematology. New York, N.Y.: Raven Press; 1988, pp. 297–323.
8. Zipursky, A., Brown, E. and Palko, J., The erythrocyte differential count in the newborn infant, *Am. J. Pediatr. Hematol. Oncol.* 1983; **5**: 45–51.
9. Iolascon, A., Faienza, M.F., Moretti, A., Perrotta, S. and Miraglia del Giudice, E., UGT1 promoter polymorphism accounts for increased neonatal appearance of hereditary spherocytosis, *Blood* 1998; **91**: 1093.
10. Becker, P.S. and Lux, S.E., Disorders of the red cell membrane. In: Nathan, D.G. and Oski, F.A., eds. Hematology of Infancy and Childhood. Philadelphia: W.B. Saunders; 1993, pp. 529–633.
11. Trucco, J.I. and Brown, A.K., Neonatal manifestations of hereditary spherocytosis, *Am. J. Dis. Child.* 1967; **113**: 263–270.
12. Keimowitz, R. and Desforges, J.F., Infantile pyknocytosis, *N. Engl. J. Med.* 1965; **273**: 1152–1155.
13. Ackerman, B.D., Infantile pyknocytosis in Mexican-American infants, *Am. J. Dis. Child.* 1969; **117**: 417–423.
14. Beutler, E., G6PD deficiency, *Blood* 1994; **84**: 3613–3636.
15. Valaes, T., Severe neonatal jaundice associated with glucose-6-phosphate dehydrogenase deficiency: pathogenesis and global epidemiology, *Acta. Paediatr. Suppl.* 1994; **394**: 58–76.
16. MacDonald, M.G., Hidden risks: Early discharge and bilirubin toxicity due to glucose-6-phosphate dehydrogenase deficiency, *Pediatrics* 1995; **96**: 734–738.
17. Luzzatto, L., G6PD deficiency and hemolytic anemia. In: Nathan, D.G. and Oski, F.A., eds. Hematology of Infancy and Childhood. Philadelphia: W.B. Saunders, 1993, pp. 674–695.
18. Mentzer, W.C. Jr., Pyruvate kinase deficiency and disorders of glycolysis. In: Nathan, D.G. and Oski, F.A., eds. Hematology of Infancy and Childhood. Philadelphia: W.B. Saunders, 1993, pp. 634–673.
19. Valaes, T., Doxiadis, S.A. and Fessas, Ph., Acute hemolysis due to naphthalene inhalation, *J. Pediatr.* 1963; **63**: 904–915.
20. Naiman, J.L. and Kosoy, M.H., Red cell glucose-6-phosphate dehydrogenase deficiency: a newly recognized cause of neonatal jaundice and kernicterus in Canada, *J. Canad. Med. Assoc.* 1964: **91**: 1243–1249.
21. Meloni, T. and Cagnazzo, G., Phenobarbital for prevention of hyperbilirubinemia in glucose-6-phosphate dehydrogenase-deficient newborn infants, *J. Pediatr.* 1973; **82**: 1048–1051.
22. Meloni, S. and Costa, S., Haptoglobin, hemopexin, hemoglobin and hematocrit in newborns with erythrocyte glucose-6-phosphate dehydrogenase deficiency, *Acta. Haematol.* (Basel) 1975; **54**: 284–288.
23. Kaplan, M., Rubaltelli, F.F., Hammerman, C., Vilei, M.T., Leiter, C., Abramov, A. and Muraca, M., Conjugated bilirubin in neonates with glucose-6-phosphate dehydrogenase deficiency, *J. Pediatr.* 1996; **128**: 695–697.
24. Kaplan, M., Vreman, H.J., Hammerman, C., Leiter, C., Abramov, A. and Stevenson, D.K., Contribution of haemolysis to jaundice in Sephardic Jewish glucose-6-phosphate dehydrogenase deficient neonates, *Br. J. Haematol.* 1996; **93**: 822–827.
25. Kaplan, M., Renbaum, P., Levy-Lahad, E., Hammerman, C., Lahad, A. and Beutler, E., Gilbert syndrome and glucose-6-phosphate dehydrogenase deficiency: a dose-dependent genetic interaction crucial to neonatal hyperbilirubinemia, *Proc. Natl. Acad. Sci. USA* 1997; **94**: 12128–12132.
26. Oski, F.A., Disorders of red cell metabolism. In: Oski, F.A. and Naiman, J.L., eds. Hematologic Problems in the Newborn. Philadelphia: W.B. Saunders, 1982, pp. 97–136.
27. Matthay, K.K. and Mentzer, W.C., Erythrocyte enzymopathies in the newborn, *Clin. Hematol.* 1981; **10**: 31–55.
28. Oski, F.A., Nathan, D.G., Sidel, V.W. and Diamond, L.K., Extreme hemolysis and red-cell distortion in erythrocyte pyruvate kinase deficiency. I. Morphology, erythrokinetics and family enzyme studies, *New Engl. J. Med.* 1964; **270**: 1023–1030.
29. Schmaier, A., Maurer, H.M., Johnston, C.L., *et al.*, Alpha thalassemia screening in neonates by mean corpuscular volume and mean corpuscular hemoglobin concentration, *J. Pediatr.* 1973; **83**: 794–797.
30. Pearson, H.A., Disorders of hemoglobin synthesis and metabolism. In: Oski, F.A. and Naiman, J.L., eds. Hematologic Problems in the Newborn. Philadelphia: W.B. Saunders, 1982, pp. 245–282.

64

Jon F. Watchko

31. Oort, M., Heerspink, W., Roos, D., Flavell, R.A. and Bernini, L.F., Haemolytic disease of the newborn and chronic anaemia induced by gamma-beta thalassemia in a Dutch family, *Br. J. Haematol.* 1981; **48**: 251–262.
32. Chavez, G., Mulinare, J. and Edmonds, L.D., Epidemiology of Rh hemolytic disease of the newborn in the United States, *JAMA* 1991; **24**: 3270–3274.
33. Gottvall, T., Hilden, J. and Selbing, A., Evaluation of standard parameters to predict exchange transfusions in the erythroblastotic newborn, *Acta. Obstet. Gynecol. Scand.* 1994; **73**: 300–306.
34. Solola, A., Sibal, B. and Mason, J., Irregular antibodies: an assessment of routine prenatal screening, *Obstet. Gynecol.* 1983; **61**: 25–30.
35. Naiman, J.L., Erythroblastosis fetalis. In: Oski, F.A. and Naiman, J.L., eds. Hematologic Problems in the Newborn. Philadelphia: W.B. Saunders, 1982, pp. 326–332.
36. Ozolek, J.A., Watchko, J.F. and Mimouni, F., Prevalence and lack of clinical significance of blood group incompatibility in mothers with blood type A or B, *J. Pediatr.* 1994; **125**: 87–91.
37. Voak, D. and Bowley, C.C., A detailed serological study on the prediction and diagnosis of ABO haemolytic disease of the newborn (ABO HD), *Vox. Sang.* 1969; **17**: 321–348.
38. Halbrecht, I., Role of hemagglutinins anti-A and anti-B in pathogenesis of jaundice of the newborn (icterus neonatorum precox), *Am. J. Dis. Child.* 1944; **68**: 248–249.
39. Mollison, P.L., Blood Transfusion in Clinical Medicine. Oxford: Blackwell Scientific Publications Ltd., 1983, p. 691.
40. Hubinont, P.O., Bricoult, A. and Ghysdael, P., ABO mother-infant incompatibilities, *Am. J. Obstet. Gynecol.* 1960; **9**: 593–600.
41. Leistikow, E.A., Collin, M.F., Savastano, G.D., de Sierra, T. and Leistikow, B.N., Wasted health care dollars. Routine cord blood type and Coombs' testing, *Arch. Pediatr. Adolesc. Med.* 1995; **149**: 1147–1151.
42. Quinn, M.W., Weindling, A.M. and Davidson, D.C., Does ABO incompatibility matter? *Arch. Dis. Child.* 1988; **63**: 1258–1260.
43. Judd, W.J., Luban, N.L.C., Ness, P.M. *et al.*, Prenatal and perinatal immunohematology: recommendations for serologic management of the fetus, newborn infant and obstetric patient, *Transfusion* 1990; **30**: 175–183.
44. Gourley, G.R., Perinatal bilirubin metabolism. In: Gluckman, P.D. and Heymann, M.A., eds. Perinatal and Pediatric Pathophysiology. A Clinical Perspective. Boston: Hodder and Stoughton, 1993, pp. 437–439.
45. Odell, G.B., Neonatal Hyperbilirubinemia. New York: Grune and Stratton, 1980.
46. Gartner, L.M., Lee, K.-S., Vaisman, S. *et al.*, Development of bilirubin transport and metabolism in the newborn rhesus monkey, *J. Pediatr.* 1977; **90**: 513–531.
47. Poland, R.D. and Odell, G.B., Physiologic jaundice: The enterohepatic circulation of bilirubin, *N. Engl. J. Med.* 1971; **284**: 1–6.
48. Gartner, U., Goeser, T. and Wolkoff, A.W., Effect of fasting on the uptake of bilirubin and sulfobromopthalein by the isolated perfused rat liver, *Gastroenterology* 1997; **113**: 1707–1713.
49. Fevery, J., Fasting hyperbilirubinemia: unraveling the mechanism involved, *Gastroenterology* 1997; **113**: 1798–1799.
50. Wright, K., Tarr, P.I., Hickman, R.O. and Guthrie, R.D., Hyperbilirubinemia secondary to delayed absorption of intraperitoneal blood following intrauterine transfusion, *J. Pediatr.* 1982; **100**: 302–304.
51. Rajagopalan, I. and Katz, B.Z., Hyperbilirubinemia secondary to hemolysis of intrauterine intraperitoneal blood transfusion, *Clin. Pediatr.* 1984; **23**: 511–512.
52. Ritter, J.K., Chen,F., Sheen, Y., Tran, H.M., Kimura, S., Yeatman, M.T. and Owens, I.S., A novel complex locus UGT1 encodes human bilirubin, phenol and other UDP-glucuronosyltransferase isoenzymes with identical carboxyl termini, *J. Biol. Chem.* 1992; **267**: 3257–3261.
53. Ritter, J.K., Crawford, J.M. and Owens, I.S., Cloning of two human liver bilirubin UDP-glucuronosyltransferase cDNA's with expression in COS-1 cells, *J. Biol. Chem.* 1991; **266**: 1043–1047.
54. Clarke, D.J., Moghrabi, N., Monaghan, G., Cassidy, A, Boxer, M., Hume, R. and Burchell, B., Genetic defects of the UDP-glucoronosyltransferase-1 (UGT1) gene that cause familial non-haemolytic unconjugated hyperbilirubinemias, *Clinica. Chimica. Acta.* 1997; **266**: 63–74.
55. Kawade, N. and Onishi, S., The prenatal and postnatal development of UDP glucuronyltransferase activity towards bilirubin and the effect of premature birth on this activity in human liver, *Biochem. J.* 1981; **196**: 257–260.

56. Coughtrie, M.W., Burchell, B. *et al.*, The inadequacy of perinatal glucuronidation: immunoblot analysis of the developmental expression of individual UDP-glucuronosyltransferase isoenzymes in rat and human liver microsomes, *Mol. Pharmacol.* 1988; **34**: 729–735.
57. Valaes, T., Bilirubin metabolism: review and discussion of inborn errors, *Clin. Perinatol.* 1976; **3**: 177–209.
58. Crigler, J.F. Jr., and Najjar, V.A., Congenital familial nonhemolytic jaundice with kernicterus, *Pediatrics* 1952; **10**: 169–180.
59. Labrune, P., Myara, A., Hadchouel, M., Ronchi, F., Bernard, O., Trivin, F., Roy-Chowdhury, N., Roy-Chowdhury, J., Munnich, A. and Odievre, M., Genetic heterogeneity of Crigler–Najjar syndrome type I: a study of 14 cases, *Hum. Genet.* 1994; **94**: 693–197.
60. Bosma, P.J., Roy-Chowdhury, N., Goldhoorn, B.G., Hofker, M.H., Oude Elferink, R.P.J., Jansen, P.L.M. and Roy-Chowdhury, J., Sequence of exons and the flanking regions of human bilirubin UDP-glucuronosyltransferase gene complex and identification of a genetic mutation in a patient with Crigler–Najjar syndrome, type I, *Hepatology* 1992; **15**: 941–947.
61. Ritter, J.K., Yeatman, M.T., Ferreira, P. and Owens, I.S., Identification of a genetic alteration in the code for bilirubin UDP-glucuronosyltransferase in the UDT1 gene complex of a Crigler–Najjar type I patient, *J. Clin. Invest.* 1992; **90**: 150–155.
62. Bosma, P.J., Roy-Chowdhury, J., Huang, T., Lahari, P., Oude Elferink, R.P.J., Van Es, H.H.G., Lederstein, M., Whitington, P.F., Jansen, P.L.M. and Roy-Chowdhury, N., Mechanism of inherited deficiencies of multiple UDP-glucuronosyltransferase isoforms in two patients with Crigler–Najjar syndrome, type I, *FASEB J.* 1992; **6**: 2859–2863.
63. Shevell, M.I., Bernard, B., Adelson, J.W., Doody, D.P., Laberge, J.M. and Guttman, F.M., Crigler–Najjar syndrome type I: Treatment by home phototherapy followed by orthotopic hepatic transplantation, *J. Pediatr.* 1987; **110**: 429–431.
64. Fox, I.J., Roy Chowdhury, J., Kaufman, S.S., Goertzen, T.C., Roy Chowdury, N., Warkentin, P.I., Dorko, K., Sauter, B.V. and Strom, S.C., Treatment of the Crigler–Najjar syndrome type I with hepatocyte transplantation, *N. Engl. J. Med.* 1998; **338**: 1422–1426.
65. Roy Chowdury, J., Roy Chowdury, N., Strom, S.C., Kaufman, S.S., Horslen, S. and Fox, I.J., Human hepatocyte transplantation: gene therapy and more? *Pediatrics* 1998; **102**: 647–648.
66. Kim, B.H., Takahashi, M., Tada, K., Bosma, P.J., Roy Chowdury, J. and Roy Chowdury, N., Cell and gene therapy for inherited deficiency of bilirubin glucuronidation, *J. Perinatol.* 1996; **16**: S67–S72.
67. Moghrabi, N., Clarke, D.J., Boxer, M. and Burchell, B., Identification of an A-to-G missense mutation in exon 2 of the UGT1 gene complex that causes Crigler–Najjar syndrome type 2, *Genomics* 1993; **18**: 171–173.
68. Gilbert, A. and Lereboullet, P., La cholemia simple familiale, *Semaine Med.* 1901; **21**: 241–243.
69. Gourley, G.R., Disorders of bilirubin metabolism. In: Suchy, F.J., ed. Liver Disease in Children. St Louis: Mosby-Yearbook, 1994; 401–413.
70. Powell, L.W., Hemingway, E., Billing, B.H. and Sherlock, S., Idiopathic unconjugated hyperbilirubinemia (Gilbert's syndrome): a study of 42 families, *N. Engl. J. Med.* 1967; **277**: 1108–1112.
71. Bosma, P.J., Roy Chowdhury, J., Bakker, C., Gantla, S. De Bor, A., Oostra, B.A., Lindhout, D.,Tytgat, G.N.J.,Jansen, P.L.M., Oude Eleferink, R.P.J. and Roy Chowdhury, N., The genetic basis of the reduced expression of bilirubin UDP-glucuronosyltransferase 1 in Gilbert's syndrome, *N. Engl. J. Med.* 1995; **333**: 1171–1175.
72. Oski, F.A., Unconjugated hyperbilirubinemia. In: Avery, M.E and Taeusch, H.W., eds. Diseases of the Newborn. Philadelphia: W.B. Saunders, 1984, pp. 630–632.
73. Bancroft, J.D. and Gourley, G.R., Gilbert syndrome is associated with neonatal jaundice. *Hepatology* 1995; **22**: 374A.
74. Bancroft, J.D., Kreamer, B. and Gourley, G.R., Gilbert syndrome is associated with neonatal jaundice, *Pediatr. Res.* 1996; **39**: 304A.
75. Bancroft, J.D., Kreamer, B. and Gourley, G.R., Gilbert syndrome accelerates development of neonatal jaundice, *J. Pediatr.* 1998; **132**: 656–660.
76. Roy Chowdhury, N., Deocharan, B., Bejjanki, H.R., Gantla, S., Roy Chowdhury, J., Koliopoulos, C., Petmezaki, S. and Valaes, T., The presence of a Gilbert-type promoter abnormality increases the level of neonatal hyperbilirubinemia, *Hepatology* 1997; **26**: 370A.
77. Sampietro, M., Lupica, L., Perrero, L., Comino, A., Di Montemuros, F.M., Capellini, M.D. and Fiorelli, G., The expression of uridine diphosphate glucuronosyltransferase gene is a major determinant of bilirubin level in heterozygous beta-thalassemia and in glucose-6-phosphate dehydrogenase deficiency, *Br. J. Haematol.* 1997; **99**: 437–439.

78. Galanello, R., Perseu, L., Melis, M.A., Cipollina, L., Barella, S., Giagu, N., Turco, M.P., Maccioni, O. and Cao, A., Hyperbilirubinemia in heterozygous beta-thalasemmia is related to co-inherited Gilbert's sydnrome, *Br. J. Haematol.* 1997; **99**: 433–436.
79. Monaghan, G., McLellan, A, McGeehan, A., Volti, S.L., Mollica, F., Salemi, I., Din, Z., Cassidy, A., Hume, R. and Burchell, B., Gilbert's syndrome is a contributory factor in prolonged unconjugated hyperbilirubinemia of the newborn, *J. Pediatr.* 1999; **134**: 441–446.
80. Maisels, M.J. and Newman, T.B., Kernicterus in otherwise healthy, breast-fed term newborns, *Pediatrics* 1995; **96**: 730–733.
81. Beutler, E., Gelbart, T. and Demina, D., Racial variability in the UDP-glucuronosyltransferase 1 (UDGT1A1) promoter: A balanced polymorphism for regulation of bilirubin metabolism? *Proc. Natl. Acad. Sci. USA* 1998; **95**: 8170–8174.
82. Newman, T.B., Easterling, M.J., Goldman, E.S. and Stevenson, D.K., Laboratory evaluation of jaundice in newborns: frequency, cost and yield, *Am. J. Dis. Child.* 1990; **144**: 364–368.
83. Newman, T.B., Easterling, M.J., Goldman, E.S. and Stevenson, D.K., Laboratory evaluation of jaundice in newborns: Corrections, *Am. J. Dis. Child.* 1992; **146**: 1420–1421.
84. Maisels, M.J., Jaundice. In: Avery, G.B., Fletcher, M.A. and MacDonald, M.G., eds. Neonatology. Pathophysiology and Management of the Newborn. Philadelphia: J.B. Lippincott, 1999, pp. 765–819.

5 Neonatal Jaundice in Glucose-6-Phosphate Dehydrogenase Deficiency

Timos Valaes

Professor of Pediatrics, Tufts University School of Medicine, Boston, Massachusetts, USA

Glucose-6-phosphate dehydrogenase (G6PD) deficiency is the commonest clinically significant enzyme defect. The populations of the Mediterranean littoral, the Middle East, the Arabian peninsula, South-East Asia and Africa are predominantly affected and about 4,500,000 affected infants are born each year.[1,2] Immigration and inter-marriage in the last few centuries have transformed G6PD deficiency into a global problem. The G6PD gene (Gd) is located in the X chromosome and hemizygous Gd⁻ males have the full enzyme deficiency and are easily diagnosed with screening tests. As a result of X chromosome inactivation, however, Gd^+/Gd^- females have two red cell populations – normal and G6PD deficient – of varying proportions and enzyme activity in the peripheral blood ranging from <5% to >95% of the normal. Their heterozygocity can be missed even with the most sensitive tests.[1-3] The activity of the normal G6PD enzyme declines as red cell age advances, a process that is accentuated in G6PD deficiency. In fact in Class III mutants (moderate deficiency) the young red cells have enough residual enzyme activity to make them resistant to the hemolytic effect of drugs[3]. The situation is more complex in Class II mutants (severe deficiency) and even more so in the extremely rare Class I mutants (severe deficiency and life-long hemolysis and anemia). However, even in these mutants the propensity for hemolysis is influenced by red cell age. With the exception of the neonatal period, in individuals carrying a Class II or III Gd⁻ mutant, hemolytic crises are triggered by exogenous agents or infection. There is uncertainty regarding the list of proscribed drugs and chemicals.[1-3] Inclusion in the list has been based on clinical observations, as confirmation by *in vivo* tests is difficult to obtain, and no *in vitro* test has proved to be consistently reliable. It is left to the alert and inquisitive physician to discover the drugs and chemicals that trigger hemolysis.

Address for correspondence: 53 Demetrakopoulou Street, VOULA 166 73 Greece, Tel/Fax: 8991702

G6PD DEFICIENCY IN THE NEONATE

In relation to other age groups the neonatal period is characterized by a higher frequency and severity of the clinical manifestations of G6PD deficiency. Moreover, jaundice rather than anemia dominates the clinical picture.[4-9] The explanation lies in the uniqueness of bilirubin metabolism (see Chapter 1) and red cell metabolism in the neonate.[10-12] Due to the rapid expansion of the fetal red cell mass toward the end of gestation, at birth the age distribution of the red cells is shifted to the left (younger red cells). This explains the elevated G6PD activity found in cord blood. At the other end of the spectrum, about 10% of the red cells in normal neonates have as short a life-span as 1% of the oldest cells in the adult.[13] In addition, G6PD normal neonatal red cells exhibit reduced resistance to oxidative stress.[11,14-17] These characteristics of the red cells at birth are exaggerated in G6PD deficiency.[12]

HEMOLYSIS TRIGGERED BY EXOGENOUS AGENTS

Hemolysis can be triggered in a G6PD deficient neonate by exposure to certain oxidative agents either directly or indirectly. If a mother is exposed to a hemolytic agent, transfer to the infant can occur transplacentally or via the breast milk. In transplacental exposure evidence of hemolysis is present at birth.[18-20] Ingestion of fava beans by a breast feeding mother can cause favism in her G6PD deficient baby.[21] Agents used for umbilical cord antisepsis such as triple dye, mentholated powder and sulfanilamide powder have been implicated in causing exaggerated jaundice in G6PD deficient neonates.[22,23] Inhalation of naphthalene by exposure to moth balls has caused a severe hemolytic crisis and even kernicterus.[24-26] In cases of early exposure, anemia, Heinz body formation and red cell dysmorphology are not always present but are conspicuous in those exposed after the first week of life. Water soluble vitamin K analogues, in doses several fold higher than the recommended 1 mg, have been associated with severe hemolysis and kernicterus in G6PD deficient neonates.[4] Although rare, naphthalene inhalation by normal babies has also produced hemolysis[25] and high doses of vitamin K analogues caused an epidemic of hemolysis and kernicterus in (presumed G6PD normal) preterm infants in the 1950's.[27-30] We do not know how many other household chemicals such as deodorizing or disinfectant solutions or sprays, can trigger hemolysis when inhaled by susceptible neonates. Inquiring about the possibility of such an exposure should be part of the evaluation of unexplained severe neonatal jaundice, particularly of late onset.[12]

SPONTANEOUS SEVERE NEONATAL JAUNDICE IN G6PD DEFICIENCY

Severe neonatal jaundice can occur spontaneously (with no exposure to a hemolytic agent or infection) in G6PD deficient Class II Gd$^-$ newborns, but we do not know if this also occurs in populations with Class III Gd$^-$ (mostly of African origin).[12] When compared with controls, G6PD deficient neonates generally have higher bilirubin levels in the cord blood and over the next 6–7 days. The frequency distribution of bilirubin levels is unimodal, shifted to the right (higher), and there is a more pronounced tail in the region of high values. The proportion of G6PD deficient neonates that develop severe jaundice is 2–4 times higher than controls and the incidence of severe jaundice in G6PD deficient neonates is related to the background incidence of (non-specific) neonatal bilirubinemia in the population.[12] It is noteworthy that overt anemia, reticulocytosis and morphologic evidence of hemolysis is seldom found in these infants.[4,12] This suggests that hemolysis is self-limited, involves an older fraction of the red cell population and is extravascular, as is the case with G6PD normal senescent erythrocytes.

In G6PD deficient neonates most of the individual bilirubinemia curves are monophasic and similar in shape to that of controls. Nevertheless, in 10 to 15% of the deficient neonates a biphasic curve with a secondary period of accelerating bilirubin increase has been documented and it is mainly in this group that intervention is required to avert bilirubin toxicity. This group also illustrates the unpredictability of the course of bilirubinemia in G6PD deficiency. This unpredictability explains the paradox that in the last 40 years, as the management of severe neonatal jaundice has improved, the relative importance of G6PD deficiency as a cause of kernicterus has increased.[12] In the Greek population, before the introduction of exchange transfusion, the incidence of kernicterus in males was 112 to 278 per 10,000 G6PD deficient and 6 to 11 per 10,000 normal neonates. In recent years exchange transfusion and phototherapy have eliminated kernicterus from all other causes except G6PD deficiency (5 per 10,000 G6PD deficient males) in spite of liberal use of phototherapy and a post-delivery hospital stay of 4–5 days.[31]

Kaplan and coworkers have suggested that in G6PD deficient infants who develop spontaneous hyperbilirubinemia, the problem is an inability to conjugate bilirubin rather than an increase in bilirubin production (from hemolysis).[32] In my opinion, the studies supporting this view have serious methodological errors and, with the exception of the interraction between G6PD deficiency and Gilbert syndrome (see below), the idea that ineffective conjugation, rather than hemolysis, is an important determinant of hyperbilirubinemia in G6PD deficient neonates, has not been established.

INTERACTION BETWEEN G6PD DEFICIENCY AND GILBERT SYNDROME

Family analysis strongly suggested that in conjunction with G6PD deficiency a second independently transmitted genetic factor was responsible for the development of severe neonatal jaundice in some sibships.[33] Anecdotal evidence and theoretical considerations linked Gilbert's syndrome with this second genetic factor.[12,34] The description of a DNA marker for Gilbert's syndrome in the promoter region of the UDPGT1 gene[35] made it possible to test the hypothesis that the decreased conjugating capacity characteristic of Gilbert's syndrome will be expressed in the neonatal period by influencing the level and duration of bilirubinemia. The presence of the abnormal allele in the heterozygous and more so in the homozygous state produced a modest increase in the mean TSB levels in the first 2–4 days of life[36,37] and was associated with very prolonged jaundice in breast-fed babies (more than 28 days).[38] The interaction of Gilbert's syndrome with G6PD deficiency was confirmed by an extensive study in Israel.[39] The presence of the Gilbert's syndrome variant allele increased the incidence of severe jaundice (TSB ≥ 15.0 mg/dl) in the G6PD deficient neonates in a dose related fashion, while the effect in the G6PD normal group was not significant. Moreover, there was no difference in the incidence of severe jaundice between G6PD deficient and G6PD normal neonates homozygous for the normal promoter allele. It is interesting that the presence of severe jaundice in neonates with hereditary spherocytosis is also related to an interaction with the Gilbert's syndrome allele.[40]

These examples demonstrate that if the precarious balance in the neonatal period is disturbed by a shift to higher bilirubin production rates combined with a shift to lower bilirubin elimination rates, the risk of significant hyperbilirubinemia is multiplied. Currently, the data are insufficient to discuss the implications of the above gene to gene interactions for the balanced polymorphism in the Gd and the Gilbert's syndrome locus.

In populations in which G6PD deficiency and the associated severe neonatal jaundice are common, early identification of the affected neonates by cord blood testing, close monitoring for jaundice and prompt intervention have succeeded in eliminating kernicterus. Awareness of the problem and a high level of suspicion based on the racial and ethnic background of the parents (of mothers for male neonates, of either parent for females) might help to identify a rare case in other populations. In recent years, kernicterus associated with G6PD deficiency has been reported in the USA.[41] Early post partum discharge has increased the possibility of exposure to hemolytic chemicals at home and placed the responsibility of detecting severe neonatal jaundice on the parents, something they are ill-equipped to do. In multiracial and multiethnic societies, kernicterus associated with G6PD deficiency will occur when least expected and only an awareness of the problem and a high level of suspicion will reduce the number of cases.

The risk of kernicterus in G6PD-deficient infants appears to be comparable with that associated with Rh disease.[4,6,42] Thus, in the presence of G6PD deficiency, more aggressive treatment of hyperbilirubinemia is indicated.

References

1. Beutler, E., G6PD deficiency, *Blood* 1994; **84**: 3613–3636.
2. WHO working group, Glucose-6-phosphate dehydrogenase deficiency, *Bul WHO* 1989; **67**: 601–611.
3. Luzzatto, L., G6PD deficiency and hemolytic anemia. In: Nathan, D.G. and Oski, F.A., eds. *Hematology of infancy and childhood.* 4th ed. WB Saunders: Philadelphia, 1993; 674–695.
4. Doxiadis, S.A. and Valaes, T., The clinical picture of glucose-6-phosphate dehydrogenase deficiency in early infancy, *Arch. Dis. Child.* 1964; **39**: 545–553.
5. Yeu, P.C.K. and Strickland, M., Glucose-6-phosphate dehydrogenase deficiency and neonatal jaundice in Chinese male infants in Hong Kong, *Lancet* 1965; **7**: 350–351.
6. Brown, W.R. and Wong, H.B., Hyperbilirubinemia and kernicterus in glucose-6-phosphate dehydrogenase-deficient infants in Singapore, *Pediatrics* 1968; **41**: 1055–1062.
7. Milbauer, B., Peled, N. and Svirsky, S., Neonatal hyperbilirubinemia and glucose-6-phosphate dehydrogenase deficiency, *Israel J. Med. Sci.* 1973; **9**: 11547–11552.

8. Kaplan, M. and Abramov, A., Neonatal hyperbilirubinemia associated with glucose-6-phosphate dehydrogenase deficiency in Sephardic Jewish neonates: Incidence, severity, and the effect of phototherapy, *Pediatrics* 1992; **90**: 401–405.
9. Meloni, T., Cutillo, S., Testa, U. and Luzzatto, L. Neonatal jaundice and severity of glucose-6-phosphate dehydrogenase deficiency in Sardinian babies, *Early Human Develop*. 1987; **15**: 317–322.
10. Valaes, T., Bilirubin and red cell metabolism in relation to neonatal jaundice, *Postgrad. Med. J.* 1969; **45**: 86–106.
11. Oski, F.A., Neonatal hematology: The erythrocyte and its disorders. In: Nathan, D.G. and Oski, F.A., eds. *Hematology of infancy and childhood*. 4th ed. WB Saunders: Philadelphia, 1993; 18–43.
12. Valaes, T., Severe neonatal jaundice associated with glucose-6-phosphate dehydrogenase deficiency: pathogenesis and global epidemiology, *Acta. Paediatr*. 1994; **83**: Suppl 394: 58–76.
13. Bratteby, L.-E., Garby, L., Groth, T., Schneider, W. and Wadman, B., Studies of erythro-kinetics in infancy. XIII. The mean life span and the life span frequency function of red blood cells formed during foetal life, *Acta. Paediatr. Scand.* 1968; **57**: 311–320.
14. Zinkham, W.H. and Childs, B., Effect of Vitamin K and naphthalene metabolites on glutathione metabolism of erythrocytes from normal newborns and patients with naphthalene hemolytic anemia, *Am. J. Dis. Child.* 1957; **94**: 420–423.
15. Gross, R.T., Bracci, R., Rudolph, N., Schroeder, E. and Kochen, J.A., Hydrogen peroxide toxicity and detoxification in the erythrocytes of newborn infants, *Blood* 1967; **29**: 481–493.
16. Lubin, B. and Oski, F.A., Red cell metabolism in the newborn infant IV. Irreversible oxidant-induced injury, *J. Pediatr.* 1972; **81**: 698–704.
17. Shahal, Y., Bauminger, E.R., Zmora, E., Katz, M., Major, D., Horn, S. and Meyerstein, N., Oxidative Stress in newborn erythrocytes, *Pediatr. Res.* 1991; **29**: 119–129.
18. Mentzer, W.C. Jr., and Collier, E., Hydrops fetalis associated with erythrocyte G6PD deficiency and maternal ingestion of fava beans and ascorbic acid, *J. Pediat.* 1975; **86**: 565–567.
19. Brown, A.K. and Cevik, N., Hemolysis and jaundice in the newborn following maternal treatment with sulfamethoxypyridazine (Kynex), *Pediatrics* 1965; **36**: 742–744.
20. Glass, L., Rajegowda, B.K., Bowen, E. and Evans, H.E., Exposure to quinine and jaundice in a glucose-6-phosphate dehydrogenase deficient newborn, *J. Pediatr.* 1982; **82**: 734–735.
21. Emanuel, B. and Schoenfeld, A., Favism in a nursing infant, *J. Pediatr.* 1961; **58**: 263–266.
22. Freier, S., Mayer, K., Levene, C. and Abrahamov A., Neonatal jaundice associated with familiar G6PD deficiency in Israel, *Arch. Dis. Child.*, 1965; **40**: 280–283.
23. Olowe, S.A., Ransome-Kuti, O., The risk of jaundice in G6PD deficient babies exposed to menthol: *Acta. Paediatr. Scand.* 1980; **69**: 341–345.
24. Zinkham, W.H. and Childs, B., A defect of glutathione metabolism in erythrocytes from patients with a naphthalene – induced hemolytic anemia, *Pediatrics* 1958; **22**: 461–471.
25. Valaes, T., Doxiadis, S.A. and Fessas, Ph., Acute hemolysis due to naphthalene inhalation, *J. Pediatr.* 1963; **63**: 904–915.
26. Naiman, J.L. and Kosoy, M.H., Red cell glucose-6-phosphate dehydrogenase deficiency: A newly recognized cause of neonatal jaundice and kernicterus in Canada, *J. Canad Med. Ass.* 1964; **91**: 1243–1249.
27. Crosse, V.M., Meyer, T.C. and Gerard, J.W., Kernicterus and prematurity, *Arch. Dis. Child.* 1955; **30**: 501–508.
28. Allison, A.C., Danger of vitamin K to newborn, *Lancet* 1955; **1**: 669.
29. Gasser, C., Heinz body anemia and related phenomena, *J. Pediatr.* 1959; **54**: 673–690.
30. Lucey, J.F. and Dolan, R.G., Hyperbilirubinemia of newborn infants associated with the parenteral administration of a vitamin K analogue to the mothers, *Pediatrics* 1959; **23**: 553–560.
31. Valaes, T., Koliopoulos, C. and Koltsidopoulos A., The impact of phototherapy in the management of neonatal hyperbilirubinemia: Comparison of historical cohorts, *Acta. Paediatr.* 1996; **85**: 273–276.
32. Kaplan, M. and Hammerman, C., Severe neonatal hyperbilirubinemia: A potential complication of glucose-6-phosphate dehydrogenase deficiency, *Clin. Perinatol.* 1998; **25**: 575–590.
33. Fessas, Ph., Doxiadis, S.A. and Valaes, T., Neonatal jaundice in glucose-6-phosphated dehydrogenase deficient infants, *Brit. Med. J.* 1962; **2**: 1359–1362.
34. Valaes, T., Bilirubin metabolism: Review and discussion of inborn errors, *Clin. Perinatol.* 1976; **3**: 177–209.
35. Bosma, P.J., Roy-Chowdhury, J., Bakker, C. *et al.*, The genetic basis of the reduced expression of bilirubin UDP-glucuronosyltransferase 1 in Gilbert's syndrome, *N. Eng. J. Med.* 1995; **333**: 1171–1175.

36. Roy-Chowdhury, N., Deochrevan, B., Bejjanki, H.R. *et al.*, The presence of a Gilbert-type promoter abnormality increases the level of neonatal hyperbilirubinemia, *Hepatology* 1997 AASLD Abstr 370A.
37. Bancroft, J.D., Kreamer, B. and Gourley, G.R., Gilbert syndrome accelerates development of neonatal jaundice, *J. Pediatr.* 1998; **132**: 656–660.
38. Monaghan, G., McLellan, A., McGeehan, A. *et al.*, Gilbert's syndrome is a contributory factor in prolonged unconjugated hyperbilirubinemia of the newborn, *J. Pediatr.* 1999; **134**: 441–446.
39. Kaplan, M., Renbaum, P., Levi-Lahad, E. *et al.*, Gilbert syndrome and glucose-6-phosphate dehydrogenase deficiency: a dose dependent genetic interaction crucial to neonatal hyperbilirubinemia, *Proc. Natl. Acad Sci. USA* 1997; **94**: 12128–12132.
40. Iolascon, A., Faienza, M.F., Moretti, A. *et al.*, UG T1 promoter polymorphism accounts for increased neonatal appearance of hereditary spherocytosis, *Blood* 1998; **91**: 1093.
41. MacDonald, M.G., Hidden Risks: Early discharge and bilirubin toxicity due to glucose-6-phosphate dehydrogenase deficiency, *Pediatrics* 1995; **96**: 734–738.
42. Slusher, T.M., Vreman, H.J., McLaren, D. *et al.*, Glucose-6-phosphate dehydrogenase deficiency and carboxy hemoglobin concentrations associated with bilirubin related morbidity and death in Nigerian infants, *J. Pediatr.* 1995; **126**: 102–108.

Bilirubin Toxicity

6 The Neuropathology of Kernicterus: Definitions and Debate

Mamdouha Ahdab-Barmada

The WHY-NMD Institute for the Study of Neuromuscular Disorders, Pittsburgh, Pennsylvania, USA

INTRODUCTION

Bilirubin-associated damage to the central nervous system (CNS) remains a puzzling problem.[1–8] Clinical observations and experimental studies reveal a complexity that is far greater than suggested by an *a priori* cause and effect relation between the presence of bilirubin in the brain and the onset of neuronal damage.[9–22] For example, yellow staining of the brain does not necessarily imply bilirubin-related injury,[23–26] and bilirubin-associated CNS lesions may occur at low levels of serum bilirubin when other risk factors are present.[27,28] Attempts at neuropathologic and biochemical definition of bilirubin-associated damage in the mature and premature human infant, in experimental animals, and in *in vitro* systems are all fraught with continued controversy; this at a time when the management of neonatal hyperbilirubinemia remains a challenge for clinicians concerned with undertreatment[2,9] and overtreatment.[1,11–12] Revisiting our understanding of the neuropathology of kernicterus is a prerequisite for clarifying these conundrums and serves as the focus of this review.

HISTORICAL PERSPECTIVES

In 1847, Hervieux[29] first described yellow staining of the cerebral basal ganglia at autopsy in deeply jaundiced newborns. Orth confirmed these observations in 1875,[30] as he searched for bilirubin crystals in jaundiced brains. He also noted diffuse yellow staining of the meninges and periventricular areas in the brains of infants dying with jaundice. Later, Schmorl coined the term "kernicterus"[31] and differentiated two types of yellow staining of the brain in icteric newborns: (i) a diffuse yellow color of the meninges, cerebrospinal fluid and periventricular tissues, and (ii) a deeper yellow-orange color of the subcortical neuronal clusters including the basal ganglia, subthalamic nucleus, hippocampus, dentate nucleus, olive, nuclei of the cranial nerves and grey matter of the spinal cord.

In 1948, Becker and Vogel[32] provided a careful review of all reported cases of kernicterus, including those described by Orth and Schmorl. They tabulated the brain structures in which gross icteric discoloration was found and recorded the areas of histologic microscopic damage for each case.[32,33] Although they found no correlation between the extent of pathologic change and the intensity and duration of jaundice they emphasized that "the pathological distinction of kernicterus is the yellow discoloration of the nuclear structures of the brain". Moreover, the authors cautioned that "the most disputed aspect of the problem is the question of the 'histologic' damage to the nerve cells".[32] They acknowledged that they did not know whether neurons were injured primarily by bacterial, ischemic, traumatic or toxic factors, then selectively impregnated by the increased levels of bile pigment circulating in the blood; or whether the bile pigment itself was responsible for the observed nerve cell alterations. Dereymacker[34] confirmed these findings and outlined well-defined anatomical characteristics and clinical correlates of kernicterus in 1949.

Becker and Vogel felt that, by itself, anoxia was not sufficient to explain the lesions observed in the neurons. They also noted, on occasion, that marked yellow discoloration of brain nuclei would occur even though the anemia associated with erythroblastosis fetalis was mild during life. They suggested that red blood cell hemolysis might liberate substances capable of changing blood pH, and thus the polarity of the membrane of nerve cells, permitting penetration by the bile pigment. Nerve cells continuously in contact with such abnormal metabolic products would suffer irreversible damage.

Zuelzer and Mudgett,[35] in an analysis of 55 of their own cases stressed the role of prematurity, sepsis and infection as important risk factors for kernicterus, and concluded that kernicterus represents "a special situation in which injury to the nervous system is made visible" by the deposited yellow pigment. Claireaux, Cole and Lathe characterized the pigment seen in the brain as indirect reacting unconjugated bilirubin, confirmed that it remained yellow after fixation, while conjugated bilirubin in liver tissue became green upon fixation in formalin. They also described "a bilirubin-retaining lipid" in the yellow stained brain nuclei that was absent from tissue extracted from the non-specific diffusely yellow discolored areas of brain tissue.[40]

Although criteria were proposed for a specific definition of kernicterus that included clinical and pathologic parameters,[37–39,41,42] not all clinicopathological studies subscribed to these specific definitions. Thus, any yellow staining of brain tissue at autopsy, including diffusely discolored white matter, meninges or periventricular tissues of fresh, non-fixed brain, was labeled kernicterus, with or without any prominent nuclear staining of deep ganglia.[23–26] This non-selective approach increased confusion and helped to obscure the concept of kernicterus as a disease entity. Despite attempts to return to more stringent pathological criteria for the diagnosis of kernicterus,[27,49–56] the associated ischemic, hyperoxic, hypoglycemic and septic lesions found in the brains of sick premature neonates.[43–48] continued to confound the issue.[23,24,26,27] Kernicterus, however, is a definable and established entity, the neuropathology of which is detailed in the following sections.

ANATOMICAL, CYTOLOGICAL AND HISTOLOGICAL CHARACTERISTICS OF KERNICTERUS

Gross Anatomy

Yellow staining of the brain occurs upon exposure to elevated levels of bilirubin. Three patterns of yellow discoloration within the central nervous system have been described, each presumably related to a different pathogenesis. The pathogenesis of bilirubin associated neurotoxicity remains incompletely understood and is the focus of a separate chapter in this text (Chapter 7). The three typical brain bilirubin staining patterns include:

1. *Diffuse yellow staining of areas that normally lack blood–brain barrier*: These include the leptomeninges, ependyma, choroid plexuses, cerebrospinal fluid, and circumventricular organs which are readily stained whenever bilirubin levels are increased in the serum of newborns and adults. The circumventricular organs comprise the pituitary and pineal glands, pituitary stalk and median eminence, organum vasculosum of the lamina terminalis, subfornical organ, subhabenular organ and area postrema in the medulla.

2. *Diffuse yellow staining of brain tissue in areas where blood–brain barrier integrity has become compromised*: This encompasses the following conditions: hypoxic-ischemic encephalopathy, edematous cerebral and cerebellar cortex lining deep sulci, periventricular leukomalacia, focal neuronal necrosis, ischemic cerebral infarcts, septic infarcts, and traumatic lesions. Experimental disturbances of the blood–brain barrier (e.g., with urea or hyperosmolar solutions) could also be included in this category. In patterns 1 and 2, the bilirubin that penetrates and stains brain tissues may be conjugated or unconjugated, and is often bound to albumin. Bilirubin staining in this instance does not usually indicate binding to brain tissue and is easily lost when the tissue is immersed in formalin for a prolonged period. (e.g., for 24 hours or longer.)[27,42]

3. *Yellow staining of specific neuronal groups (kernicterus)*: The bilirubin staining in this instance is often characterized by an intense canary yellow to yellow-orange color as contrasted with the paler, sometimes greenish staining observed in patterns 1 and 2, and remains bright yellow following formalin fixation of the brain. It does not oxidize to green nor does it fade, despite prolonged immersion in formalin for weeks or even years.[27,38,39,41,42,49,53] It often remains in neurons, at least partially, through processing into paraffin.[27,53,55] This selective and persistent staining of nuclear clusters in the brain is believed to represent active uptake and lipid-binding of unconjugated bilirubin pigment by neurons. The yellow staining of these neuronal clusters is remarkably selective, with certain nuclei being involved consistently more often than others. This pattern of bilirubin staining has been described with only minor variations in (i) mature newborns with erythroblastosis fetalis and icterus gravis;[32,38,39,52,53] (ii) apparently healthy mature newborns;[57,58] (iii) asphyxiated premature or septic neonates;[27,35,36,55,56] (iv) in experimental animal models;[49,50,51,59,60] and (v) the rare adults reported with kernicterus.[61–63] The nuclei most often discolored yellow include the i) globus pallidus, ii) subthalamic nucleus,

iii) metabolic sector of the hippocampus, iv) red nuclei, v) oculomotor nuclei, vi) cranial nerve nuclei in the floor of the fourth ventricle including those of nerves VI, VII, VIII, cochlear and vestibular nuclei, vii) cerebellar roof nuclei, viii) dentate nuclei, ix) inferior olivary nuclei, x) gracili nucleus, xi) cuneatus nuclei, and xii) spinal anterior horns (Figures 6.1(a), (b) and (c)).

It is important to note that the cerebral cortex and putamen, although usually exquisitely sensitive to ischemic insults, do not stain yellow in the formalin-fixed brain tissue of a premature infant with kernicterus (Figure 6.1(a)). Similarly, the Sommer's sector of Ammon's horn which is typically sensitive to ischemic insults is not usually stained while the "metabolic sector" or H4-H3,[64] is bright yellow. A diffuse yellow staining of Ammon's horn is observed sometimes when the tissue is softened, infarcted and ischemic. Passive diffusion of bilirubin pigment into necrotic tissues is usually lost when the tissue is fixed in formalin, while true kernicterus, which represents uptake and retention of pigment by neurons, does not fade with fixation of tissues. An exception to this rule involves uptake and lipid-binding of bilirubin within macrophages in areas of cerebral cortical and white matter infarction, rendering it resistant to passive diffusion within formalin solution, and further confusing gross evaluation. However, this pattern may be clarified with histologic

(a)

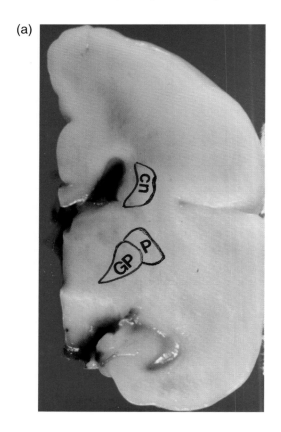

(b)

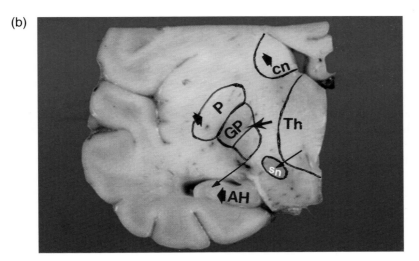

(c)

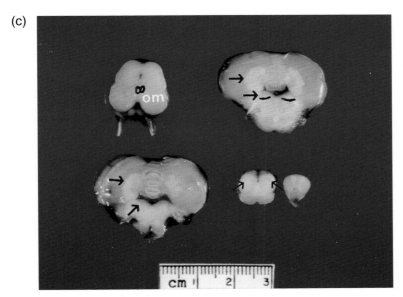

Figure 6.1. (a) Coronal section of the right hemisphere of the brain in a 25 week gestation kernicteric premature infant, at the level of mammillary bodies. Selective deep orange-yellow staining of the globus pallidus (GP), and pale yellow discoloration of surrounding brain. Note unstained putamen (P) and caudate (cn). Formalin fixed two weeks. X1.5; (b) Coronal section of the left hemisphere of a 34 week gestation premature kernicteric infant, at the level of Ammon's horn. Bright yellow staining (thin arrows) of globus pallidus (GP), subthalamic nucleus (Sn) and Ammon's hom (AH) metabolic sector, with unstained Sommer's sector, putamen (P) and caudate nucleus (cn) (fat arrows). Pale yellow discoloration of thalamus (Th). No staining of cerebral cortex. Formalin fixed two weeks. X1.5; and (c) Transverse sections of brainstem and cerebellum illustrating yellow staining of oculomotor nuclei (OM) in the midbrain, and vestibular nuclei (arrow) in pons and medulla, while cerebellar dentate nuclei (arrow) only show pale yellow discoloration. Formalin fixed two weeks.

study of tissues, when the yellow pigment is noted in macrophages rather than in neurons.

In kernicterus, there is exquisite and selective staining of susceptible brain nuclei, a pattern of staining that is distinctly different from the pattern of selective damage associated with hypoxia, ischemia, or hyperoxia.[65-67] Thus, it is essential to distinguish between the non-specific pattern of yellow staining of the brain that occurs with elevated bilirubin levels, or with preceding damage to focal areas of brain (and which washes away during prolonged formalin fixation of the brain) and the persistent yellow staining of grey nuclei (kernicterus) which may occur at high or low levels of bilirubin, without preceding damage to the grey nuclei. This latter type of yellow staining persists in fixed tissues for weeks to years. Such clinicopathologic findings enable us to correlate the type and pattern of yellow staining with the appropriate clinical syndrome.

Histological and Cytological Alterations

Careful reviews have outlined histological and cytological alterations in jaundiced newborns.[25,27,32,37-39,41,52,56] Some of the changes described appear to represent non-specific alterations due to edema, ischemia and autolysis, other changes appear consistently in icteric infants at high or low bilirubin levels, in experimental animal studies and *in vitro* studies.

Non-specific changes have been characterized as early and late. Early non-specific changes may include microvacuolation of the neuropil and myelinated tracts (Figure 6.2). This was the predominant change described in cases of diffuse yellow staining of premature brains by Turkel *et al*.[24,25] Such findings are seen in jaundiced neonates dying in the first week of life. Late non-specific changes include neuronal loss and astrocytosis that may be widespread in infants with severe associated hypoxic-ischemic encephalopathy.

Specific neuronal changes in kernicterus are summarized in Table 6.1. Early (2–5 days) neuronal changes indicative of kernicterus include yellow pigment in the neuronal cytoplasm of frozen or even paraffin sections (Figure 6.3). This finding is more frequent in infants dying in the first week of life, but has been described in brains of infants surviving weeks to years. Other early changes may include: (i) a moth-eaten appearance of neuronal and nuclear membranes (Figure 6.2) with prominent cytoplasmic microvacuolation at the cell membrane; (ii) dense and pyknotic nuclei; (iii) loss of Nissl substance and basophilic cytoplasm; (iv) Periodic-acid-Schiff (PAS) positive membrane-bound aggregates; and (v) cellular dissolution.

Subacute neuronal changes in kernicterus may include: (i) a finely spongy neuropil within involved nuclei, (ii) hypertrophic bare astrocytic nuclei; (iii) cellular dissolution of some neurons, with loss of cytoplasmic and nuclear membranes; (iv) basophilic neurons with increased nuclear density, etched and hazy nuclear and cytoplasmic membranes; and (v) early granular mineralization of neuronal cytoplasmic membranes.

Late neuronal changes in kernicterus include: (i) neuronal loss with prominent reactive "metabolic" (as opposed to fibrillary) astrocytosis (bare Alzheimer's type II

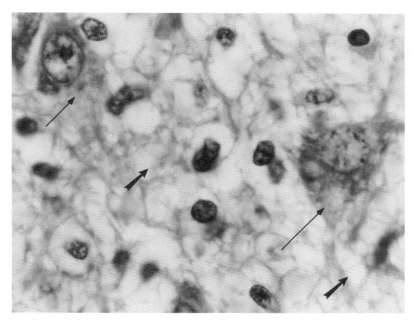

Figure 6.2. Microvacuolation of neuropil (large arrows) and of neuronal cytoplasmic membranes (thin arrows at moth-eaten foci). Oil immersion, paraffin processed, H&E stained section of oculomotor nuclei.

Table 6.1. Neuropathologic findings of kernicterus.

Early (2–5 days)	Subacute (6–10 days)	Late (> 10 days)
Yellow pigment in neuronal cytoplasm	Spongy neuropil within involved nuclei	Neuronal loss with astrocytosis
Moth-eaten appearance of neuronal and nuclear membranes	Hypertrophic, bare astrocytic nuclei	Granular mineralizations of residual neuronal membranes in affected nuclei
Pyknotic nucleus	Basophilic neurons with increased nuclear density	Demyelinization of optic tracts, and fornix
Loss of Nissl substance	Cellular dissolution of some neurons	Dysmyelination and degeneration of globus pallidus and subthalamic nucleus
Basophilic cytoplasm	Granular mineralization of neuronal cytoplasmic membranes	
PAS positive membrane bound aggregates within neurons		

astrocytic nuclei); (ii) granular mineralization of residual neuronal membranes in affected nuclei; (iii) occasional fully mineralized nerve cells and proximal axonal segments; (iv) demyelination of optic tracts and fornix described in long term

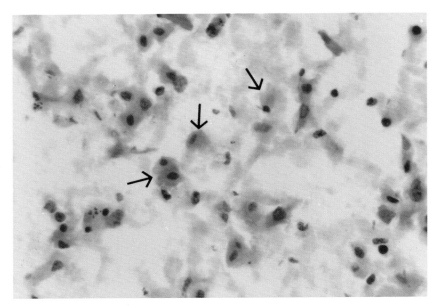

Figure 6.3. Frozen section of hippocampal cortex of a premature newborn infant with kernicterus. Note edema of neuropil and yellow pigment (thin arrow) filling many relatively well preserved pyramidal neurons. Formalin fixed two weeks. Oil immersion, H&E stained.

survivors of early icterus gravis; and (v) dysmyelination and degeneration of globus pallidus and subthalamic nucleus.[53,68–70]

Ultrastructural Changes

These changes have been described in detail in experimental animals[51,71–74] and noted in the brains of kernicteric infants.[27] Such changes include: (i) patchy loss of segments of neuronal nuclear and cytoplasmic membrane, replaced by early myelin figures (Figure 6.4); (ii) marked membrane alterations with prominent lipid whorls and dense bodies (Figure 6.5); and (iii) dense bodies scattered within the cytoplasm that possibly represent degenerated mitochondria with accumulated glycogen and calcium granules.

Selective Vulnerability of Bilirubin-Associated Brain Lesions

Microscopic changes grossly parallel the sites of bilirubin deposits in the brain. However, if areas of bright yellow staining such as the globus pallidus, subthalamic nucleus, red nucleus, roof nuclei and cranial nerve nuclei show prominent neuronal damage, dentate nuclei and inferior olivary nuclei are less often and less severely affected.[27,75] In other areas, damage may be restricted to one type of neuron, sparing surrounding neurons: thus, despite lack of gross staining, there is a typical selective damage to one layer of cells, i.e., Purkinje cells in the cerebellar cortex, while granular

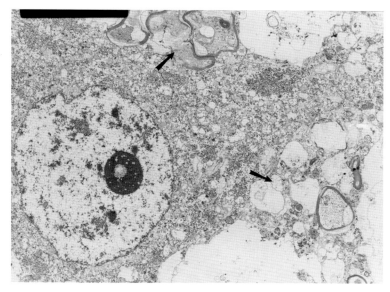

Figure 6.4. Ultrastructural appearance of a neuron with early focal degeneration of cytoplasmic membrane, possibly at the site of axo-somatic synapses (arrows), replaced by early myelin figures. Epon-embedded. Uranyl acetate and lead citrate stained. X7725

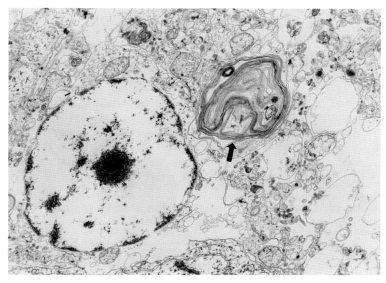

Figure 6.5. Ultrastructural appearance of slightly more extensive neuronal and nuclear membrane alterations, replaced focally by lipid whorls (large arrow) and dense bodies. Epon-embedded. Uranylacetate and lead citrate stained. X16500.

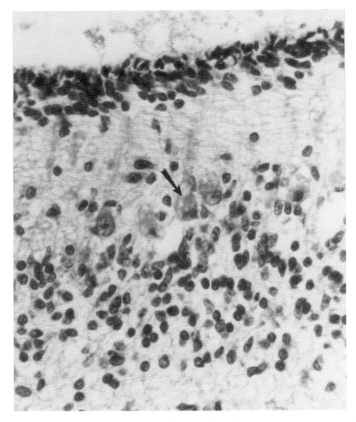

Figure 6.6. Cerebellar cortex in a premature kernicteric infant. Note early selective vacuolation of cytoplasmic membranes of Purkinje cells (arrow), while granular neurons are relatively spared. Paraffin section. H&E stained. X450.

neurons are spared (Figure 6.6). Neuronal damage can be exquisitely selective, i.e., neurons in the reticular portion of the substantia nigra will always show changes while neurons in the compacta portion only show ischemic damage whenever it occurs.[27,51] Patterns of bilirubin staining of nuclear clusters is thus different from patterns seen with ischemic[65,66] or hyperoxic[67] neuronal damage.

   Apparently astrocytes and oligodendroglial cells are not affected by the contiguous neuronal necrosis, in contrast to the reactive proliferation observed with ischemic neuronal necrosis. As stressed by Mair,[75] there is no hyperplasia or hypertrophy of the astrocytes, no microglial reaction, no perivascular cellular reaction and no vascular wall damage within nuclei affected by kernicterus. However, astrocytes "primed" by hypoxic-ischemic insults to the brain, will contain accumulated glycolipids within their cytoplasm, which may in turn, trap bilirubin pigment and thus later impair glial metabolism.

Post-Icteric Encephalopathy

Histological sequelae of kernicterus have been described in rare instances where there was prolonged survival following neonatal jaundice.[33,39,41,76,77] A common histologic pattern observed in post-icteric encephalopathy consists of a selective involvement of the globus pallidus and subthalamic nucleus most prominently, often the hippocampus, and sometimes other susceptible nuclei typically stained in acute kernicterus. Malamud[53] emphasized the selective topographical triad in post-icteric encephalopathy which is pathognomonic of bilirubin toxicity, i.e., the globus pallidus, subthalamic nucleus and hippocampus. This same pattern of involvement has recently been described in magnetic resonance imaging studies of children with post-kernicteric encephalopathy, i.e., abnormal bilateral high intensity signals in the globus pallidus,[78,79,80] internal capsule,[78] and thalamus.[78] Of interest in this regard is that these nuclei are those that contain the most mature extrapyramidal cells in the newborn brain; such cells contain large quantities of gangliosides at birth and are already involved in neurotransmitter secretion. Bilirubin pigment trapped within such cells could act as a possible oxidant leading to cellular degeneration. The specific topographic pattern involved in posticteric encephalopathy is similar to that described in dentatorubropallidoluysian atrophy, an autosomal dominant progressive degenerative disease of the dentatorubral and pallidoluysian systems.[81] Thus, the finding of impairment of synaptosomal dopamine release in the presence of bilirubin[82] becomes pertinent, reproducing some of the genetically impaired neurotransmitter metabolism reported in the aforementioned familial syndrome.

CONCLUSION

Bilirubin toxicity to the central nervous system (CNS) may occur when indirect bilirubin levels are elevated. Kernicterus reflects bilirubin pigment incorporation into gangliosides or phospholipids of mature neurons, with either rapid or slowly progressive damage to neurons depending on the amount of pigment trapped within cell. It is characterized by a consistent, unique topographic pattern of nuclear involvement. The combination of both selective bright yellow-orange staining of certain brain nuclei, with evidence of neuronal damage and degeneration within such nuclei, is necessary to ascribe the neuropathologic diagnosis of kernicterus to postmortem brain tissue.[27,56] Strict application of such criteria with an emphasis on the necessity of microscopic evidence of neuronal damage will help to reduce confusion regarding the diagnosis and pathophysiology of kernicterus.

Reference

1. Valaes, T., Kollopoulos, C. and Koltsidopoulos, A., The impact of phototherapy in the management of neonatal hyperbilirubinemia-comparison of historical cohorts, *Acta. Paediatr.* 1996; **85**; 273–276.
2. Ives, N.K., Kernicterus in preterm infants; Lest we forget (to turn on the lights), *Pediatrics* 1992; **90**; 757–759.

3. Newman, T.B. and Maisels, M.J., Bilirubin and brain damage: What do we do now? *Pediatrics* 1989; **83**; 1062–1065.
4. Newman, T.B. and Maisels, M.J., Does hyperbilirubinemia damage the brain of healthy newborn infants? *Clin. Perinatol.* 1990; **17**: 331–358.
5. Watchko, J.F. and Oski F.A., Kernicterus in preterm newborns: past, present, and future, *Pediatrics* 1992; **90**: 707–715.
6. Watchko, J.F. and Claassen, D., Kernicterus in premature infants: Current prevalence and relationship to NICHD phototherapy study exchange criteria, *Pediatrics* 1994; **93**: 996–999.
7. Oktay, R., Satar, M. and Atici, A., The risk of bilirubin encephalopathy in neonatal hyperbilirubinemia, *Turk. J. Pediatr.* 1996; **38**: 199–204.
8. Valaes, T., Severe neonatal jaundice associated with glucose-6-phosphate dehydrogenase deficiency: pathogenesis and global epidemiology, *Acta. Paediatr.* 1994; **83** (Suppl): 58–76.
9. Wennberg, R.P., Bilirubin recommendations present problems: New guideline simplistic and untested, *Pediatrics* 1992; **89**: 821–822.
10. Newman, T.B. and Klebanoff, M.A., Neonatal hyperbilirubinemia and long-term outcome: Another look at the collaborative perinatal project, *Pediatrics* 1993; **92**: 651–657.
11. Hein, H.A., Why do we keep using phototherapy in healthy newborns? *Pediatrics* 1984; **73**: 881–882.
12. Watchko, J.F. and Oski F.A., Bilirubin 20 mg/dl = vigintiphobia, *Pediatrics* 1983; **71**: 660–663.
13. Scheidt, P.C., Graubard, B.I., Nelson, K.B. *et al.*, Intelligence at six years in relation to neonatal bilirubin level: Follow-up of The National Institute of Child Health and Human Development Clinical Trial of Phototherapy, *Pediatrics* 1991; **87**: 797–805.
14. Graziani, L.J., Mitchells, D.G., Kornhauser, M. *et al.*, Neurodevelopment of preterm infants: Neonatal neurosonographic and serum bilirubin studies, *Pediatrics* 1992; **89**: 229–234.
15. O'Shea, T.M., Dillard, R.G., Klinepeter, K.L. *et al.*, Serum bilirubin levels, intracranial hemorrhage, and the risk of developmental problems in very low birth weight neonates, *Pediatrics* 1991; **90**: 888–892.
16. Van de Bor, M., van Zeben-van der Aa, T.M., Verloove-Vanhorick, S.P. *et al.*, Hyperbilirubinemia in preterm infants and neurodevelopmental outcome at 2 years of age: Results of a national collaborative survey, *Pediatrics* 1989; **83**: 915–920.
17. Van de Bor, M., Ens-Dokkum, M., Schreuder, A.M. *et al.*, Hyperbilirubinemia in low birth weight infants and outcome at 5 years of age, *Pediatrics* 1992; **89**: 359–364.
18. De Vries, L.S.; Lary, S. and Dubowitz, L.M.S., Relationship of serum bilirubin levels to ototoxicity and deafness in high-risk low-birth-weight infants, *Pediatrics* 1985; **76**: 351–354.
19. Bergman, I., Hirsch, R.P., Fria, T.J. *et al.*, Cause of hearing loss in the high-risk premature infant, *J. Pediatrics* 1985; **106**: 95–101.
20. Doyle, L.W., Keirs, E., Kitchen, W.H. *et al.*, Audiologic assessment of extremely low birth weight infants – a preliminary report, *Pediatrics* 1992; **90**: 744–749
21. Worley, G., Erwin, C.W., Goldstein, R.F. *et al.*, Delayed development of sensorineural hearing loss after neonatal hyperbilirubinemia: A case report with brain magnetic resonance imaging, *Develop. Med. Child Neurol.* 1996; **38**: 271–278.
22. Silver, S., Sohmer, H. and Kapitulnik, J., Postnatal development of somatosensory evoked potentials in jaundiced Gunn rats and effects of sulfadimethoxine administration, *Pediatr. Res.* 1996; **40**: 209–214.
23. Kim, M.H., Yoon, J.I., Sher, J. *et al.*, Lack of predictive indices in kernicterus: A comparison of clinical and pathological factors in infants with or without kernicterus, *Pediatrics* 1980; **66**: 852–858.
24. Turkel, S.B., Miller, C.A., Guttenberg, M.E. *et al.*, A clinical pathological reappraisal of kernicterus, *Pediatrics* 1982; **69**: 267–272.
25. Turkel, S.B., Autopsy findings associated with neonatal hyperbilirubinemia, *Clin. Perinatol.* 1990; **17**: 381–397.
26. Ritter, D.A., Kenny, J.D., Norton, J. *et al.*, A prospective study of free bilirubin and other risk factors in the development of kernicterus in premature infants, *Pediatrics* 1982; **69**: 260–267.
27. Ahdab-Barmada, M. and Moossy, J., The neuropathology of kernicterus in the premature neonate: Diagnostic problems, *J. Neuropath. Exp. Neurol.* 1984; **43**: 45–56.
28. Perlman, J.M., Rogers, B.B. and Burns, D., Kernicteric findings at autopsy in two sick near term infants, *Pediatrics* 1997; **99**: 612–615.
29. Hervieux, J., De l'icterè des nouveaux-nés, *MD. thesis*, Paris, 1847.
30. Orth, T., Uber das vorkommen von bilirubinkrystallen bei neugeborenen kindern, *Virchows Archiv. Pathol.*, 1875; **63**: 447–462.

31. Schmorl, G., Zur Kenntniss des ikterus neonatorum., *Verh Dtsch. Pathol Gesellsch* 1904; **6**: 109–115.
32. Becker, P.F.L. and Vogel, P., Kernicterus: A review with a report of the findings in a study of seven cases, *J. Neuropathol. Exp. Neurol.* 1948; **7**: 190–215.
33. Zimmerman, H.M. and Yannet, H., Kernicterus: Jaundice of the nuclear masses of the brain, *Am. J. Dis. Child.* 1933; **45**: 740–759.
34. Dereymacker, A. Contribution a l'Etude Clinique, Anatomique et Experimentale de l'Ictere Nucleaire du Nouveau-ne. Masson, Paris, 1949.
35. Zuelzer, W.W. and Mudgett, R.T., Kemicterus: Etiologic study based on an analysis of 55 cases, *Pediatrics* 1950; **6**; 452–474.
36. Claireaux, A., Haemolytic disease of the newborn. Part II. Nuclear Jaundice (Kernicterus), *Arch. Dis. Child.* 1950; **25**: 71–80.
37. Gerrard, J., Kernicterus, *Brain* 1952; **75**: 526–571.
38. Bertrand, 1. Bessis, M. and Segarra-Obiol, J.M. l'Ictere Nucleaire, Masson Paris, 1952.
39. Haymaker, W., Margoles, C., Pentschew, A. *et al.*, Pathology of kernicterus and posticteric encephalopathy. In: Swinyard C.A., ed. Kernicterus and its importance in cerebral palsy. A conference presented by The American Academy for Cerebral Palsy. Eleventh Annual Meeting. New Orleans, LA. Springfield: Thomas, 21–228, 1961.
40. Claireaux, A.E., Cole, P.G. and Lathe G.H., Icterus of the brain in the newborn, *Lancet* 1953; **2**: 1226–1236.
41. Larroche, J.C., Kernicterus. In: Handbook of Clinical Neurology. Volume 6. Vinken, P.J. and Bruyn, G.W. eds. North Holland Publishing Co., Amsterdam 1968, pp. 491–516.
42. Larroche, J.C., Perinatal brain damage. Bilirubin and brain damage. In Adams, J., Corsellis, J.A.N. and Duchar, L.W., eds. Greenfield's neuropathology. 4th ed. Edward Arnold Publish., London, 1984.
43. Aidin, R., Comer, B. and Tovey, G. Kernicterus and prematurity, *Lancet* **1**: 1153–1154, 1954.
44. Crosse, V.M., Meyer, T.C. and Gerrard, J.W., Kernicterus and prematurity, *Arch. Dis. Child.* 1955; **30**: 501–508.
45. Harris, R.C., Lucey, J.F. and MacLean, R.J., Kernicterus in premature infants associated with low concentration of bilirubin in the plasma, *Pediatrics* 1958; **21**: 875–884.
46. Gartner, L.M., Snyder, R.N., Chabon, R.S. *et al.*, Kernicterus: High incidence in premature infants with low serum bilirubin concentrations, *Pediatrics* 1970; **45**: 906–917.
47. Seidman, D.S. and Stevenson, D.K., The issues of hyperbilirubinemia, *Pediatrics* 1995; **96**: 543–544, (Letter and Reply).
48. Valaes, T. and Gellis, S.S., Is kernicterus always the definitive evidence of bilirubin toxicity? *Pediatrics* 1981; **67**: 940–941.
49. Blanc, W.A. and Johnson, L., Studies on kernicterus, *J. Neuropathol. Exp. Neurol.* 1959; **18**: 165–189.
50. Johnson, L., Sarmiento F., Blanc, W.A. *et al.*, Kernicterus in rats with inherited deficiency of glucuronyl transferase, *Am. J. Dis. Child.* 1960; **97**: 591–608.
51. Jew, J.Y. and Sandquist, D., CNS changes in hyperbilirubinemia. Functional implications, *Arch. Neurol.* 1979; **16**: 149–154.
52. Claireaux, A.F., Pathology of human kernicterus. In: Sass-Kortsak, A., ed. Kernicterus. Toronto: University of Toronto Press, 1959; 140–149.
53. Malamud, N., Pathogenesis of kernicterus in the light of its sequelae. In: Kernicterus and its importance in cerebral palsy. Springfield, Ill., Charles C. Thomas, 1961; 230–245.
54. Chen, H.C., Kernicterus in the Chinese newborn. A morphological and spectrophotometric study, *J. Neuropathol. Exp. Neurol.* 1964; **23**: 527–549.
55. Larroche, J.C. In: Developmental pathology of the neonate. Amsterdam: Excerpta Medica, 1977; 447–454.
56. Ahdab-Barmada, M. Neonatal kernicterus: Neuropathologic diagnosis. In: Levine, R.L., Maisels, M.J., eds. Hyperbilirubinemia in the newborn. Report of the 85th Ross Conference on Pediatric Research. Columbus, OH, Ross Laboratories, 1983, pp. 2–8.
57. Penn, A.A., Enzmann, D.R., Hahn, J.S. *et al.*, Kernicterus in a full-term infant, *Pediatrics* 1994; **93**: 1003–1006.
58. Maisels, M.J. and Newman, T.B., Kernicterus in otherwise healthy, breast-fed newborns, *Pediatrics* 1995; **96**: 730–733.
59. Rozdilsky, B. and Olszewski, J., Experimental study of the toxicity of bilirubin in newborn animals, *J. Neuropathol. Exp. Neurol.* 1961; **20**: 193–205.

60. Schutta, H.S. and Johnson L., Clinical signs and morphologic abnormalities in Gunn rats treated with sulfadimethoxine, *J. Pediatr.* 1969; **75**: 1070–1079.
61. Whitington G.L., Congenital nonhemolytic icterus with damage to the central nervous system. Report of a case in a Negro child, *Pediatrics* **18**: 1960; 437–440.
62. Blumenschein, S.D., Kallen, R.T., Storey, B. *et al.*, Familial nonhemolytic jaundice with late onset of neurological damage, *Pediatrics* 1968; **42**: 786–791.
63. Ho, K.C., Hodach, R., Varma R. *et al.*, Kernicterus and central pontine myelinolysis in a 14 year-old boy with fulminating viral hepatitis, *Ann. Neurol.* 1980; **8**: 633–636.
64. Rose, M., Gyrus limbicus anterior und Regio retrosplenialis (Cortex holoprotoptychos Rose, quinquestratificatus) Vergleichende Architektonik bei Tier und Mensch, *J.F. Psychol. Neurol.* 1927; **35**: 65–173.
65. Towbin, A., Cerebral hypoxic damage in fetus and newborn. Basic patterns and their clinical significance, *Arch. Neurol.* 1969; **20**: 35–43.
66. Leech, R.W. and Alvord, E.C. Jr., Anoxic-ischemic encephalopathy in the human neonatal period, *Arch. Neurol.* 1977; **34**: 109–113.
67. Ahdab-Barmada, M., Moossy, J. and Painter, M., Pontosubicular necrosis and hyperoxemia, *Pediatrics* 1980; **66**: 840–847.
68. Lund, M., Kernicterus. A clinical and pathological study of two late cases, *Acta. Psych. Scand.* 1955; **80**: 265–280.
69. Van Bogaert, L., Aspects cliniques et pathologiques des sequelles tardives des l'Ictere nucleaire, *Acta. Neurologica. Belgica.* 1949; **49**: 961–964.
70. Soecken, G., Kernicterus und morbus heamolyticus neonatorum, *Arch. Kinderheilk.* (Berl) 1957; **5**: 1–94.
71. Schutta, T.T.S., Johnson, L. and Neville, H.E., Mitochondrial abnormalities in bilirubin encephalopathy, *J. Neuropathol. Exp. Neurol.* 1970; **29**: 296–305.
72. Batty, H.K. and Millhouse, O.E., Ultrastructure of the Gunn rat substantia nigra. II Mitochondrial changes, *Acta. Neuropathol.* (Berl) 1976; **34**: 7–19.
73. Schutta, H.S. and Johnson, L., Electron microscopic observation on acute bilirubin encephalopathy in Gunn rats induced by sulfadimethoxine, *Lab. Invest.* 1971; **24**: 82–89.
74. Jew, J.Y. and Williams, T.H., Ultrastructural aspects of bilirubin encephalopathy in cochlear nuclei of the Gunn rat, *J. Anat.* 1977; **124**: 599–614.
75. Mair, W.G.P., Cerebral changes in kernicterus. IV Internat, *Congr. Neuropath.* 1961; **4**: 83–89.
76. Hoffman, W. and Hanssmann, M., Icterus gravis neonatorum. Folgezustande und pathogenese, *Mschr. Kinderheilk.* 1926; **33**: 193–224.
77. Friede R.L., Kernicterus (Bilirubin encephalopathy). In: Developmental Neuropathology. Berlin, NY, Springer-Verlag, 2nd ed., 1989, pp. 115–121.
78. Penn, A.A., Enzmann, D.R., Hahn, J.S. and Stevenson, D.K., Kernicterus in a full term infant, *Pediatrics* 1994; **93**: 1003–1006.
79. Martich-Kriss, V., Kollias, S.S. and Ball, W.S., MR findings in kernicterus, *Ann. Neuroradiol.* 1995; **16**: 819–821.
80. Yokochi, K., Magnetic resonance imaging in children with kernicterus, *Acta. Paediatr.* 1995; **84**: 937–939.
81. Warner, T.T., Williams, L.D. and Walker, R.W., A clinical and molecular genetic study of dentatorubropallidoluysian atrophyin in four European families, *Ann. Neurol.* 1995; **37**: 452–459.
82. Cashore, W.J., The neurotoxicity of bilirubin, *Clin. Perinatol.* 1990; **17**: 437–447.

7 The Pathophysiology of Bilirubin Toxicity

Thor Willy Ruud Hansen

Section on Neonatology, Department of Pediatrics, Rikshospitalet, Oslo, Norway.

The scientific study of neonatal jaundice celebrated its sesquicentennial in 1997. In 1847 Hervieux made this common clinical phenomenon in newborns the subject of his doctoral thesis.[1] A generation later Orth[2] described yellow staining of the basal ganglia and in 1904 Schmorl coined the term *kernicterus* (jaundice of the basal ganglia).[3] The term kernicterus has since been used to describe three scenarios: 1) an acute syndrome characterized by lethargy, poor feeding, hypertonia with opisthotonus, fever and a high pitched cry in very jaundiced infants; 2) the neuropathological findings in infants who died during or following an acute illness as just described (see Chapter 6); and 3) a chronic condition seen in survivors of the acute syndrome, characterized by choreoathetosis, asymmetric spasticity, paresis of upward gaze, neurogenic hearing loss, and occasionally mental retardation.

Subsequent observations have shown that hyperbilirubinemia may exert effects on the nervous system short of kernicterus. Thus, infants who are markedly jaundiced are frequently drowsy, lethargic and less interested in feeding. Auditory and visual evoked responses measured in such infants evidence altered neuronal function.[4-6] These clinical and neurophysiological correlates of hyperbilirubinemia appear to be reversible. Some authors designate these effects as hyperbilirubinemic encephalopathy[7] although agreement on the definition of this term vis-a-vis kernicterus has not been reached. Many investigators believe that kernicterus and bilirubin encephalopathy are points on a continuum, though this hypothesis remains to be proven.

During the past 40 years, many studies have explored the pathogenesis of bilirubin neurotoxicity and as a result a wealth of information on how bilirubin gets into brain, how it is distributed there, and what effects it has on cells and cellular processes has accrued. Despite this progress, there is as yet no agreement on the basic mechanism(s) of bilirubin neurotoxicity. In the following discussion many of these findings will be reviewed and an argument made that the observed effects of bilirubin on the central nervous system are best understood in terms of bilirubin binding characteristics and of bilirubin's effects on basic cell regulatory mechanisms.

89

BILIRUBIN CHEMISTRY AND SOLUBILITY

Bilirubin is the end product of heme catabolism and is formed through oxidation-reduction reactions. The main isomer in the human organism is biliruin-IXα (Z,Z), that exists either as a charged dianion, or as the bilirubin acid. In the former case the presence of eight hydrophilic moieties imparts some water solubility at neutral pH, while in the latter case the formation of intramolecular hydrogen bonds[8–10] results in near insolubility in water.[8] Thus at pH 7.4 the solubility of bilirubin (4–7 nM) is for practical purposes equal to the concentration of the dianion. The non-α and the photo-isomers of bilirubin are more soluble, but occur only in trace amounts under physiologic conditions (in the absence of phototherapy).[9]

The overwhelming body of evidence suggests that it is the hydrophobic bilirubin-IXα (Z,Z) isomer which is responsible for the toxic effects, while the water-soluble isomers are non-toxic.[11,12] Bilirubin becomes water-soluble when it is bound to glucuronic acid during conjugation in the hepatocytes, and when bound to albumin for transport in serum. In both circumstances, bilirubin is non-toxic.[13,14] It is noteworthy that bilirubin binding to these molecules appears to occur on lysine residues,[15,16] the implications of which will be discussed later in this chapter.

BILIRUBIN BINDING AND THE "FREE BILIRUBIN THEORY"

Bilirubin binding to albumin was first described by Bennhold[17] and subsequent studies have shown that albumin has a primary, high affinity binding site for bilirubin with the capacity for binding up to one molecule of bilirubin per molecule of albumin. Secondary binding sites evince lower affinities for bilirubin.[9,18] Because of the high binding affinity of albumin for bilirubin (10^7-10^8 mol^{-1}), equilibrium concentrations of unbound ("free") bilirubin in plasma are very low.[19] Even in the presence of high unconjugated bilirubin levels in the markedly jaundiced neonate, concentrations of unbound bilirubin are only in the low nanomolar range as measured with the peroxidase method.[20–22] The same is true in experimental animal models of jaundice.[23–24]

The importance of bilirubin binding (or lack thereof) with respect to the pathogenesis of bilirubin neurotoxicity has been a focus of considerable debate among investigators. According to the "free bilirubin theory", free or unbound bilirubin can cross the blood–brain barrier and cell membranes, and produce neuronal injury.[25] The free bilirubin theory also assumes that variations in the serum bilirubin concentration of unbound are important for neurotoxicity. Thus, when the bilirubin/albumin ratio exceeds unity, or the binding capacity of albumin is decreased because of altered albumin characteristics[26,27] or because of the presence of binding competitors,[28–30] unbound bilirubin concentrations will increase, and more bilirubin will be shifted into tissues by the laws of equilibrium. The water-soluble isomers, in contrast, are not able to cross lipid-containing membranes, and in the absence of a specific transporter are excluded from brain and from cells. Albumin-bound bilirubin is essentially excluded from the brain by virtue of the size of the albumin molecule,[24] though some entry of albumin into the central nervous system may occur in the immature organism or when the blood–brain barrier is damaged (see discussion below).

Measurements of Unbound Bilirubin and Bilirubin Binding

Many laboratory tests have been devised to measure the reserve albumin binding capacity for bilirubin, as well as unbound bilirubin itself.[31] Though these tests have been research tools of considerable interest, they have been of limited clinical utility with the possible exception of the peroxidase-oxidation method.[21,22] By and large, it has been difficult to demonstrate strong correlations between bilirubin binding measurements and evidence of neurotoxicity.[32,33] Some have perceived this lack of correlation as evidence against the "free bilirubin theory", but this may not be correct for several reasons. First, increases in unbound bilirubin concentrations are likely to be short-lived because equilibration with tissues such as brain appears to be quite rapid.[34–36] Second, our methods for measuring bilirubin neurotoxicity are not very sensitive or specific. It is therefore not surprising that a correlation between fleeting elevations in unbound bilirubin concentrations and gross neurologic outcome measures has been hard to establish. Furthermore, neither bilirubin binding tests nor measurements of unbound bilirubin concentrations take into account a third possible variable, that of inter-individual differences in vulnerability to bilirubin neurotoxicity. As will be discussed later, evidence is emerging that brain cells may be able to detoxify bilirubin, and that this capacity may be subject to variation depending on both intrinsic and extrinsic factors.

BILIRUBIN AND THE BLOOD–BRAIN BARRIER

In order to exert its neurotoxic effects, bilirubin must enter the central nervous system, i.e., cross the blood–brain barrier. As previously mentioned, the lipophilicity of the bilirubin molecule may account for its ability to do so.[37] A cartoon illustrating some of the concepts regarding bilirubin entry into brain, as well as its disposition within and clearance from brain, is shown in Figure 7.1. In the presence of an intact blood–brain barrier bilirubin appears to enter the brain as the unbound molecule. If the capacity of serum albumin to bind bilirubin is reduced, the increase in serum unbound bilirubin drives more bilirubin into the brain. If the integrity of the blood–brain barrier is broken, or if brain blood flow is increased, both unbound as well as albumin-bound bilirubin may enter the brain in increased amounts.

Immaturity of the Blood–Brain Barrier

Immaturity of the blood–brain barrier has been hypothesized to contribute to, or exacerbate, he effects of bilirubin on the newborn brain. The concept of an "immature" blood–brain barrier at birth may have originated from early studies using bilirubin itself as a marker of blood–brain barrier integrity.[38,39] Indeed, even recent reports suggest that the newborn blood–brain barrier is more permeable to

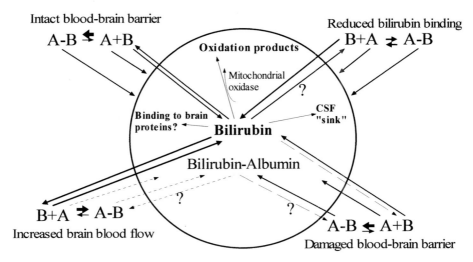

Figure 7.1. Mechanisms of bilirubin entry into, disposition in, and clearance from brain. The unbound bilirubin molecule (B) is able to enter the brain through an intact blood–brain barrier. Albumin (A) and albumin-bound bilirubin (A-B), however, do not cross the intact blood–brain barrier. If the ability of albumin to bind bilirubin is reduced by intrinsic or extrinsic factors, the equilibrium balance is shifted in the direction of more unbound bilirubin. The entry of unbound bilirubin into brain is increased, while albumin and albumin-bound bilirubin still do not enter. If the blood-brain barrier is damaged or compromised, albumin and albumin-bound bilirubin may be able to enter the brain. There is some evidence that albumin-bound bilirubin may be cleared more slowly from the brain, at least in the presence of an opened blood–brain barrier. If brain blood flow is increased, the acute entry of unbound bilirubin into brain is increased. Increased brain blood flow also appears to be accompanied by some entry of albumin-bound bilirubin into brain, at least when the increase in brain blood flow is caused by respiratory acidosis.

Bilirubin is cleared from brain primarily by transfer back into the circulation. However, bilirubin is also oxidized by an enzyme on the inner mitochondrial membrane of brain cells. It is also possible that some bilirubin is cleared through the cerebrospial fluid. Bilirubin in the brain is probably bound to structural elements, but there is no conclusive evidence as to how such binding occurs.

bilirubin than older more mature subjects despite equivalent restricted permeability to albumin in young and old age groups.[40,41] The lack of albumin passage across the blood–brain barrier in young animals has been confirmed by others[24] and is consistent with electron microscopic investigations of cerebral capillary tight junctions demonstrating early establishment of paracellular barrier integrity in most mammalian species including humans.[42] Transcellular transport properties of the fetal and neonatal blood–brain barrier, nevertheless, do differ from the adult so as to meet the specialized needs of the developing brain and this aspect of maturation continues postnatally.[43,44]

Entry of Albumin and Albumin-Bound Bilirubin into Brain

The question of whether or not albumin enters the brain in immature organisms[24,40,41,45] is interesting relative to hyperbilirubinemia, because albumin in *in vitro* studies has been shown to block the toxic effects of bilirubin when it is present in molar concentrations that equal or exceed that of bilirubin.[13,14] Whether this is true in brain tissue, or whether other cerebral proteins may play a similar protective role, is not clear. A series of studies evidence disrupted brain metabolism and activity when the blood–brain barrier is opened and both albumin-bound and unbound bilirubin enter the central nervous system.[46–48] Wennberg and Hance[47] report that such changes were best predicted by brain bilirubin content, i.e., the degree of blood–brain barrier opening, and that an enhanced degree of bilirubin binding to albumin appeared to be protective. The results of these studies, although far from conclusive, suggest that bilirubin bound to albumin is not neurotoxic.

Increasing the Blood–Brain Barrier Permeability to Bilirubin

Increased permeability of the blood–brain barrier to bilirubin has been produced experimentally in animals through irradiation,[49] asphyxia,[50,51] hyperosmolality,[24,52,53] and hypercarbia.[23,24,54] These studies all demonstrated that brain bilirubin concentrations are increased following opening of the blood–brain barrier. Interestingly, during hypercarbia, most but not all of the bilirubin enters the brain as the unbound molecule.[24] In contrast, during hyperosmolality entry of albumin is significant, and a large proportion of the bilirubin that enters brain in this instance is probably albumin-bound. Thus, the mechanisms of bilirubin entry may be different in hypercarbia and in hyperosmolality. The increased entry of unbound bilirubin into brain in hypercarbia may best be understood in terms of increased blood flow, although the entry of albumin-bound bilirubin in this condition indicates enhanced blood–brain barrier permeability as well.

   Several *in vitro* studies have shown that bilirubin affects membrane function, causing increased permeability.[5,14,55,56] Bilirubin has also been shown to be toxic to glial cells,[57,58] which might conceivably affect blood–brain barrier function. A logical question is thus whether hyperbilirubinemia per se affects the function of the blood–brain barrier. This hypothesis has been addressed experimentally, and the results indicate that bilirubin does indeed increase blood–brain barrier permeability to some extent. Gulati and co-workers found that the blood–brain barrier of jaundiced neonates was more permeable to a dye than that of non-jaundiced but otherwise comparable infants.[59] Moreover, Roger and colleagues demonstrated that pre-exposure to bilirubin increased the blood–brain barrier permeability to bilirubin in immature rats, and this appeared to be more pronounced in areas known to be more heavily stained in kernicterus.[41] This phenomenon might be compatible with clinical data suggesting that not only the level of serum bilirubin, but also the duration of hyperbilirubinemia exposure may contribute to the risk of neurologic sequelae.[60]

REGIONAL AND SUB-CELLULAR LOCALIZATION OF BILIRUBIN IN BRAIN

Orth appears to have been the first to point out the characteristic staining pattern of kernicterus, with particularly intensive staining of the nuclear region, the wall of the third and fourth ventricles, the hippocampus, and the cerebellum.[2] Schmorl distinguished between a diffuse yellow discoloration of the entire brain seen in most infants who died with jaundice, and a form in which circumscribed areas of intense discoloration were superimposed on a pale yellow background.[3] Claireaux and colleagues were the first to extract bilirubin from the brains of infants who had died with severe jaundice and found increased concentrations (35 nmol/g) in the nuclear regions as compared with the remainder of the brain (8 nmol/g).[61] The mechanism(s) underlying this pattern of bilirubin distribution in the brain is (are) not clear.

The initial descriptions of kernicterus leave no doubt that these infants suffered from Rhesus isoimmunization leading some to speculate that hemolysis plays a role in the regional deposition of bilirubin within the central nervous system. However, the idea that hemolysis, beyond its role in increasing bilirubin production, is a key risk factor for kernicterus, is open to question. A number of early studies documented kernicterus in infants who had severe jaundice in the absence of hemolysis[62–64] as well as in patients with Crigler–Najjar syndrome,[65–66] a non-hemolytic disease. Thus hemolysis is probably not an important contributor to the staining pattern of kernicterus.

Theoretically regional differences in brain bilirubin deposition might relate to local differences in brain bilirubin uptake, tissue binding, metabolism, or excretion. Several animal studies have demonstrated bilirubin concentration patterns in brain which were compatible with kernicterus.[47,49,52,54,67] However, as these studies involved intravenous infusions of bilirubin lasting up to several hours, it may not be possible to distinguish between the relative contribution of bilirubin uptake, local metabolism, and excretion. More recent studies using acute (5 min) infusions of bilirubin into young adult rats[34–36] have not revealed staining patterns compatible with kernicterus. Roger and colleagues[41] suggest that exposure of an immature blood–brain barrier to bilirubin may alter the blood–brain barrier in such a way that the subsequent permeability to bilirubin is enhanced in brain regions which are known to be more heavily stained in kernicterus. It is possible that such regional changes in blood–brain barrier permeability could explain the kernicterus staining phenomenon. However, the mechanism for such an effect of on blood–brain barrier permeability is not known.

The question of the subcellular localization of bilirubin *in vivo* may be important relative to the mechanism of toxicity. Thus early studies which showed that bilirubin inhibited oxidative phosphorylation suggested that mitochondria would be the target for bilirubin toxicity in the cell.[68,69] *In vitro* studies in cell cultures seem to support this theory.[70] Neuropathological studies of victims of kernicterus using electron microscopy also demonstrate changes in the appearance of mitochondria,[71,72] though this does not necessarily indicate that the mitochondria is the primary target of toxicity. Future studies to determine the subcellular localization of bilirubin *in vivo* are warranted.

CLEARANCE OF BILIRUBIN FROM BRAIN

Brain-to-Blood Transfer

The reported half-life of bilirubin in the central nervous system varies from 13 min[36] to 1.7 h.[53] Brain bilirubin may be excreted or diffuse back into the circulation, it may be excreted or diffuse into the cerebrospinal fluid, or it may be removed from brain through local metabolism. Data from Levine *et al*[53] showed that the clearance of bilirubin from brain and from serum closely paralleled each other, suggesting that brain-to-blood transfer of bilirubin is the major clearance route. However, recent data from our own lab showed that bilirubin clearance from brain was more rapid than from serum,[73] pointing to the existence of additional mechanisms for clearing bilirubin from brain.

Clearance of Bilirubin into Cerebrospinal Fluid

Bilirubin is found in the CSF of jaundiced infants[74-76] and such levels are increased when the blood–brain barrier is opened[76,77] or if the CSF contains blood and/or elevated protein concentrations.[74,75] Meisel and co-workers reported CSF bilirubin levels of $\sim$5 µmol/l in infants with mean serum levels of $\sim$220 µmol/l, thus showing a concentration gradient from blood to CSF.[74] However, while these CSF concentrations agree in general terms with brain concentrations found in experimental animals, it is not clear whether the flux is from brain to CSF or in the opposite direction. It is therefore difficult to ascertain whether excretion through the CSF is a significant mechanism for removal of bilirubin from the brain.

Oxidation of Bilirubin in the Brain

Brodersen and Bartels were the first to demonstrate the existence of a bilirubin-oxidizing enzyme on inner mitochondrial membranes from brain, as well as from other organs.[78] In spite of the obvious relevance of this observation to the understanding of bilirubin neurotoxicity, this phenomenon has only recently been examined further. Hansen and colleagues confirmed that brain mitochondrial membranes are able to oxidize bilirubin at a rate of 100–300 pmol/min/mg protein, a level that may constitute a biologically relevant mechanism for bilirubin clearance from the brain.[79] The responsible enzyme has lower specific activity in mitochondria from neuronal cells as compared to a mixed glial/neuronal source,[80] an observation which could possibly account for why bilirubin appears to be more toxic to neurons than glia. Of further interest are the observations that i) the specific activity of this enzyme increases significantly with postnatal age,[80] and ii) different strains of rats evince genetically based differences in the activity of the bilirubin-oxidizing enzyme in brain.[81] Whether these developmental and/or individual variations in bilirubin-oxidizing enzyme activity contribute to differences in vulnerability to bilirubin associated brain injury is a source of conjecture and warrants futher investigation.

The identity of the bilirubin-oxidizing enzyme in brain is not known. Although Brodersen and Bartels[78] as well as others[82] have referred to the enzyme as bilirubin oxidase, it's identity with the commercially available bilirubin oxidase (EC 1.3.3.5) has not been documented and appears doubtful based on preliminary data from our laboratory (Hansen, T.W.R., Allen, J.W., unpublished data). Based on its apparent localization on the inner mitochondrial membrane, at least three enzymes or enzyme groups have received consideration as candidates for this function and are currently being studied: malate dehydrogenase, monoamine oxidase, and the cytochrome oxidases. The localization of the enzyme on the inner mitochondrial membrane is also interesting in light of the hypothesis that bilirubin toxicity is due to inhibition/ uncoupling of oxidative phosphorylation.[68,69] Though it is not clear that this phenomenon is operative in the pathogenesis of bilirubin neurotoxicity, the possible existence of an autoprotective mechanism on the very respiratory chain that bilirubin is supposed to perturb, is intriguing.

CELLULAR AND MOLECULAR MECHANISM OF TOXICITY

The Inhibitory Effects of Bilirubin

The first experimental studies that addressed the question of the cellular mechanism of bilirubin toxicity were performed more than forty years ago and suggested that bilirubin exerted its effect by inhibiting respiration and uncoupling oxidative phosphorylation.[68,69] The implications of these *in vitro* observations for the *in vivo* situation have been debated, and there is still no agreement that respiratory inhibition is the basic mechanism for bilirubin toxicity.[46,86] A multitude of other bilirubin effects have been documented. With very few exceptions these effects have been inhibitory in nature and include: decreased neuronal viability,[83–85] decreased membrane potential and increased membrane permeability,[55,56] decreased protein synthesis,[56,86–88], decreased DNA synthesis/repair and increased DNA damage,[56,84,89,90] decreased synaptic activation and increased post-synaptic excitability,[91] decreased neurotransmitter synthesis/uptake/release,[92] and enzyme inhibition.[87,93–101]

A cartoon of bilirubin effects in cells is shown in Figure 7.2. Though most of the processes shown in this figure are dependent to some degree upon the availability of energy-rich phosphates, many *in vitro* effects of bilirubin, particularly those of enzyme inhibition, have been documented in assay systems devoid of respiratory activity. Further, inhibition by bilirubin of energy-dependent functions may not necessarily be mediated through interference with energy metabolism. For example, neurotransmitter metabolism and release are inhibited by bilirubin.[92] Moreover, we have recently shown that bilirubin inhibits neurotransmitter release in permeabilized synaptosomes.[102] In this model streptolysin permeabilizes the synaptic membrane so that the membrane potential disappears, while the presence of excess ATP makes the process independent of endogenous energy metabolism. Thus the effects of bilirubin in this model cannot depend on increased membrane permeability, nor on inhibition of mitochondrial respiration, but must be mediated through other mechanisms.

Inhibition of Protein Phosphorylation

Reversible phosphorylation/dephosphorylation of proteins has been found to be a key mechanism for the regulation of both neuronal and non-neuronal cellular functions.[103] Hypothetically, bilirubin might interfere with many different cellular regulatory reactions of the protein phosphorylation type as shown in Figure 7.3. We have

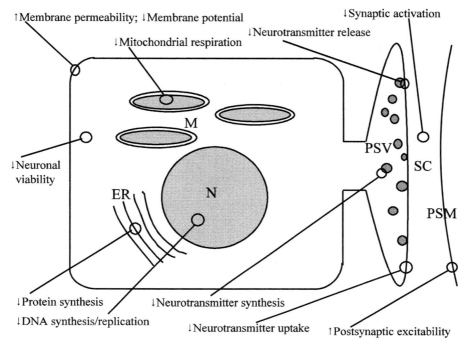

↑Membrane permeability; ↓Membrane potential

↓Mitochondrial respiration

↓Synaptic activation

↓Neurotransmitter release

M

↓Neuronal viability

ER

N

PSV

SC

PSM

↓Protein synthesis

↓DNA synthesis/replication

↓Neurotransmitter synthesis

↓Neurotransmitter uptake

↑Postsynaptic excitability

Figure 7.2. Effects of bilirubin on neurons and neuronal metabolic processes. Bilirubin has been shown to affect a large number of cellular functions and processes, both *in vivo* and *in vitro*. These include decreased neuronal viability; increased membrane permeability and decreased membrane potential; uncoupling of oxidative phosphorylation; inhibition of neurotransmitter release, synthesis, and uptake; inhibition of synaptic activation; increased postsynaptic excitability; decreased protein synthesis; and decreased synthesis and replication of DNA. Other bilirubin-affected functions not indicated in the cartoon include inhibition of enzyme function and protein phosphorylation. M = mitochondria; N = nucleus; ER = endoplasmic reticulum; PSV = presynaptic vesicles; SC = synaptic cleft; and PSM = postsynaptic membrane.

previously shown that bilirubin inhibits phosphorylation of the synaptic vesicle-associated protein synapsin I *in situ* in isolated, intact nerve terminals (synaptosomes) in a time- and dose-dependent manner.[100] Because phosphorylation of synapsin I is believed to be involved in the regulation of neurotransmitter release,[104] these findings suggested that some of the effects of bilirubin on the brain, specifically inhibition of synaptic activation,[91] could partly be caused by inhibition of protein phosphorylation. However, the mechanism whereby bilirubin interferes with protein phosphorylation[68,69,96,100,105] remains unclear.

Recent studies have demonstrated an inhibitory effect of bilirubin on the phosphorylation of a variety of substrate proteins catalyzed by purified protein kinases *in vitro* in assays devoid of ATP-generating organelles.[159] Moreover, kinetic analysis of the effects of bilirubin on the activity of the isolated catalytic sub-unit of cAMP-dependent protein kinase (PKA), using [^{32}P]ATP and a synthetic peptide (consisting of residues[57–72] of the protein termed "phospholemman")[106] as substrates, indicated

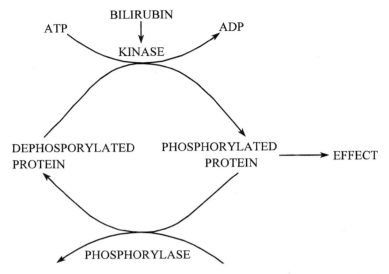

Figure 7.3. Proposed mechanism for inhibition of protein/peptide phosphorylation. Bilirubin inhibits most of the phosphorylation reactions that have been tested. This effect does not appear to depend on substrate characteristics, and is therefore thought to be due to an interaction between bilirubin and the kinase. In most cellular processes which are regulated by protein phosphorylation, the phosphorylated substrate "turns on" the process. As an example, neurotransmitter release is increased in the presence of phosphorylated synapsin I and decreased in the presence of dephosphorylated synapsin I. In the presence of bilirubin, production of the phosphorylated protein would be inhibited and the end effect would be decreased. Many of the inhibitory effects of bilirubin in biological systems might be caused by this type of mechanism.

that bilirubin has a non-competitive mechanism of action. We are at present studying the question of whether the inhibitory effects of bilirubin on protein/peptide phosphorylation depend on characteristics of the enzyme or the substrate.[107]

The Role of Lysine Binding

Bilirubin is known to bind to lysine both on albumin and ligandin, two key proteins in bilirubin transport and metabolism.[14,16,108,109] Lysine appears to be present in many molecules/structures that participate in reactions or biological phenomena which bilirubin has been shown to inhibit/influence. Thus, lysine is an invariant presence on sub-domain II of the protein kinase family.[110] Lysine is also found on histone, myosin light chain, glycogen synthase, membranes, as well as many enzymes (Na^+/K^+-ATPase, Ca^{++}/Mg^{++}-ATPase, UDP-glucose phosphorylase, mRNA capping enzyme, myosin light chain kinase, glycogen synthase, and several others).[111–119] Work in our group has recently shown that polylysine blocks the inhibitory effect of bilirubin on phospholemman phosphorylation by PKA.[120] A synthetic, lysine-containing decapeptide which mimics part of sub-domain II on the protein kinase family also partially blocked the inhibitory effect of bilirubin, while decapeptides in which lysine had been substituted for alanine and arginine respectively did not have this effect.[120] GSH transferase is inhibited by bilirubin.[16] Chemical modification of Lys-44 on GSH transferase by 2,4,6-trinitrobenzene sulphonate results in a time-dependent inactivation of the enzyme, a process that is enhanced by bilirubin.[16] This would appear to argue further for the important role of lysine binding in the mediation of bilirubin toxicity.

Of special interest is Na^+/K^+-ATPase, an enzyme which is inhibited by bilirubin,[94,121] and in which modification of lysine in α-sub-units strongly reduces the enzyme's activity.[115,116] This lysine is involved in ATP binding to the enzyme,[115] a notable observation in light of our documentation of inhibition of many phosphorylation reactions.[101] Lysine is also found at or near the ATP-binding site of Ca^{++}/Mg^{++}-ATPase,[117] and at active sites of UDP-glucose phosphorylase,[118] aspartate aminotransferase,[122] mRNA capping enzyme,[123] RNA and DNA ligases,[124] phosphoenolpyruvate carboxykinase,[125] lactate monooxygenase,[126] triosephosphate isomerase,[128] myosin light chain kinase,[127] aldose reductase,[129] UDP-galactose 4-epimerase,[130] mRNA guanyltransferase,[119] and glycogen synthase.[131] Though the interaction with bilirubin has not been studied for all of these enzymes, many of the reactions involved are inhibited by bilirubin. Taken together these observations suggest a potential role of lysine binding in the mediation of bilirubin toxicity, a mechanism that warrants further investigation.

CONCLUSION

Bilirubin is toxic to brain as well as to many other tissues. It probably enters the brain mainly as an unbound ("free") molecule as long as the blood–brain barrier is intact, but may enter bound to albumin when the blood–brain barrier is opened. The current evidence suggests that bilirubin is toxic when unbound, but the data are more controversial with regard to the effects of albumin-bound bilirubin in brain. Bilirubin entry into brain is facilitated by the presence of endogenous or exogenous compounds that compete for the binding site to albumin, by increased brain blood flow, and by opening of the blood–brain barrier. Bilirubin itself may increase the permeability of the blood–brain barrier and thus facilitate its own entry into the central nervous system. The mechanism(s) that underlies why bilirubin preferentially localizes to the basal ganglia and cerebellum to produce kernicterus remains unknown. Bilirubin is cleared from brain partly through bilirubin transfer to blood through the blood–brain barrier and possibly through the CSF. Evidence is also accumulating that bilirubin may be metabolized locally in the brain by a mitochondrial enzyme. Neuronal dysfunction in the context of hyperbilirubinemia may be mediated by inhibiting protein phosphorylation, possibly through bilirubin binding to lysine residues. Our understanding of the basic mechanism for bilirubin neurotoxicity, however, is far from complete and remains an area of intense investigation.

References

1. Hervieux, J., De l'ictère des nouveau-nés, *These Med.* Paris, 1847.
2. Orth, I., Ueber das Vorkommen von Bilirubinkrystallen bei neugeborenen Kindern, *Virch. Arch. Pathol. Anat.* 1875; **63**: 447–462.

3. Schmorl, G., Zur Kenntnis des Ikterus Neonatorum, *Verh. Dtsch. Pathol. Ges.* 1904; **6**: 109–115.
4. Levi. G., Sohmer, H. and Kapitulnik, J., Auditory nerve and brain stem responses in homozygous jaundiced Gunn rats, *Arch. Otorhinolaryngol.* 1981; **232**: 139–143.
5. Nwaesei, C.G., Van Aerde, J., Boyden, M. and Perlman, M., Changes in auditory braistem responses in hyperbilirubinemic infants before and after exchange transfusion, *Pediatrics* 1984; **74**: 800–803.
6. Chen, Y.J. and Kang, W.M., Effects of bilirubin on visual evoked potentials in term infants, *Eur. J. Pediatr.* 1995; **154**: 662–666.
7. Hansen, T.W.R. and Bratlid, D., Bilirubin and brain toxicity, *Acta. Paediatr. Scand.* 1986, **75**: 513–522.
8. Brodersen, R., Bilirubin. Solubility and interaction with albumin and phospholipids, *J. Biol. Chem.* 1979; **254**: 2364–2369.
9. Brodersen, R., Physical chemistry of bilirubin: binding to macromolecules and membranes. In: Heirwegh, K.P.M. and Brown, S.B., eds. *Bilirubin Chemistry.* Boca Raton: CRC press, Inc, 1982, pp. 75–123.
10. Brodersen. R., Flodgaards. H. and Hansen, J.K., Intramolecular hydrogen bonding in bilirubin, *Acta. Chem. Scand.* 1967; **21**: 2284–2285.
11. Silberberg, D.H., Johnson, L., Schutta, H. and Ritter, L., Effects of photodegradation products of bilirubin on myelinating cerebellum cultures, *J. Pediatr.* 1970; **77**: 613–618.
12. Thaler, M.M., Toxic effects of bilirubin and its photo-decomposition products, *Birth Defects: Original Article Series* 1970; **6**: 128–130.
13. Bratlid, D., Albumin binding and toxicity of bilirubin (Thesis). Oslo: Universitetsforlaget; 1973.
14. Cowger, M.L., Mechanism of bilirubin toxicity on tissue culture cells: Factors that affect toxicity, reversibility by albumin, and comparison with other respiratory poisons and surfactants, *Biochem. Med.* 1971; **5**: 1–16.
15. Jacobsen, C., Lysine residue 240 of human serum albumin is involved in high-affinity binding of bilirubin, *Biochem. J.* 1978; **171**: 453–459.
16. Xia, C., Meyer, D.J., Chen, H., Reinemer, P., Huber, R. and Ketterer, B., Chemical modification of GSH transferase P1-1 confirms the presence of Arg-13, Lys-44 and one carboxylate group in the GSH binding domain of the active site, *Biochem. J.* 1993; **293**: 357–362.
17. Bennhold, H., Über die Funktion der Serumeiweisskörper im tierischen Organismus, *Verh. Dtsch. Ges. Inn. Med.* 1929; **42**: 211–213.
18. Brodersen, R., Cashore, W.J., Wennberg, R.P., Ahlfors, C.E., Rasmussen, L.F. and Shusterman, D., Kinetics in bilirubin oxidation with peroxidase as applied to studies of bilirubin–albumin binding, *Scand. J. Clin. Lab. Invest.* 1979; **39**: 143–150.
19. Brodersen, R., Binding of bilirubin to albumin, *Crit. Rev. Clin. Lab. Sci.* 1980; **11**: 305–399.
20. Jacobsen, J. and Wennberg, R.P., Determination of unbound bilirubin in the serum of newborns, *Clin. Chem.* 1974; **20**: 783–789.
21. Shimabuku, R. and Nakamura, H., Total and unbound bilirubin determination using an automated peroxidase micromethod, *Kobe. J. Med. Sci.* 1982; **28**: 91–104.
22. Nakamura, H., Takada, S., Shimabuku, R., Matsuo, M., Matsuo, T. and Negishi, H., Auditory nerve and brainstem responses in newborn infants with hyperemia, *Pediatrics* 1985; **75**: 703–708.
23. Bratlid, D., Cashore, W.J. and Oh, W., Effect of acidosis on bilirubin deposition in rat brain, *Pediatrics* 1994; **73**: 431–434.
24. Hansen, T.W.R., Øyasaeter, S., Stiris, T. and Bratlid, D., Effects of sulfisoxazole, hypercarbia, and hyperosmolality on entry of bilirubin and albumin into young rat brain regions, *Biol. Neonate* 1989; **56**: 22–30.
25. Wennberg, R.P., Ahlfors, C.E. and Rasmussen, L.F., The pathochemistry of kernicterus, *Early. Hum. Dev.* 1979; **3/4**: 353–372.
26. Cashore, W.J., Horwich, A., Laterra, J. and Oh, W., Effect of postnatal age and clinical status of newborn infants on bilirubin-binding capacity, *Biol. Neonate* 1977; **32**: 304–309.
27. Cashore, W.J., Horwich, A., Karotkin, E.H. and Oh, W., Influence of gestational age and clinical status on bilirubin-binding capacity in newborn infants, *Am. J. Dis. Child.* 1977; **131**: 898–901.
28. Bratlid, D., Pharmacologic aspects of neonatal hyperbilirubinemia. *Birth Defects: Original article series* 1976; **12**: 184–189.
29. Odell, G.B., Studies in kernicterus. I. The protein binding of bilirubin, *J. Clin. Invest.* 1959; **38**: 823–833.
30. Blanc, W.A. and Johnson, L., Studies on kernicterus. Relationship with sulfonamide intoxication, report on kernicterus in rats with glucuronyl transferase deficiency, and review of pathogenesis, *J. Neuropathol. Exp. Neurol.* 1959; **18**: 165–189.
31. Cashore, W.J., Bilirubin binding tests. In: Levine, R.L. and Maisels, M.J., eds. Hyperbilirubinemia in the newborn. Report of the 85th Ross Conference on Pediatric Research, 1983, pp. 101–110.

32. Lee, K-S. and Gartner, L.M., Bilirubin binding by plasma proteins: A critical evaluation of methods and clinical implications, *Reviews in Perinatal. Medicine.* 1978; **2**: 319–343.
33. Poland, R.L., Cepeda, E.E. and Garg, G., Comparison of four bilirubin binding tests, *Pediatr. Res.* 1984; **18**: 340A.
34. Hansen, T.W.R. and Cashore, W.J., Rates of bilirubin clearance from rat brain regions, *Biol. Neonate* 1995; **68**: 135–140.
35. Hansen, T.W.R., Acute entry of bilirubin into rat brain regions, *Biol. Neonate.* 1995; **67**: 203–207.
36. Hansen, T.W.R., Bilirubin entry into and clearance from rat brain during hypercarbia and hyperosmolality, *Pediatr. Res.* 1996; **39**: 72–76.
37. Ives, N.K. and Gardiner, R.M., Blood brain barrier permeability to bilirubin in the rat studied using intracarotid bolus injection and *in situ* brain perfusion techniques, *Pediatr. Res.* 1990; **27**: 436–441.
38. Stern. L. and Peyrot, R., Le fonctionnement de la barrière hemato-encepalique aux divers stages du developpement chéz diverses especes animales, *CR Soc. Biol.* 1927; **96**: 1124–1126.
39. Stern, L. and Peyrot, R., La resistance de la barrière hemato-encephalique au passage des colloids du sang dans liquide cephaloachidien aux divers stages de developpement chez les diverses especes animales, *CR Soc. Biol.* 1927; **96**: 1149–1152.
40. Lee, C., Oh, W., Stonestreet, B.S. and Cashore, W.J., Permeability of the blood brain barrier for ^{125}I-albumin-bound bilirubin in newborn piglets, *Pediatr. Res.* 1989; **25**: 452–456.
41. Roger, C., Koziel, V., Vert, P. and Nehlig, A., Autoradiographic mapping of local cerebral permeability to bilirubin in immature rats: effect of hyperbilirubinemia, *Pediatr. Res.* 1996; **39**: 64–71.
42. Johanson, C.E., Ontogeny and phylogeny of the blood brain barrier. In: Neuwelt, E.A. ed. Implications of the blood brain barrier and its manipulation. Basic Science Aspects. New York: Plenum; 1983, p. 158.
43. Sternberger, N.H. and Sternberger, L.A., Blood brain barrier protein recognized by monoclonal antibody, *Proc. Natl. Acad. Sci. USA* 1987; **84**: 8169–8173.
44. Braun, L.D., Cornford, E.M. and Oldendorf, W.H., Newborn rabbit blood brain barrier is selectively impermeable and differs substantially from the adult, *J. Neurochem.* 1980; **34**: 147–152.
45. Ohsugi, M., Sato, H. and Yamamura, H., Transfer of bilirubin covalently bound to ^{125}I-albumin from blood to brain in the Gunn rat newborn, *Biol. Neonate* 1992; **62**: 47–54.
46. Ives, N.K., Bolas, B.M. and Gardiner, R.M., The effects of bilirubin on brain energy metabolism during hyperosmolar opening of the blood brain barrier: an *in vivo* study using ^{31}P nuclear magnetic resonance spectroscopy, *Pediatr. Res.* 1989; **26**: 356–361.
47. Wennberg, R.P. and Hance, A.J., Experimental bilirubin encephalopathy: importance of total bilirubin, protein binding, and blood brain barrier, *Pediatr. Res.* 1986; **20**: 789–792.
48. Hansen, T.W.R., Sagvolden, T. and Bratlid, D., Open-field behavior of rats previously subjected to short-term hyperbilirubinemia with or without blood brain barrier manipulations, *Brain. Res.* 1987; **424**: 26–36.
49. Day, R., Kernicterus problem: experimental *in vivo* and *in vitro* staining of brain tissue with bilirubin [Abstract], *Am. J. Dis. Child.* 1947; **73**: 241–242.
50. Lucey, J.F., Hibbard, E., Behrman, R.E., Esqivuel de Gallardo, F.O. and Windle, W.F., Kernicterus in asphyxiated newborn monkeys, *Exp. Neurol.* 1964; **9**: 43–58.
51. Mayor, F.J., Pagés, M., Diez-Guerra. J., Valdivieso, F. and Mayor, F., Effect of postnatal anoxia on bilirubin levels in rat brain, *Pediatr. Res.* 1985; **19**: 231–236.
52. Levine, R.L., Fredericks, W.R. and Rapoport, S.I., Entry of bilirubin into the brain due to opening of the blood brain barrier, *Pediatrics* 1982; **69**: 255–259.
53. Levine, R.L., Fredricks, W.R. and Rapoport, S.I., Clearance of bilirubin from rat brain after reversible osmotic opening of the blood brain barrier, *Pediatr. Res.* 1985; **19**: 1040–1043.
54. Burgess, G.H., Oh, W., Bratlid. D., Brubakk, A.-M., Cashore, W.J. and Stonestreet, B.S., The effects of brain blood flow on brain bilirubin deposition in newborn piglets, *Pediatr. Res.* 1985; **19**: 691–696.
55. Mayor, F.J., Diez-Guerra, J., Valdivieso, F. and Mayor, F., Effect of bilirubin on the membrane potential of rat brain synaptosomes, *J. Neurochern.* 1986; **47**: 363–369.
56. Amit, Y., Chan, G., Fedunec, S., Pomansky, M.J. and Schiff, D., Bilirubin toxicity in a neuroblastoma cell line N-115: 1. Effects on Na$^+$/K$^+$ ATPase, [^{3}H]-thymidine uptake, l[^{35}S]-methionine incorporation, and mitochondrial function, *Pediatr. Res.* 1989; **25**: 364–368.
57. Sugita, K., Sato, T. and Nakajima, H., Effects of pH and hypoglycemia on bilirubin cytotoxicity *in vitro*, *Biol. Neonate.* 1987; **52**: 22–25.
58. Amit, Y. and Brenner, T., Age-dependent sensitivity of cultured rat glial cells to bilirubin toxicity, *Exp. Neurol.* 1993; **121**: 248–255.

59. Gulati, A., Mahesh, A.K. and Misra, P.K., Blood brain barrier permeability studies in control and icteric neonates, *Pediatr. Res.* 1990; **27**: 206A.
60. Nilsen, S.T., Finne, P.H., Bergsjø, P. and Stamnes, T.O., Males with neonatal hyperbilirubinemia examined at 18 years of age, *Acta. Paediatr. Scand.* 1984; **73**: 176–180.
61. Claireaux, A.E., Cole, P.G. and Lathe, G.H., Icterus of the brain in the newborn, *Lancet* 1953; **2**: 1226–1230.
62. Aidin, R., Corner, B. and Tovey, G., Kernicterus and prematurity, *Lancet* 1950; **1**: 1153–1154.
63. Govan, A.D.T. and Scott, J.M., Kernicterus and prematurity, *Lancet* 1953; **1**: 611–614.
64. Boon, W.H., Kernicterus not associated with haemolytic disease, *Arch. Dis. Child.* 1957; **32**: 85–90.
65. Crigler, J.F. Jr. and Najjar, V.A., Congenital familial nonhemolytic jaundice with kernicterus, *Pediatrics* 1952; **10**: 169–180.
66. Rosenthal, I.M., Zimmerman, H.J. and Hardy, N., Congenital nonhemolytic jaundice with disease of the central nervous system, *Pediatrics* 1956; **18**: 378–386.
67. Rose, A.L. and Wisniewski, H., Acute bilirubin encephalopathy induced with sulfa-dimethoxine in Gunn rats, *J. Neuropathol. Exp. Neurol.* 1979; **38**: 152–164.
68. Day, R.L., Inhibition of brain respiration *in vitro* by bilirubin: Reversal of inhibition by various means, *Am. J. Dis. Child.* 1954; **88**: 504–506.
69. Zetterström, R. and Ernster, L., Bilirubin, an uncoupler of oxidative phosphorylation in isolated mitochondria, *Nature* 1956; **178**: 1335–1337.
70. Amit, Y., Poznansky, M.J. and Schiff, D., Bilirubin toxicity in a neuroblastoma cell line N-115: II. Delayed effects and recovery, *Pediatr. Res.* 1989; **25**: 369–372.
71. Schutta, H.S. and Johnson, L., Electron microscopic observations on acute bilirubin encephalopathy in Gunn rats induced by sulfadimethoxine, *Lab. Invest.* 1971; **24**: 82–89.
72. Schutta, H.S., Johnson, L. and Neville, B.E., Mitochondrial abnormalities in bilirubin encephalopathy, *J. Neuropathol. Exp. Neurol.* 1970; **29**: 296–304.
73. Hansen, T.W.R. and Allen, J.W., Hemolytic anemia does not increase entry into, nor alter rate of clearance of bilirubin from rat brain, *Biol. Neonate.* 1996; **69**: 268–274.
74. Meisel, P., Jährig, D. and Jährig, K., Bilirubin im Liquor cerebrospinalis Neugeborener. Vergleichende Untersuchungen des Liquor cerebrospinalis bei Bilirubin mie und ZNS-Affektionen, *Kinderartzi. Prax.* 1981; **49**: 633–642.
75. Meisel, P., Jährig, D. and Jährig, K., Bilirubin im Liquor cerebrospinalis Neugeborener. II.Einflussfaktoren auf den Bilirubinbingehalt des Liquor cerebrospinalis, *Kinderarztl. Prax.* 1982; **50**: 370–378.
76. Weyrauch, P.-C., Jährig, K. and Wiersbitsky, S., Ergebnisse der Liquoruntersuchungen bei Neugeborenen, *Kinderarzti. Prax.* 1973; **41**: 447–454.
77. Lee, T.-C. and Y-Tsia, D.Y., Experimental studies on blood-spinal fluid barrier for bilirubin, *J. Lab. Clin. Med.* 1959; **54**: 512–524.
78. Brodersen, R. and Bartels, P., Enzymatic oxidation of bilirubin, *Eur. J. Biochem.* 1969; **10**: 468–473.
79. Hansen, T.W.R. and Allen, J.W., Bilirubin oxidizing activity in rat brain, *Biol. Neonate* 1996; **70**: 289–295.
80. Hansen, T.W.R. and Allen, J.W., Oxidation of bilirubin by brain mitochondrial membranes – dependence on cell type and postnatal age, *Biochem. Molec. Med.* 1997; **60**: 155–160.
81. Hansen, T.W.R., Tommarello, S. and Allen, J.W., Oxidation of bilirubin by brain mitochondrial membranes – genetic variability, *Biochem. Molec. Med.* 1997; **62**: 128–131.
82. Yokosuka, O. and Billing, B., Enzymatic oxidation of bilirubin by intestinal mucosa, *Biochim. Biophys. Acta.* 1987; **923**: 268–274.
83. O'Callaghan, J.P. and Miller, D.B., Cerebellar hypoplasia in the Gunn rat is associated with changes in neurotypic and gliotypic proteins, *J. Pharmacol. Exp. Ther.* 1985; **234**: 522–533.
84. Schiff, D., Chan, G. and Poznansky, M.J., Bilirubin toxicity in neural cell lines N115 and NBR10A, *Pediatr. Res.* 1985; **19**: 908–911.
85. Notter, M.F.D. and Kendig, J.W., Differential sensitivity of neural cells to bilirubin toxicity, *Exp. Neurol.* 1986; **94**: 670–682.
86. Cowger, M.L., Igo, R.P. and Labbe, R.F., The mechanism of bilirubin toxicity studied with purified respiratory enzyme and tissue culture systems, *Biochemistry* 1965; **4**: 2763–2770.
87. Greenfield, S. and Nandi Majumdar, A.P., Bilirubin encephalopathy: Effect on protein synthesis in the brain of the Gunn rat, *J. Neurol. Sci.* 1974; **22**: 83–89.
88. Katoh-Semba, R. and Kashiwamata, S., Rates of protein synthesis and degradation in Gunn rat cerebellum with bilirubin-induced cerebellar hypoplasia, *Neurochem. Pathol.* 1984; **2**: 31–37.

89. Rosenstein, B.S. and Ducore, J.M., Enhancement by bilirubin of DNA damage induced in human cells exposed to phototherapy light, *Pediatr. Res.* 1984; **18**: 3–6.
90. Rosenstein, B.S., Ducore, J.M. and Cummings, S.W., The mechanism of bilirubin-photosensitized DNA strand breakage in human cells exposed to phototherapy light, *Mutat. Res.* 1983; **112**: 397–406.
91. Hansen, T.W.R., Paulsen, O., Gjerstad, L. and Bratlid, D., Short-term exposure to bilirubin reduces synaptic activation in rat transverse hippocampal slices, *Pediatr. Res.* 1988; **23**: 453–456.
92. Ochoa, E.L.M., Wennberg, R.P., An, Y., Tandon, F.T., Takashima, T., Nguyen, T. and Chui, T., Interactions of bilirubin with isolated presynaptic nerve terminals: functional effects on the uptake and release of neurotransmitters, *Cell. Mol. Neurobiol.* 1993; **13**: 69–86.
93. Karp, W.B., Biochemical alterations in neonatal hyperbilirubinemia and bilirubin encephalopathy: A review, *Pediatrics* 1979; **64**: 361–368.
94. Kashiwamata, S., Asai, M. and Semba, R.K., Effect of bilirubin on the Arrhenius plots for Na, K-ATPase activities of young and adult rat cerebra, *J. Neurochem.* 1981; **36**: 826–829.
95. Ogasawara, N., Watanabe, T. and Goto, H., Bilirubin: A potent inhibitor of NAD+-linked isocitrate dehydrogenase, *Biochim. Biophys. Acta.* 1973; **327**: 233–237.
96. Constantopoulos, A. and Matsaniotis, N., Bilirubin inhibition of protein kinase: its prevention by cyclic AMP, *Cytobios.* 1976; **17**: 17–20.
97. Flitman, R. and Worth, M.E., Inhibition of hepatic alcohol dehydrogenase by bilirubin, *J. Biol. Chem.* 966; **241**: 669–672.
98. Kashiwamata, S., Niwa, F., Katoh, R. and Higashida, H., Malate dehydrogenase of bovine cerebrum: inhibition by bilirubin, *J. Neurochem.* 1975; **24**: 189–191.
99. McLoughlin, D.J. and Howell, M.L., Bilirubin inhibition of enzymes involved in the mitochondrial malate-aspartate shuttle, *Biochim. Biophys. Acta.* 1987; **893**: 7–12.
100. Hansen, T.W.R., Bratlid, D. and Walaas, S.I., Bilirubin decreases phosphorylation of synapsin I, a synaptic vesicle-associated neuronal phosphoprotein, in intact synaptosomes from rat cerebral cortex, *Pediatr. Res.* 1988; **23**: 219–223.
101. Hansen, T.W.R., Mathiesen, S.B.W. and Walaas, S.I., Bilirubin has widespread inhibitory effects on protein phosphorylation, *Pediatr. Res.* 1996; **39**: 1072–1077.
102. Hansen, T.W.R., Mathiesen, S.B.W., Setland, I. and Walaas, S.I., Bilirubin inhibits Ca^{++}-dependent release of norepinephrine from permeabilized nerve terminals, *Neuro. Chem. Res.* 1999; **24**: 733–738.
103. Walaas, S.I. and Greengard, P., Protein phosphorylation and neuronal function, *Pharmacol. Rev.* 1991; **43**: 299–349.
104. Greengard, P., Valtorta, F., Czernik, A.J. and Benfenati, F., Synaptic vesicle phosphoproteins and regulation of synaptic function, *Science* 1993; **259**: 780–785.
105. Morphis, L., Constantopoulos, A. and Matsaniotis, N., Bilirubin induced modulation of cerebral protein phosphorylation in neonate rabbits *in vivo*, *Science* 1982; **218**: 156–158.
106. Palmer, C.J., Scott, B.T. and Jones, L.R., Purification and complete sequence determination of the major plasma membrane substrate for cAMP-dependent protein kinase and protein kinase C in myocardium, *J. Biol. Chem.* 1991; **266**: 11126–11130.
107. Hansen, T.W.R., Mathiesen, S.B.W., Østvold, A.C. and Walaas, S.I., Bilirubin inhibits casein kinase 2 by a non-competitive mechanism, *Pediatr. Res.* 1997; **41**: 152A.
108. Jacobsen, C., Chemical modification of the high-affinity bilirubin-binding site of human serum albumin, *Eur. J. Biochem.* 1972; **27**: 513–519.
109. Lo Bello, M., Pastore, A., Petruzelli, R., Parker, M.W., Wilce, M.C.J., Federici, G. and Ricci, G., Conformational states of human placental glutathione transferase as probed by limited proteolysis, *Biochem. Biophys. Res. Comm.* 1993; **194**: 804–810.
110. Hanks, S.K., Quinn, A.M. and Hunter, T., The protein kinase family: conserved features and deduced phylogeny of the catalytic domains, *Science* 1988; **241**: 42–52.
111. Pearson, R.B. and Kemp, B.E., Chemical modification of lysine and arginine residues in the myosin regulatory light chain inhibits phosphorylation, *Biochim. Biophys. Acta.* 1986; **870**: 312–319.
112. Lambert, S.F. and Thomas, J.O., Lysine-containing DNA-binding regions on the surface of the histone octamer in the nucleosome core particle, *Eur. J. Biochem.* 1986; **160**: 191–201.
113. Mahrenholz, A.M., Wang, Y.H. and Roach, P.J., Catalytic site of rabbit glycogen synthase isozymes. Identification of an active site lysine close to the amino terminus of the subunit, *J. Biol. Chem.* 1988; **263**: 10561–10567.
114. Miles, L.A., Dahlberg, C.M., Plescia, J., Felez, J., Kato, K. and Plow, E.F., Role of Cell-surface lysines in plasminogen binding to cells: identification of alpha-enolase as a candidate plasminogen receptor, *Biochemistry* 1991; **30**: 1682–1691.

115. Kaya, S., Tsuda, T., Haiwara, K., Fukui, T. and Taniguchi, K., Pyridoxal 5'-phosphate probes at Lys-480 can sense the binding of ATP and the formation of phosphoenzymes in Na$^+$K$^+$-ATPase, *J. Biol. Chem.* 1994; **269**: 7419–7422.

116. Pedemonte, C.H., Kirley, T.L., Treuheit, M.J. and Kaplan, J.H., Inactivation of the Na,K-ATPase by modification of Lys-501 with 4-acetamido-4''-isothiocyanatostilbene-2,2'disulfonic acid(SITS), *FEBS Lett.* 1992; **314**: 97–100.

117. Stefanova, I.I.I., Mata, A.M., East, J.M., Gore, M.G. and Lee, A.G., Reactivity of lysyl residues on the (Ca(2+)-Mg(2+))-ATPase to 7-amino-4-methylcoumarin-3-acetic acid syccinimidyl ester, *Biochemistry* 1993; **32**: 356–362.

118. Fukui, T., Kazuta, Y., Katsube, T., Tagaya, M. and Tanizawa, K., Exploring the active site in UDP glucose pyrophosphorylase by affinity labeling and site-directed mutagenesis, *Biotechnol. Appl. Biochem.* 1993; **18**: 209–216.

119. Niles, E.G. and Christen, L., Identification of the vaccinia virus mRNA guanyltransferase active site lysine, *J. Biol. Chem.* 1993; **268**: 24986–24989.

120. Hansen, T.W.R., Mathiesen, S.B.W. and Walaas, S.I., Modulation of the effect of bilirubin on protein phosphorylation by lysine-containing peptides, *Pediatr. Res.* 1997; **42**: 615–617.

121. Kashiwamata, S., Goto, S., Semba, R.K. and Suzuki, F.N., Inhibition by bilirubin of (Na$^+$/K$^+$)-activated adenosine triphosphatase and K$^+$-activated p-nitrophenyl-phosphatase activities of NaI-treated microsomes from young rat cerebrum, *J. Biol. Chem.* 1979; **254**: 4577–4588.

122. Kim, D.W., Yoshimura, T., Esaki, N., Satoh, E. and Soda, K., Studies of the active-site lysyl residue of thermostable aspartate aminotransferase: combination of site-directed mutagenesis and chemical modification, *J. Biochem.* [Tokyo] 1994; **115**: 93–97.

123. Schwer, B. and Shuman, S., Mutational analysis of yeast mRNA capping enzyme, *Proc. Natl. Acad. Sci. USA* 1994; **91**: 4328–4332.

124. Cong, P. and Shuman, S., Covalent catalysis in nucleotidyl transfer. A KTDG motif essential for enzyme-GMP complex formation by mRNA capping enzyme is conserved at the active sites of RNA and DNA ligases, *J. Biol. Chem.* 1993; **268**: 7256–7260.

125. Bazaes, S., Silva, R., Goldie, H., Cardemil, E. and Jabalquinto, A.M., Reactivity of cysteinyl, arginyl, and lysyl residues of Escherichia coli phosphoenolpyruvate carboxykinase against group-specific chemical agents, *J. Protein. Chem.* 1993; **12**: 571–577.

126. Muh, U., Massey, V. and Williams, C.H. Jr., Lactate monooxygenase. 1. Expression of the mycobacterial gene in Escherichia coli and site-directed mutagenesis of lysine 266, *J. Biol. Chem.* 1994; **269**: 7982–7988.

127. Komatsu, H. and Ikebe, A., Affinity labeling of smooth-muscle myosin light-chain kinase with 5'[p-(fluoro sulphonyl)benzoyl]adenosine, *Biochem. J.* 1993; **296**: 53–58.

128. Lodi, P.J., Chang, L.C., Knowles, J.R. and Koinives, E.A., Triosephosphate isomerase requires a positively active site: the role of lysine-12, *Biochemistry* 1994; **33**: 2809–2814.

129. Tarle, I., Borhani, D.W., Wilson, D.K., Quiocho, F.A. and Petrash, J.M., Probing the active site of human a1dose reductase. Site-directed mutagenesis of Asp-43, Tyr-48, Lys-77, and His-110, *J. Biol. Chem.* 1993; **268**: 25687–25693.

130. Swanson, B.A. and Freu, P.A., Identification of lysine 153 as a functionally important residue in UDP-galactose 4-epimerase from Escherichia coli, *Biochemistry* 1993; **32**: 13231–13236.

131. Furukawa, K., Tagaya, M., Tanizawa, K. and Fukui, T., Role of the conserved Lys-X-Gly-Gly sequence at the ADP-glucose-binding site in Escherichia coli glycogen synthase, *J. Biol. Chem.* 1993; **268**: 23837–23842.

8 Evoked Potentials and Bilirubin

Steven M. Shapiro

Division of Child Neurology, Medical College of Virginia, Virginia Commonwealth University, Richmond, Virginia, USA

EVOKED POTENTIALS AND BILIRUBIN

The use of noninvasive electrophysiological measures to predict the onset of conditions that lead to brain damage can help guide preventative therapies and also assess the role of bilirubin encephalopathy in the development of sensory systems and cognitive dysfunction. Evoked potentials (EPs) are electrical potentials obtained in response to a stimulus, and in clinical use are surface recorded, computer averaged responses to repeated auditory, visual or somatosensory stimuli. EPs measure neuronal function of the sensory system being stimulated. EPs of the auditory system have been most extensively studied in hyperbilirubinemia, but limited studies of visual and somatosensory EPs are available. Evoked potentials are highly sensitive to abnormalities of neuronal function such as conduction delay, desynchronization, and loss of cells which occur in a number of pathological conditions involving brain injury, metabolic disorders and demyelination.[1-3]

Brainstem Auditory Evoked Potentials (BAEPs) and Bilirubin

Localization of bilirubin-induced pathology in the auditory nervous system

The neuropathology of elevated bilirubin is based primarily on studies completed in the 1950's, on patients with the extreme form of bilirubin neurotoxicity, kernicterus. Clinical studies show audiometric evidence for a predominantly high-frequency sensorineural hearing loss that is usually bilateral and symmetric, with recruitment and abnormal loudness growth functions.[4-11] Central auditory nervous system abnormalities, either alone or in combination with sensory loss, are suggested by reports of decreased binaural fusion, auditory aphasia and imperception, word deafness, and numerous instances of patients labeled as "deaf" when objective tests

Address for correspondence: Division of Child Neurology, 7th Floor, Randolph Manor Hall, P.O. Box 980211, Richmond, Virginia 23298-0211, 804-828-0442, Fax: 804-828-6690, Tdd: 1-800-828-1120

show normal thresholds.[6, 8–12] Autopsy studies of infants with classic kernicterus,[13–15] and more recent studies in premature, low birth weight infants with "low-bilirubin kernicterus"[16] have shown *central auditory pathology*, with involvement of brainstem auditory structures including the dorsal and ventral cochlear nuclei, superior olivary complex, nuclei of the lateral lemniscus, and inferior colliculi, but no significant abnormalities of the eighth nerve[13] or inner ear structures.[17,18] However, the specificity of these findings for bilirubin toxicity has been questioned, since most studies were done in patients who had concurrent risk factors, e.g., hypoxia-ischemia, acidosis, and aminoglycoside exposure.

While the classical clinical syndrome includes deafness, studies have shown an association between moderate-to-severe sensorineural hearing loss and elevated bilirubin levels in the newborn in the absence of kernicterus.[19–21] Both the amount and duration of hyperbilirubinemia are risk factors.[19,20] More recently, evidence has been presented that the development of sensorineural loss associated with hyperbilirubinemia may be delayed and progressive.[22]

Another clinical entity, termed "auditory neuropathy," has recently been described and functionally defined as the presence of normal otoacoustic emissions (OEAs) with absent or abnormal BAEPs.[23,24] Adults with auditory neuropathy have difficulty processing sounds and speech and distinguishing speech from noise. OEAs assess the mechanical integrity of the inner ear and are widely used for hearing screening in infants.[25,26] OEAs are normal with hearing loss or auditory dysfunction due to lesions in the receptors (inner hair cells), auditory nerve or central auditory pathways. Reports of children with auditory neuropathy after documented hyperbilirubinemia raise the possibility of an association between bilirubin neurotoxicity and auditory neuropathy. Chisin *et al.* studied children with hearing loss following hyperbilirubinemia.[27] They used cochlear microphonic recordings to assess inner ear function similar to OEAs, and found absent BAEPs in the presence of normal inner ear function, which would now be labelled auditory neuropathy. Stein *et al.*, reported that 3 of 4 infants and children diagnosed with auditory neuropathy had hyperbilirubinemia as neonates.[28] These investigators are now following 8 children with auditory neuropathy, 6 of whom had elevated bilirubin levels, 4 of 6 requiring exchange transfusion. Berlin *et al.*, cite 5 infants with auditory neuropathy, at least two of whom had hyperbilirubinemia,[29] and Rance *et al.*, reported that 10 of 20 infants with auditory neuropathy had high bilirubin levels, including 6 of 12 infants identified in a screening program using both BAEPs and OEAs.[30] While the number of patients with auditory neuropathy is small, collectively, the data suggest that about half of the cases of auditory neuropathy may be related to hyperbilirubinemia.

Brainstem auditory evoked potentials (BAEPs)

Brainstem auditory evoked potentials (BAEPs), also known as brainstem auditory evoked responses (BAERs) and auditory brainstem responses (ABRs), are electrical potentials evoked by auditory stimulation and recorded non-invasively from the scalp. A series of characteristic waves can be distinguished from the background electrical activity electroencephalogram (EEG) by averaging the EEG response to

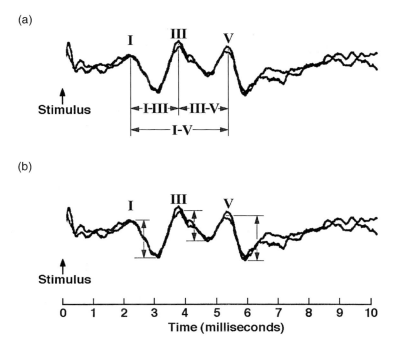

Figure 8.1. Replicated BAEP waves obtained from a 5 day old infant to 45 dB HL* monaural click stimuli at 29.3 clicks/second, amplified from electrodes on the vertex and ipsilateral mastoid, filtered from 30–3000 Hz. (a) Illustration of waves I, III and V, and I–III, III–V and I–V interwave intervals. Latencies are the time from the onset of the stimulus to the peak of the vertex positive wave. Interwave intervals are derived from subtracting wave latencies to obtain the time between peaks. Wave I is generated by neurons in the distal auditory nerve, wave III by neurons in the ipsilateral cochlear nucleus of the brainstem, and wave V by predominantly contralateral axons in the lateral lemniscus which project into the inferior colliculi in the midbrain.[35–38] (b) Peak to trough amplitude measurements of the same wave shown in (a). Since amplitude varies widely from individual to individual, amplitude ratios, e.g., the ratio of the amplitude of wave V to wave I (V:I amplitude ratio), are more commonly used when assessing wave amplitude. * dBHL= decibels hearing level.

many stimuli, each epoch of EEG recorded being triggered by and time-locked to the stimulus. The BAEP waves arise from neural generators in the auditory nerve and brainstem fiber tracts and nuclei.[31–38] Each wave of the BAEP is generated by a small subpopulation of synchronously firing neural elements; thus each component of the BAEP wave reflects the activation of specific but temporally overlapping anatomical regions of the brainstem. The BAEP measures neuronal function and, because of the prominent and early involvement of the auditory nervous system as a result of bilirubin neurotoxicity, it is a highly sensitive measure of the onset of neuronal dysfunction.

The most important waves clinically in humans are the so-called Jewett waves I, III and V (Figure 8.1). Wave I arises from neural generators in the proximal part of the auditory nerve, wave III from the vicinity of the cochlear nuclear in the ipsilateral pons in the lower brainstem, and wave V from axons of the ascending lateral lemniscus in the midbrain as they enter the inferior colliculus, predominantly contralateral to the side of stimulus.[35–38]

BAEP methods not in common use clinically, e.g., binaural interaction BAEPs, middle and later latency (cortical) evoked potentials, have been used in humans with conditions other than neonatal hyperbilirubinemia[39–41] and in animal models of bilirubin encephalopathy and kernicterus.[42,43]

The time between BAEP wave peaks reflects the time it takes for nerve impulses to travel from one anatomical location to another (Figure 8.1). Changes in the neural pathways cause delayed or abnormal conduction of impulses, and manifest as increased interwave intervals, i.e. the times between specific BAEP waves. Desynchronization or loss of nerve cell activity also produces changes in the amplitudes and morphology of the BAEP waves. Thus, alterations of interwave interval or wave amplitude may reflect neuronal dysfunction.

Brainstem auditory evoked potentials (BAEPs) and bilirubin

BAEPs were first applied to bilirubin encephalopathy in studies of older children and adults with chronic kernicteric bilirubin encephalopathy.[27,44] Abnormal function of the auditory nerve and the brainstem were found with BAEPs, even in patients from whom normal cochlear microphonic recordings were obtained,[27] implying normal functioning of outer hair cells of the inner ear.

Recently, BAEPs have been applied to the study of bilirubin toxicity in hyperbilirubinemic human newborns.[27,44–47] Increases in interwave intervals (the time between BAEP peaks, a measure of central auditory function) and decreases in amplitudes were found.[45–48] These abnormalities were reversed when exchange transfusions were used to treat hyperbilirubinemia.[47,49,50] BAEP changes (interwave intervals) correlate directly and significantly with serum levels of total indirect and unbound bilirubin in the newborn period.[46,51]

Physiologic measures have been studied systematically in animal models of hyperbilirubinemia. Gunn rats[52–54] and premature monkeys first infused with bilirubin and then sulfonamide[55] have shown reproducible BAEP abnormalities. Hyperbilirubinemic Gunn rats have functional abnormalities of the central nervous system as measured with BAEPs.[53,54,56] Their BAEPs have prolongation of the I–II and I–III interwave intervals (equivalent to the I–III and I–V interwave intervals in human) and amplitude reductions of waves II and III.[53,54] These abnormalities correlate with the known sites of bilirubin damage in the auditory brainstem pathways,[57–60] specifically in the cochlear nuclei and other, lower brainstem (pontine) nuclei. When jaundiced rats are given sulfonamide to displace albumin-bound bilirubin from the blood, the bilirubin enters brain tissue[61] producing changes in the BAEP. These changes include striking increases in I–II interwave intervals and decreased wave amplitudes, and are reproducible, and at least partially reversible.[52,62] Another central auditory function, binaural interaction, as measured with BAEPs,[63] has been shown to be abnormal in this model.[42] This abnormality is probably related to neuropathological damage to the superior olivary complex, an area involved with the interaural processing of sound. The superior olivary complex is damaged in human kernicterus[16] and studies in jaundiced Gunn rats reveal neuroanatomical and immunohistochemical abnormalities that correspond to BAEP abnormalities.[59,60] Recent evidence that dysfunction of BAEP binaural interaction precedes conventional BAEP changes in acute bilirubin toxicity indicates that these areas may be especially susceptible to bilirubin toxicity, and measurement of binaural interaction BAEPs may increase our ability to detect early neuronal alterations in bilirubin toxicity.[43]

In summary, hyperbilirubinemia continues to be a threat to the auditory nervous system. Neonates at highest risk for encephalopathy may be more precisely identified by using electrophysiological means such as BAEPs.

Visual and Somatosensory Evoked Potentials and Bilirubin

Somatosensory evoked potentials (SSEPs)

SSEPs are obtained by recording EEG responses to peripheral electrical stimulation. In the newborn this has usually involved electrical stimulation of the median nerve at the wrist or the posterior tibial nerve above the ankle.

Silver et al.[64] studied SSEPs in jaundiced Gunn rats and found no effects in young rats but delay and amplitude reduction of cortical waves in young adult rats. When acute bilirubin toxicity in young rats was produced following sulfadimethoxine administration (thus displacing bilirubin from blood into brain tissue), changes in the peripheral but not central component were seen. Shapiro et al.[65] failed to replicate these results. Young jaundiced rats made bilirubin toxic with sulfadimethoxine showed no SSEP abnormalities, despite having typical bilirubin-induced abnormalities of BAEPs.

Bonger-Schokking et al.[66] studied SSEPs in hyperbilirubinemic human infants when their bilirubin levels peaked, and 2–3 days and 5 weeks after the peak levels occurred. They found that increases in central conduction time correlated with bilirubin levels. However, technical issues with this study raise some concerns about the reliability of their results. For example, they averaged an unusually small number of stimuli, claiming that repeated stimulation altered their responses. Their claim has not been replicated in other laboratories, which average many more stimuli to obtain reliable results. Rubboli et al.[67] studied 5 children and adolescents with Crigler–Najjar syndrome type I. Three of five patients had no abnormalities of multimodality evoked potentials, although the 2 more symptomatic children were not tested. Thus, the relationship of SSEPs to hyperbilirubinemia is yet to be determined.

Visual evoked potentials (VEPs)

VEPs have been studied in Gunn rats and in human infants. They measure the EEG response (by electrodes on the occipital scalp) to a light flash of graded intensity and frequency. Silver et al.[68] studied the postnatal development of flash VEPs in jaundiced Gunn rats and found prolonged wave latencies and reduced amplitude during the 3rd week of life when the bilirubin level was at its maximum. VEP latencies were also predictive of subsequent mortality. When sulfadimethoxine was administered to produce acute bilirubin toxicity,[69] prolongation of VEP latencies occurred within hours, and wave amplitudes decreased. There was also prolongation of the later component ("b" wave latency) of the electroretinogram, but this occurred several hours after the VEP changes.

Two premature infants with bilirubin levels of 207 and 200 μmol/l (12.1 and 11.7 mg/dl) had flash VEPs and BAEPs before and after exchange transfusion.[70] Latencies of VEPs and central components of BAEPs improved after the transfusion. Serial VEPs were performed in a group of 72 hyperbilirubinemic infants and 22 controls.[71] Hyperbilirubinemic infants were grouped into low, moderate, and severe groups, the latter having 21 infants with bilirubins ranging from 344 to 510 μmol/l (20.1–29.8 mg/dl). The latencies of VEP waves were prolonged in the moderate and severe groups for up to 8 weeks after birth. Amplitudes were reduced only at one week of age.

Although difficulties with visual perception have been reported in children who were hyperbilirubinemic as newborns,[72,73] these may be largely explained by nuclear and supranuclear disturbances of gaze. Pathologic studies of classical kernicterus[15] show relative sparing of the visual pathways that are assessed by VEPs.

The acute changes in VEPs seen with acute bilirubin toxicity in Gunn rats[69] and in the two infants who received exchange transfusions[70] suggest massive entry of bilirubin into the central nervous system, beyond the retina. The significance of prolonged VEP latencies in hyperbilirubinemic infants during the first 8 weeks of life remains to be determined.

References

1. Hecox, K.E., Cone, B. and Blaw, M.E., Brainstem auditory evoked response in the diagnosis of pediatric neurologic diseases, 1981; **31**: 832–839.
2. Starr, A., Sensory evoked potentials in clinical disorders of the nervous system, *Ann. Rev. Neurosci.* 1978; **1**: 103–127.
3. Greenberg, R.P. and Ducker, T.B., Evoked potentials in the clinical neurologies, *J. Neurosurg.* 1982; **56**: 1–18.
4. Crabtree, N. and Gerrard, J., Perceptive deafness associated with severe neonatal deafness. A report of sixteen cases, *J. Laryngol. Otol.* 1950; **64**: 482–506.
5. Flottorp, G., Morley, D.E. and Skatvedt, M., The localization of hearing impairment in athetoids, *Acta. Otolaryngol.* 1957; **48**: 404–414.
6. Hardy, W.G., *Auditory deficits of the kernicterus child.* In: Swinyard, C.A., ed. Kernicterus and its Importance in Cerebral Palsy. Springfield, Ill: Thomas, Charles, C., 1961; 21–228.
7. Keaster, J. and Hyman, C.B., I. H. Hearing problems subsequent to neonatal hemolytic disease or hyperbilirubinemia, *Am. J. Dis. Child.* 1969; **117**: 406–410.
8. Matkin, N.D. and Carhart, R., Auditory profiles associated with Rh incompatibility, *Arch. Otolaryngol.* 1966; **84**: 502–513.
9. Perlstein, M.A., The late clinical syndrome of posticteric encephalopathy, *Pediatr. Clin. North. Am.* 1960; **7**: 665–687.
10. Rosen, J., Deaf or 'aphasic'? 4. Variations in the auditory disorders of the Rh child, *J. Speech. Hear. Dis.* 1956; **21**: 418–422.
11. Ruben, R., Lieberman, A. and Bordley, J., Some observations on cochlear potentials and nerve action potentials in children, *Laryngoscope* 1962; **72**: 545–553.
12. Byers, R.K., Paine, R.S. and Crothers, B., Extrapyramidal cerebral palsy with hearing loss following erythroblastosis, *Pediatrics* 1955; **15**: 248–254.
13. Dublin, W., Neurological lesions in erythroblastosis fetalis in relation to nuclear deafness, *Am. J. Clin. Path.* 1951; **21**: 935–939.

14. Dublin, W., *Fundamentals of Sensorineural Auditory Pathology*. Springfield, IL: Charles C. Thomas, 1976.
15. Haymaker, W., Margles, C. and Pentschew, A., *Pathology of kernicterus and posticteric encephalopathy*. In: Swinyard, C.A., ed. Kernicterus and Its Importance in Cerebral Palsy. Springfield, IL: Charles C. Thomas, 1961; 21–22.
16. Ahdab-Barmada, M. and Moossy, J., The neuropathology of kernicterus in the premature neonate: diagnostic problems, *J. Neuropath. Exp. Neurol.* 1984; **43**: 45–56.
17. Gerrard, J., Nuclear jaundice and deafness, *J. Laryngol. Otol.* 1952; **66**: 39–46.
18. Kelemen, G., Erythroblastosis fetalis. Pathologic report on the hearing organs of a newborn infant, *AMA. Arch. Otolaryngol.* 1956; **63**: 392–398.
19. Bergman, I., Hirsch, R.P., Fria, T.J., Shapiro, S.M., Holzman, I. and Painter, M.J., Cause of hearing loss in the high-risk premature infant, *J. Pediatr.* 1985; **106**(1): 5–101.
20. De Vries, L.S., Lary, S. and Dubowitz, L.M.S., Relationship of serum bilirubin levels to ototoxicity and deafness in high-risk, low birth-weight infants, *Pediatrics* 1985; **76**(3): 351–354.
21. De Vries, L.S., Lary, S., Whitelaw, A.G. and Dubowitz, L.M., Relationship of serum bilirubin levels and hearing impairment in newborn infants, *Early. Hum. Dev.* 1987; **15**(5): 269–277.
22. Worley, G., Erwin, C.W., Goldstein, R.F., Provenzale, J.M. and Ware, R.E., Delayed development of sensorineural hearing loss after neonatal hyperbilirubinemia: a case report with brain magnetic resonance imaging, *Dev. Med. Child. Neurol.* 1996; **38**(3): 271–277.
23. Deltenre, P., Mansbach, A.L., Bozet, C., Clercx, A. and Hecox, K.E., Auditory neuropathy: a report on three cases with early onsets and major neonatal illnesses, *Electroencephalogr. Clin. Neurophysiol.* 1997; **104**(1): 17–22.
24. Starr, A., Picton, T.W., Sininger, Y., Hood, L.J. and Berlin, C.I., Auditory neuropathy, *Brain* 1996; **119**(Pt 3): 741–753.
25. Decreton, S.J., Hanssens, K. and De Sloovere, M., Evoked otoacoustic emissions in infant hearing screening, *Int. J. Pediatr. Otorhinolaryngol.* 1991; **21**(3): 235–247.
26. Stevens, J.C., Webb, H.D., Hutchinson, J., Connell, J., Smith, M.F. and Buffin, J.T., Click evoked otoacoustic emissions in neonatal screening, *Ear. Hear.* 1990; **11**(2): 128–133.
27. Chisin, R., Perlman, M. and Sohmer, H., Cochlear and brain stem responses in hearing loss following neonatal hyperbilirubinemia, *Ann. Otol.* 1979; **88**: 352–357.
28. Stein, L.K., McGee, T., Tremblay, K., Kraus, N. and Cheatham, M.A., Auditory neuropathy associated with elevated bilirubin levels. Association for Research in Otolaryngology MidWinter Meetings. St. Petersberg Beach, Florida, 1997.
29. Berlin, C.I., Role of infant hearing screening in health care, *Seminars in Hearing* 1966; **17**(2): 115–124.
30. Rance, G., Beer, D.E., Cone-Wesson, B., Shepard, R.K., Dowell, R.C., King, A.M., Rickards, F.W. and Clark, G.M., Clinical findings for a group of infants and young children with auditory neuropathy. *Ear and Hearing* 1999; **20**: 238–252.
31. Huang, C.-M. and Buchwald, J.S., Interpretation of the vertex short-latency acoustic response: A study of the single neurons in the brain stem, *Brain. Res.* 1977; **137**: 291–303.
32. Jewett, D.L. and Romano, M.N., Neonatal development of auditory system potentials averaged from the scalp of rat and cat, *Brain. Res.* 1972; **36**: 101–115.
33. Melcher, J.R. and Kiang, N.Y., Generators of the brainstem auditory evoked potential in cat. III: Identified cell populations, *Hear. Res.* 1996; **93**(1–2): 52–71.
34. Starr, A. and Hamilton, A.E., Correlation between confirmed sites of neurological lesions and abnormalities of far field auditory brainstem responses, *Electroenceph. Clin. Neurophysiol.* 1976; **41**: 595–608.
35. Møller, A.R., Jannetta, P.J. and Møller, M.B., Neural generators of brainstem evoked potentials. Results from human intracranial recordings, *Ann. Otol. Rhinol. Laryngol.* 1981; **90**(6 Pt 1): 591–596.
36. Møller, A.R. and Jannetta, P.J., Interpretation of brainstem auditory evoked potentials: results from intracranial recordings in humans, *Scand. Audiol.* 1983; **12**(2): 125–133.
37. Møller, A.R., Auditory neurophysiology, *J. Clin. Neurophysiol.* 1994; **11**(3): 284–308.
38. Møller, A.R., Jho, H.D., Yokota, M. and Jannetta, P.J., Contribution from crossed and uncrossed brainstem structures to the brainstem auditory evoked potentials: a study in humans, *Laryngoscope* 1995; **105**(6): 596–605.
39. Dobie, R.A., Binaural interaction in human auditory evoked potentials, *Electroenceph. Clin. Neurophysiol.* 1980; **49**: 303–313.
40. Hosford-Dunn, H., Mendelson, T. and Salamy, A., Binaural interactions in the short-latency evoked potentials of neonates, *Audiology* 1981; **20**: 394–408.

41. Levine, R.A., Gardner, J.C., Stufflebeam, S.M. *et al.*, Binaural auditory processing in multiple sclerosis subjects, *Hear. Res.* 1993; **68**(1): 59–72.
42. Shapiro, S.M., Binaural effects in brainstem auditory evoked potentials of jaundiced rats, *Hearing. Res.* 1991; **53**: 41–48.
43. Chapin, L.T. and Shapiro, S.M., Abnormalities in binaural interaction precede abnormalities in brainstem auditory evoked potentials in jaundiced Gunn rat pups given sulfonamide, *Pediatric. Research.* 1997; **41**(4 (Part 2)): 143A.
44. Kaga, K., Kitazumi, E., Kodama, K., Auditory brain stem responses of kernicterus infants, *Int. J. Ped. Otorhinolaryngol.* 1979; **1**: 255–294.
45. Lenhardt, M.L., McArtor, R. and Bryant, B., Effects of neonatal hyperbilirubinemia on the brainstem electrical response, *J. Peds.* 1984; **104**: 281–284.
46. Nakamura, H., Takada, S., Shimabuku, R., Matsuo, M., Matsuo, T. and Negishi, H., Auditory nerve and brainstem responses in newborn infants with hyperbilirubinemia, *Pediatrics* 1985; **75**: 703–708.
47. Perlman, M., Fainmesser, P., Sohmer, H., Tamari, H., Wax, Y. and Pevsmer, B., Auditory nerve-brainstem evoked responses in hyperbilirubinemic neonates, *Pediatrics* 1983; **72**: 658–664.
48. Kotagal, S., Rudd, D., Rosenberg, C. and Horenstein, S., Brain-stem auditory evoked potentials in neonatal hyperbilirubinemia, *Neurol.* 1981; **31**: 48.
49. Nwaesei, C.G., Van Aerde, J., Boyden, M. and Perlman, M., Changes in auditory brainstem responses in hyperbilirubinemic infants before and after exchange transfusion, *Peds.* 1984; **74**: 800–803.
50. Wennberg, R.P., Ahlfors, L.E. and Bickers, R., Abnormal auditory brainstem response in a newborn infant with hyperbilirubinemia: Improvement with exchange transfusion, *J. Pediat.* 1982; **100**: 624.
51. Funato, M., Tamai, H., Shimada, S. and Nakamura, H., Vigintiphobia, unbound bilirubin, and auditory brainstem responses, *Pediatrics* 1994; **93**(1): 50–53.
52. Shapiro, S.M., Acute brainstem auditory evoked potential abnormalities in jaundiced Gunn rats given sulfonamide, *Pediatr. Res.* 1988; **23**: 306–310.
53. Shapiro, S.M. and Hecox, K.E., Developmental studies of brainstem auditory evoked potentials in jaundiced Gunn rats, *Dev. Brain. Res.* 1988; **41**: 147–157.
54. Shapiro, S.M. and Hecox, K.E., Brain stem auditory evoked potentials in jaundiced Gunn rats, *Ann. Otol. Rhinol. and Laryngol.* 1989; **98**(4): 308–317.
55. Ahlfors, C.E., Bennett, S.H., Shoemaker, C.T. *et al.*, Changes in the auditory brainstem response associated with intravenous infusion of unconjugated bilirubin into infant rhesus monkeys, *Pediatr. Res.* 1986; **20**: 511–515.
56. Uziel, A., Marot, M. and Pujol, R., The Gunn rat: an experimental model for central deafness, *Acta. Otolaryngol.* 1983; **95**: 651–656.
57. Jew, J.Y. and Williams, T.H., Ultrastructural aspects of bilirubin encephalopathy in cochlear nuclei of the Gunn rat, *J. Anat.* 1977; **124**: 599–614.
58. Jew, J.Y. and Sandquist, D., CNS changes in hyperbilirubinemia, *Arch. Neurol.* 1979; **36**: 149–154.
59. Conlee, J.W. and Shapiro, S.M., Morphological changes in the cochlear nucleus and nucleus of the trapezoid body in Gunn rat pups, *Hear. Res.* 1991; **57**(1): 23–30.
60. Shapiro, S.M. and Conlee, J.W., Brainstem auditory evoked potentials correlate with morphological changes in Gunn rat pups, *Hearing. Res.* 1991; **57**(1): 16–22.
61. Diamond, I. and Schmid, R., Experimental bilirubin encephalopathy: the mode of entry of bilirubin bilirubin-^{14}C into the CNS, *J. Clin. Invest.* 1966; **45**: 678–689.
62. Shapiro, S.M., Reversible brainstem auditory evoked potential abnormalities in jaundiced Gunn rats given sulfonamide, *Pediatr. Res.* 1993; **34**(5): 629–633.
63. Dobie, R.A., Binaural interaction in brainstem-evoked responses, *Arch. Otolaryngol.* 1979; **105**: 391–398.
64. Silver, S., Sohmer, H. and Kapitulnik, J., Postnatal development of somatosensory evoked potential in jaundiced Gunn rats and effects of sulfadimethoxine administration, *Pediatr. Res.* 1996; **40**(2): 209–214.
65. Shapiro, S.M., Somatosensory and brainstem auditory evoked potentials in an experimental model of acute bilirubin neurotoxicity, *Annals. of Neurology* 1995; **38**(3): 553.
66. Bongers-Schokking, J.J., Colon, E.J., Hoogland, R.A., Van den Brande, J.L. and de Groot, C.J., Somatosensory evoked potentials in neonatal jaundice, *Acta. Pediatrica. Scandinavia.* 1990; **79**(2): 148–155.
67. Rubboli, G., Ronchi, F., Cecchi, P. *et al.*, A neurophysiological study in children and adolescents with Crigler–Najjar syndrome type I, *Neuropediatrics* 1997; **28**(5): 281–286.
68. Silver, S., Kapitulnik, J. and Sohmer, H., Postnatal development of flash visual evoked potentials in the jaundiced Gunn rat, *Pediatr. Res.* 1991; **30**(5): 469–472.

69. Silver, S., Sohmer, H. and Kapitulnik, J., Visual evoked potential abnormalities in jaundiced Gunn rats treated with sulfadimethoxine, *Pediatr. Res.* 1995; **38**(2): 258–261.
70. Chin, K.C., Taylor, M.J. and Perlman, M., Improvement in auditory and visual evoked potentials in jaundiced preterm infants after exchange transfusion, *Arch. Dis. Child.* 1985; **60**: 714–717.
71. Chen, Y.J. and Kang, W.M., Effects of bilirubin on visual evoked potentials in term infants, *Eur. J. Pediatr.* 1995; **154**(8): 662–666.
72. Hyman, C.B., Keaster, J., Hanson, V. *et al.*, CNS abnormalities after neonatal hemolytic disease or hyperbilirubinemia. A prospective study of 405 patients, *Am. J. Dis. Child.* 1969; **117**: 395–405.
73. Naeye, R.L., Amniotic fluid infections, neonatal hyperbilirubinemia and psychomotor impairment, *Pediatrics* 1978; **62**: 497–503.

9 The Clinical Sequelae of Hyperbilirubinemia

Jon F. Watchko

Division of Neonatology and Developmental Biology, Department of Pediatrics, University of Pittsburgh School of Medicine, Pittsburgh, Pennsylvania, USA

The classically described sequelae of marked neonatal hyperbilirubinemia are neurodevelopmental in nature and were originally defined in infants with Rh isoimmunization.[1-6] These markedly jaundiced infants presented with a neurologic syndrome acutely typified by lethargy, poor feeding, and hypotonia followed by hypertonia with opisthotonus, fever, a high pitched cry and occasionally seizures,[1,2,4,6] Survivors manifested long term adverse neurodevelopmental sequelae including extrapyramidal disturbances (choreoathetosis), high-frequency sensorineural hearing loss, and palsy of vertical gaze.[3,5] These sequelae reflect both i) the predilection of bilirubin toxicity for neurons (rather than glial cells)[7] and ii) the regional topography of bilirubin induced neuronal injury which is characterized by prominent basal ganglia, cochlear, and oculomotor nuclei involvement.[8,9] Intellectual deficits, however, have been observed in only a minority of infants with chronic postkernicteric bilirubin encephalopathy,[3,5] reflecting the fact that cerebral cortical neuron involvement is not a salient feature of kernicterus.

Although the constellation of extrapyramidal movement abnormality, auditory deficit, and gaze disturbance has been correlated with severe neonatal hyperbilirubinemia, individually these sequelae are not unique to this clinical context. In fact, of all infants with choreoathetosis only about 25% have a history of marked neonatal hyperbilirubinemia.[10] Similarly, the occurrence of high frequency sensorineural hearing loss in newborns is associated with several factors, particularly in high risk neonates.[11,12] Paresis of upward gaze, although commonly observed in hyperbilirubinemic encephalopathy (~90% of cases), can be seen in any dorsal midbrain syndrome including those associated with dilatation of the third ventricle, tumor, and lipid storage disease.[13] Thus, the veracity with which a causal linkage can be established between marked hyperbilirubinemia and neurodevelopmental sequelae in individual cases may be limited.[14] Noninvasive neuroimaging has been proposed as a tool to evaluate the neurologic changes with hyperbilirubinemia[15,16] and may yet prove helpful in the assessment of individual infants. Indeed, magentic resonance imaging (MRI) studies of children with postkernicteric encephalopathy demonstrate the characteristic pattern of neuropathological lesions of kernicterus,[17,18,19] i.e.,

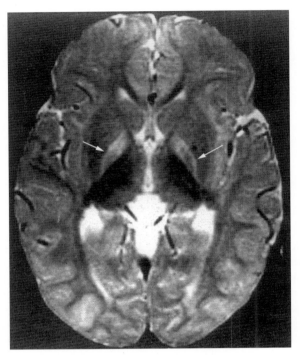

Figure 9.1. Magnetic resonance imaging scan of a male infant who had erythroblastosis fetalis and extreme hyperbilirubinemia who developed clinical signs of kernicterus as a neonate. This scan was obtained at 21 months of age and demonstrates symmetric, abnormal high intensity signals from the area of the globus pallidus (arrows). From *S. Afr. Med. J.* 1997; **87**: 146–149.

abnormal bilateral high intensity signals in the globus pallidus (Figure 9.1),[17,18,19,20] internal capsule[17] and thalamus.[17]

These MRI abnormalities, however, are not necessarily specific to hyperbilirubinemic encephalopathy.[21] Further study is necessary to define the nature of these MRI findings and establish the utility of neuroimaging in the neurologic assessment of infants at risk for hyperbilirubinemic encephalopathy. Fortunately, the classic presentation of acute bilirubin encephalopathy and its neurodevelopmental sequelae are an unusual occurrence in the present era as a result of a marked decrease in the prevalence of Rh sensitized pregnancies and the intensive management of hyperbilirubinemia in infants with hemolytic disease.

INFANTS WITH HEMOLYTIC DISEASE OF THE NEWBORN

The neurodevelopmental outcome of infants with hemolytic disease of the newborn was the focus of considerable study years ago but has received little attention as of late. Early studies date back to the pioneering work of Day and Haines who demonstrated the benefits of exchange transfusion in enhancing the intelligence quotients of children recovered from erythroblastosis fetalis.[22] Subsequently, others confirmed that exchange transfusions were effective in largely preventing long term sequelae due to hyperbilirubinemia in infants with Rh isoimmunization or hemolysis secondary to ABO incompatibility. In one such study of infants with indirect serum bilirubin levels that exceeded 20 mg/dl (342 μmol/l) [95% of which received one or more exchange transfusions], only 7 of 129 infants suffered adverse neurodevelopmental sequelae typified by sensorineural hearing loss ($n = 7$); mild athetosis ($n = 3$); or mental retardation ($n = 1$).[23] Affected infants had indirect hyperbilirubinemia in the range of 20.1 to 30.8 mg/dl (344 to 527 μmol/l) with a mean indirect bilirubin level of 27.5 mg/dl (470 μmol/l). The entire study group had an average intelligence quotient of 104.8 which did not differ from their control non-hemolytic counterparts (mean IQ 102.8).[23]

A more recent report, however, demonstrated lower intelligence quotients and more prominent neurologic abnormalities in Coombs positive hyperbilirubinemic full term infants as opposed to a hyperbilirubinemic cohort without evidence of hemolytic disease or their non-hyperbilirubinemic control group.[24] The Coombs positive cohort included infants with Rh isoimmunization and ABO incompatibility and was characterized by indirect hyperbilirubinemia in the range of 20–48 mg/dl (342–820 μmol/l) [median 22.0 mg/dl (376 μmol/l)].[24] These data reinforce longstanding evidence that hemolysis is an important risk factor for the genesis of hyperbilirubinemic encephalopathy and associated adverse neurodevelopmental sequelae in term infants. Of additional note, the latter investigation suggested that the risk of prominent neurologic abnormalities on follow-up was correlated with the duration of indirect hyperbilirubinemia >20 mg/dl (342 μmol/l), increasing in a stepwise fashion from 2.3% at <6 hours duration, to 18.7% at 6–11 hours duration, and further to 26% at 12 or more hours duration.[24] These data echo much earlier observations suggesting the duration of hyperbilirubinemia might be related to long term neurodevelopmental performance.[25] The outcome of infants with hemolysis secondary to other causes including red cell membrane defects and glucose-6-phosphate dehydrogenase deficiency remains largely undefined although their risk for hyperbilirubinemic encephalopathy appears to be commensurate with those of immune mediated hemolytic processes.[26–28]

Currently, debate continues regarding the level of hyperbilirubinemia at which neurodevelopmental sequelae are manifest in healthy full term infants without hemolysis. Similarly, our understanding of the neurotoxic potential of hyperbilirubinemia in infants born prematurely (<37 completed weeks gestation) continues to evolve. These topics have occasioned lively discussion in the pediatric literature and will be the focus of this chapter.

FULLTERM INFANTS WITHOUT HEMOLYSIS

The neurodevelopmental outcome of full term (≥37 completed weeks of gestation) jaundiced infants without hemolysis has been assessed in several developmental

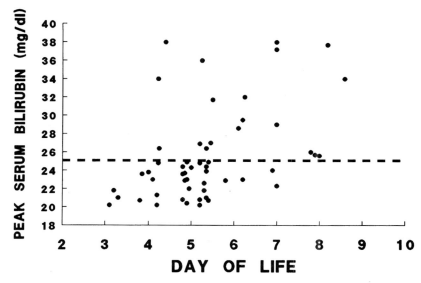

Figure 9.2. Peak serum bilirubin levels in 54 full term infants with marked hyperbilirubinemia who were normal on neurodevelopmental follow-up evaluation. From Mores *et al.*, *Acta. Paediatr.* 1959; **48**: 590–602.

follow-up studies. These investigations date back to the pioneering work of Mores and colleagues in 1959 in which they examined 54 full term infants without iso-immunization who had peak serum bilirubin levels of 20 mg/dl or greater, 19 of which had bilirubin values in excess of 25 mg/dl[29] (Figure 9.2). None were treated with exchange transfusion (the only therapeutic intervention to lower bilirubin levels at the time) and on developmental follow-up through 4 years of age, all infants were judged to be normal.

In an analogous investigation, Killander and co-workers assessed the neuro-developmental outcome of infants enrolled in their 1960 study designed to evaluate the therapeutic efficacy of a 20 mg/dl bilirubin threshold for exchange transfusion in full term infants without hemolysis.[30] Killander and colleagues alternately assigned full term infants without Rh or ABO isoimmunization to exchange transfusion or no exchange transfusion when their serum bilirubin level reached 20 mg/dl.[31] Infants from the non-exchanged group tended to have peak serum bilirubin levels in the 20–25 mg/dl range and a more protracted course of moderate hyperbilirubinemia than their exchanged counterparts.[31] The non-exchanged infants, however, did not differ from their exchanged cohort on long term neurodevelopmental follow-up,[30] and there was no case of kernicterus in either group.

A series of additional papers on the association between hyperbilirubinemia and neurodevelopmental outcome in term infants without hemolysis followed and this entire literature has been systematically analyzed.[32,33] Newman and Maisels reviewed this literature with the intent of determining the relationship between total serum bilirubin and three broad clinically relevant outcomes: i) cognitive development (as measured by intelligence quotients or developmental scores), ii) abnormal-

Table 9.1. Proportion of infants with definite neurologic abnormality vs. maximum total serum bilirubin level of primarily term infants without hemolysis.

Reference	Total serum bilirubin level		
	< 15 mg/dl (< 257 μmol/l)	≥15 mg/dl (≥257 μmol/l)	≥20 mg/dl (≥257 μmol/l)
Hardy (1971)[33]	39/2885	1/110	0/35
Mores (1959)[29]		0/54	0/54
Killander (1963)[30]		1/93	1/93
Fohl (1964)[35]	0/3	2/37	
Holmes (1968)[36]	0/46	0/34	
Culley (1970)[37]	1/97	1/24	
Bengtsson (1974)[38]	1/115	2/111	2/111
Total	41/3146	7/463	5/322
%	1.3	1.5	1.6

From *Pediatrics* 1992; **89**: 809–818, reproduced with permission from publisher.

ities on neurologic examination, and iii) hearing.[32,33] Their exhaustive analysis was notable for three important methodological considerations. First, they restricted their study to term infants without hemolysis. Second, they analyzed published data from the Collaborative Perinatal Project (CPP) including some previously unrecognized results. Third, they calculated estimates of the strength of associations, rather than relying on *P*-values. This turned out to be particularly important when evaluating the results of the CPP which yielded many statistically significant results that were clinically trivial. The results of their extensive analysis demonstrated no evidence of a clinically significant effect of bilirubin level on cognitive impairment (intelligence quotient), neurologic abnormalities (Table 9.1), or hearing loss.[32,33]

Complementing this analysis, Newman and Klebanoff re-analyzed the entire CPP to examine the association between neonatal bilirubin levels and subsequent neurodevelopmental outcome.[39] Their report differed from previously published analyses of the CPP in several ways: they i) included the latest outcome data from examinations at ages 7 and 8 years; ii) sought evidence of a threshold effect rather than assuming a linear relationship between bilirubin and outcome, and iii) assessed the effect of jaundice duration as well as maximum bilirubin level. As shown in Table 9.2, their analysis failed to demonstrate a convincing effect of any bilirubin variable on i) 7 year intelligence quotient, ii) definite neurologic abnormality, or iii) sensorineural hearing loss. Moreover, the occurrence of athetosis was not associated with peak bilirubin levels. In fact, of the 61 infants with athetosis, 57 had peak serum bilirubin levels of <10 mg/dl (<171 μmol/l) and none exceeded 20 mg/dl (342 μmol/l). Newman and Klebanoff did report, however, a statistically significant association between increasing bilirubin levels and more subtle neurologic changes (e.g., awkwardness and abnormal cremasteric reflex) [Table 9.2].

These data, when taken together, demonstrate that otherwise healthy term (≥37 completed weeks of gestation) neonates without hemolytic disease i) can develop

Table 9.2. Newman and Klebanoff collaborative perinatal project analysis: outcome vs. bilirubin level.

Intelligence quotient	
White infants	$P = 0.50$
Black infants	$P = 0.11$
Definite abnormal neurological exam	$P = 0.10$
Abnormal or suspicious neurological exam	$P < .001$
Sensorineural hearing loss	$P = 0.67$

From, *Pediatrics* 1993; **92**: 651–657.

marked hyperbilirubinemia, ii) that such hyperbilirubinemia typically does not exceed the 20–25 mg/dl range and iii) that this level of hyperbilirubinemia does not appear to place such infants at risk for long-term adverse neurodevelopmental sequelae. These are clinically relevant observations as recent data demonstrate that ~1.7% of healthy neonates can be expected to develop hyperbilirubinemia to a level exceeding 20 mg/dl and ~1.3 in 1000 a level exceeding 25 mg/dl.[40] If one assumes that there are ~4 million live births in the United States per year, then ~68,000 infants would be expected to have peak serum bilirubin levels of >20 mg/dl and ~5,200 infants peak serum bilirubin levels in excess of 25 mg/dl.

In contrast to the overall reassuring nature of this extensive body of follow-up data, a recent retrospective cohort study published from Israel reported an association between the risk of IQ below 85 and bilirubin level greater than 20 mg/dl (342 μmol/l) in term infants.[41] This association was confined to male newborns and not observed in females. Moreover, no association was found between bilirubin levels and mean IQ risk, risk of neurologic abnormality, or hearing loss. The clinical relevance of the association between the risk of IQ below 85 and bilirubin level greater than 20 mg/dl (342 μmol/l) in term male infants remains unclear and has been called into question.[33] Specifically, given that the risk of low IQs was greater in those with high bilirubin levels, but mean IQ was unaffected, the increase in low IQ must have been offset by an increase in high IQs in this same group.[33] Moreover, the significant association in one of many outcome variables in just one group could easily have been due to chance.[33]

Another recent publication, however, convincingly demonstrates that in rare instances severe hyperbilirubinemia can develop in full term otherwise healthy infants and be associated with kernicterus.[42] In this review, six cases referred to Maisels and Newman by attorneys throughout the United States between 1979 and 1991 were identified as having classic signs of acute hyperbilirubinemic encephalopathy and typical neurologic sequelae. Table 9.3 demonstrates selected clinical data on these infants including peak bilirubin levels at 4 to 10 days after birth that ranged from 39.0 to 49.7 mg/dl. All affected infants were caucasian and breast-fed, none had evidence of hemolysis, and all were treated with exchange transfusion(s).

These cases highlight the remote but definable possibility that otherwise healthy term infants without evidence of hemolysis can develop marked hyperbilirubinemia and the associated adverse longterm neurodevelopmental sequelae. What predis-

Table 9.3. Clinical data on healthy term infants without hemolysis who developed kernicterus.

Case	Weight loss (%)	Peak bilirubin total/direct (mg/dl)	Age at peak bilirubin	Hgb (g/dl)
1	11	49.7/1.1	7 days	16.2
2	22	39.0/1.8	5 days	24.0
3	1	40.3/0.8	10 days	15.8
4	20	44.7/3.4	7 days	18.4
5	?	44.7/0.0	4 days	17.8
6	18	41.4/0.6	6 days	19.5

From *Pediatrics* 1995; **96**: 730–733.

posed these infants to develop this degree of hyperbilirubinemia is unclear. The only variable common to all cases was breast-feeding, but this is not sufficient to explain the occurrence of extreme hyperbilirubinemia. Interestingly, the conjugated bilirubin fraction in 5 of the 6 affected neonates was quite low despite the marked degree of hyperbilirubinemia suggesting a defect in conjugation. The fact that the bilirubin levels returned to normal in all infants eliminates the Crigler–Najjar syndrome as a possible cause. However, other defects in conjugating capacity, e.g., Gilbert's syndrome which has recently been demonstrated to modulate neonatal hyperbilirubinemia[43,44] could theoretically contribute to the genesis of severe jaundice. This and other possible genetic determinants of neonatal hyperbilirubinemia are current areas of active clinical investigation.

In a report analagous to Maisels and Newman, Brown and Johnson reviewed 21 recent cases of kernicterus in full term and near term (36 or 37 weeks gestation) infants.[45] In their series, all but one infant had short hospital stays after delivery, all infants were breast fed (11 were reported to be dehydrated upon hospital re-admission), eight infants were <37 completed weeks of gestation, and six infants had hemolysis underlying their marked hyperbilirubinemia. Peak serum bilirubin levels were 22 mg/dl or greater in affected infants.

The recent reports of kernicterus in the near term (34–37 week gestation) infant is a disturbing development.[42,45–47] These infants are typically cared for in normal newborn nurseries and in that context caretakers may be lured into thinking that such infants are as mature as infants born at term. Indeed, infants born at 34 to 37 weeks gestation can be managed like their more mature term (≥38 weeks) counterparts in many respects: i) they are large enough to maintain their temperature in an open crib; ii) they have an established suck-swallow reflex and can take their feedings by mouth (although not necessarily breast feed vigorously); and iii) they have a mature respiratory drive and are thus not prone to apnea. However, their ability to handle bilirubin is clearly limited placing them at risk for hyperbilirubinemic encephalopathy. Physiologic hyperbilirubinemia is more marked and protracted in this gestational age group as it is in premature infants as a whole (Figure 9.3).[48]

The combination of reduced hepatic clearance and less vigorous feeding can lead to marked hyperbilirubinemia particularly with a breast feeding primiparous mother.

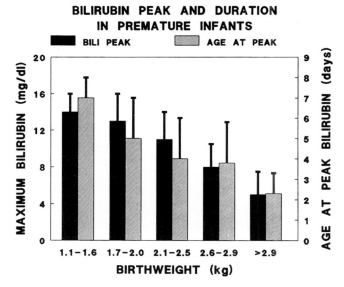

Figure 9.3. Bar graph demonstrating maximum bilirubin levels (mg/dl) and age at peak bilirubin level (days) in premature infants as a function of birthweight (kg). These data reflect the natural history of physiologic hyperbilirubinemia in the absence of any therapeutic intervention (i.e., phototherapy or exchange transfusion). From *B. M. J.* 1954; 2: 1263–1265.

Moreover, the hyperbilirubinemia may go undetected in the current era of early hospital discharge after birth, inadequate support systems for breast feeding, and a lack of timely outpatient follow-up and evaluation. These reports demonstrate that pediatricians must remain alert to the development of unexpected severe hyperbilirubinemia after hospital discharge in otherwise healthy term and near term infants.[42,45–47] This issue is discussed in further detail in Chapter 10.

Well over half of newborns will become clinically jaundiced in the first few days of life. Although in very rare circumstances full term (≥37 completed weeks of gestation) otherwise healthy newborns can develop unusually severe hyperbilirubinemia associated with neurologic sequelae,[42,45–47] the vast majority will manifest more moderate degrees of jaundice, infrequently exceeding the 20–25 mg/dl range.[40,47] Current estimates are that maximum serum bilirubin levels of >25 mg/dl occur in 1 in 770 infants and levels of >30 mg/dl in about 1 in 10,000 infants.[40,47] Peak serum bilirubin levels of less than 25 mg/dl have not been convincingly shown to cause neurologic impairment in healthy term neonates. Moreover, the evaluation and intervention for hyperbilirubinemia may not be totally innocuous.[32,33,49,50] In this context, the American Academy of Pediatrics established practice guidelines on the management of hyperbilirubinemia in the healthy term (≥37 completed weeks of gestation) newborn.[51,52] These guidelines concisely and accurately reflect the results of numerous clinical studies performed over the past several decades worldwide and offer a less aggressive therapeutic stance in the utilization of phototherapy and exchange transfusion in managing hyperbilirubinemia in such infants. To represent more accurately remaining uncertainties about when to treat jaundice in otherwise heathy term newborns without hemolytic disease, the current criteria for therapeutic intervention are given for ranges of serum bilirubin levels rather than single numbers.[51,52] These ranges also acknowledge the important role clinical judgment plays in deciding whether or not to institute phototherapy and/or exchange transfusion in the management of infants with hyperbilirubinemia. A discussion of these management guidelines is presented in Chapter 10.

PREMATURE NEONATES AND KERNICTERUS

Infants born prematurely are at increased risk for kernicterus as compared with their term counterparts. Reports from the 1950's and early 1960's not only demonstrated kernicterus in this population of newborns but also its occurrence in the absence of isoimmunization.[53,54] The latter was a novel observation and suggested that peak bilirubin levels associated with physiologic jaundice could exceed the threshold for the development of hyperbilirubinemic encephalopathy in this population of newborns. Subsequent observational studies from this period, however, demonstrated that kernicterus or the neurodevelopmental sequelae of hyperbilirubinemic encephalopathy in premature infants were typically noted only when serum bilirubin levels exceeded the 18−22 mg/dl range.[55–59] Characteristic of the debate that would evolve around the issue of neurologic outcome of premature infants with hyperbilirubinemia were two abstracts presented at the 1960 meeting of the Society for Pediatric Research. Heimer and colleagues[60] reported that increasing values of bilirubin were associated with impaired gross motor development in premature boys whereas Shiller and Silverman[61,62] failed to demonstrate any association between hyperbilirubinemia and brain damage in the low birth weight neonate. W.A. Silverman offered the following trenchant insight at the meeting:

> I would like to say that both studies reported this afternoon (ours and the one reported by the Brooklyn group) are observational studies and as such suffer from an important limitation. Wallis and Roberts recently pointed out, "If data arise from experience rather than experiment – that is fall into one class or another [eg, low bilirubin, high bilirubin] according to forces which are neither controlled by the researchers nor fully understood by them – there may be differences between groups that induce a spurious association. Only if the data arise from experiment can there be complete confidence in the absence of spurious associations" . . . The conflicting results reported this afternoon call for an experimental approach. Although we cannot assign individuals to hyper and hypobilirubinemia categories in random order, certainly a comparative randomized trial of the influence of exchange transfusion can be carried out. In view of the available evidence such a trial would be morally justified.[63]

In 1965 Wishingrad and colleagues published their results from just such an investigation and demonstrated no differences in neurologic follow-up among the exchange (18 mg/dl threshold for exchange transfusion), non-exchange (bilirubin exceeded 18 mg/dl but not exchanged), and control (premature infants whose bilirubin never exceeded 15 mg/dl) groups.[64] Other studies from this time period failed to demonstrate an association between serum bilirubin levels of less than 20 mg/dl and neurodevelopmental sequelae in the premature neonate.[59,62,65–67] It should be remembered, however, that the premature infants described in these investigations were significantly larger and more mature (32–36 weeks gestation) than the extremely low birth weight premature infants cared for in today's neonatal intensive care units.

Indeed, in the era that followed, premature infants were frequently observed to develop kernicterus at bilirubin levels considerably lower than 20 mg/dl – the so called "low bilirubin kernicterus". In a series of studies published from 1958 through 1972, kernicterus was described in premature infants at bilirubin levels ranging from 10–18 mg/dl.[68–72] This was a time of emerging new technologies and the management of smaller and more premature neonates including, for the first time, appreciable numbers of newborns with birth weights of less than 1000 g and gestational ages of less than 28 weeks. As a result, authors recommended exchange transfusions at much lower serum bilirubin levels than previously used in the very low birth weight premature infant, and these levels were utilized in the NICHD Phototherapy Study.[73] Support for lower bilirubin exchange thresholds was bolstered by the publication of the Collaborative Perinatal Project studies demonstrating an association between impaired psychomotor performance and hyperbilirubinemia (bilirubin levels >10–14 mg/dl) in low birth weight infants.[74,75]

A series of studies published in the 1980's, however, added a new dimension to the debate on the genesis of kernicterus in the premature neonate. These postmortem studies demonstrated that i) there was no statistical association between kernicterus and the clinical factors felt to place premature infants at risk for kernicterus (Table 9.4),[76,77] ii) gross bilirubin staining of the brain in the absence of associated microscopic neuronal damage of selected subcortical nuclei was frequently observed in the premature infant and this finding alone at postmortem examination did not represent

Table 9.4. Putative risk factors demonstrated not to predict the development of kernicterus in premature infants.

Birth weight*#
Gestational age*#
Peak total serum bilirubin level*#
Lowest pH#
Lowest temperature*#
Bilirubin–albumin molar ratio*
Infection*
Hypoxia*#
Hypercarbia#
Hypoglycemia*
Seizures*
Intracranial hemorrhage*

* From Kim *et al.*, *Pediatrics* 1980; **66**: 852–858.
# From, Turkel *et al.*, *Pediatrics* 1980; **66**: 502–506.

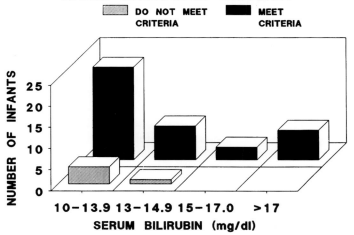

Figure 9.4. Bar graph documents the number of non-kernicteric infants expressed as a function of their NICHD Phototherapy Study exchange criteria status, and peak serum bilirubin level. Only "at risk" infants, i.e., those with peak serum bilirubin levels greater than or equal to 10 mg/dl are shown. The solid bars refer to infants who met NICHD Phototherapy Study criteria for exchange transfusion, whereas the hatched bars refer to those who did not meet such criteria. From *Pediatrics* 1994; **93**: 996–999. Reproduced by permission of Pediatrics.

true kernicterus,[9,78,79] and iii) the prevalence of kernicterus at autopsy in premature infants was declining dramatically.[78,79]

Moreover, one study further demonstrated that kernicterus was unlikely to occur even when serum bilirubin levels rose above those previously thought to place an infant at risk.[81] Fifty-six percent of non-kernicteric infants from this investigation had peak serum bilirubin levels greater than that suggested for exchange transfusion by NICHD Phototherapy Study guidelines, yet all but three were managed with phototherapy alone. Figure 9.4 shows the number of non-kernicteric study infants expressed as a function of their NICHD Phototherapy Study exchange criteria status and demonstrate that the majority of "at risk" non-kernicteric infants met exchange criteria and did so at a peak serum bilirubin level between 10 and 17 mg/dl.[81]

These data suggest that kernicterus is currently a rare event in premature infants hospitalized in NICUs. Indeed, several different institutions have reported a low prevalence of kernicterus at postmortem.[78,81,82]

HYPERBILIRUBINEMIC PREMATURE INFANTS AND SUBTLE CENTRAL NERVOUS SYSTEM INJURY

Kernicterus, however, may represent only one end of a spectrum of hyperbilirubinemic neurotoxicity in premature infants. Many have speculated that subtle central nervous system injury can result from lesser degrees of hyperbilirubinemia in this population of neonates. Studies in this vein have focused on i) cerebral palsy and ii) periventricular leukomalacia (PVL). Van de Bor and co-workers reported an association between serum bilirubin levels and cerebral palsy at two years of age in a large series of premature infants (<32 weeks gestation) as part of a National Collaborative Survey in Holland.[83] Children with minor and major handicaps had significantly higher bilirubin levels than those with normal outcomes and a consistent increase in the prevalence of handicaps was found for each 50 µmol/l (2.9 mg/dl) increase in maximal total serum bilirubin concentration.[83] On 5-year follow-up, however, the relationship between serum bilirubin level and neurodevelopmental outcome was no longer evident in the same cohort of infants except for those with intraventricular hemorrhage.[84] More recent follow-up studies performed on low birth weight neonates have failed to demonstrate a relationship between hyperbilirubinemia and cerebral palsy or early developmental delay even in infants with intraventricular hemorrhage.[85,86]

Other recent studies have raised the possibility that hyperbilirubinemia may be involved in the pathogenesis of cystic PVL.[87–89] These studies report an association between the highest serum bilirubin level and the development of cystic PVL. However, these data must be interpreted with caution because of the limitations of i) multiple significance testing (used in all three studies) with the resultant possibility of spurious conclusions, and ii) small sample size (one investigation had only 5 infants with cystic PVL).[87] With respect to the latter, a much larger study failed to demonstrate any association between cystic PVL and peak serum bilirubin level in the range of 2.3 to 22.5 mg/dl.[86] Finally, the hypothesis that hyperbilirubinemia is causally related to cystic PVL lacks a sound pathophysiologic rationale. PVL is primarily an ischemic lesion, most likely caused by hypoperfusion of the periventricular white matter. Hypotension, hypoxia, and hypocarbia are the most significant clinically related risk factors for the development of cystic PVL.[89–93] Bilirubin is not normally deposited in the periventricular region, and is primarily toxic to neurons and not the glial elements that predominate in the periventricular white matter.

PREMATURITY, HYPERBILIRUBINEMIA, AND SENSORINEURAL HEARING LOSS

Others speculate that hyperbilirubinemia may contribute to the genesis of sensorineural hearing loss (SNHL) in premature infants. SNHL as a consequence of severe hyperbilirubinemia in term infants with hemolytic disease has been well described.[3,5,94] Clinicopathologic[94] and functional evidence[96] have localized the site of auditory system damage following hyperbilirubinemia in erythroblastotic infants to the cochlear nuclei and auditory nerve. It has been noted that SNHL in erythroblastotic infants can occur in association with other neurologic sequelae characteristic of hyperbilirubinemic encephalopathy, or as the sole or outstanding residual deficit. The role of bilirubin in the genesis of SNHL in the preterm infant, however, is less clear (Table 9.5). A critical look at the literature cited to support the claim that

Table 9.5. Association between hyperbilirubinemia and sensorineural hearing loss in premature infants.

Support association	Does not support association
Naeye, 1978	Shiller & Silverman, 1961
Abramovich *et al.*, 1979	Crichton *et al.*, 1972
Anagnostakis *et al.*, 1982	van de Bor *et al.*, 1989
De Vries *et al.*, 1985	Scheidt *et al.*, 1990
Salamy *et al.*, 1989	Brown *et al.*, 1991

hyperbilirubinemia and SNHL may be causally related in premature infants, indeed, reveals a complicated picture and a tendency to overstate the dimensions of evidence.

Early studies on the long term effects of jaundice on neurodevelopmental outcome in premature infants generally failed to demonstrate a significant relationship between hyperbilirubinemia and SNHL,[62,97] even in the face of maximal serum bilirubin concentrations between 18 and 22 mg/dl.[62] At that time, ambient noise from incubators[98] and anoxia[99] were felt to be probable causes of hearing loss in such infants. Studies allegedly supporting the claim that SNHL in premature infants was causally linked to hyperbilirubinemia emerged in the late 1970's and early 1980's. One of the first such papers was that of Abramovich and co-workers.[100] Using stepwise logistic regression analysis these investigators identified recurrent apnea severe enough to require treatment with mechanical ventilation as the only significant independent predictor of SNHL. Of note, although statistically significant, recurrent apnea contributed only 5% of the variance in SNHL observed in their analysis. Hyperbilirubinemia (serum bilirubin concentration >10 mg/dl) made an additional contribution when combined with apnea but was not statistically significant as an independent variable.

Similarly, Anagnostakis and colleagues noted that infants with SNHL experienced more frequent apneic attacks associated with cyanosis than their gestationally age matched hearing intact controls.[101] They also reported that infants with SNHL ($n = 9$) were more likely to have had serum bilirubin concentrations exceeding 14 mg/dl. The latter relationship was observed in spite of their aggressive treatment of neonatal jaundice which included the use of exchange transfusion whenever serum bilirubin concentrations exceeded 1% of the babies weight expressed in grams.[101]

Devries and co-workers also reported a relationship between serum bilirubin levels >14 mg/dl and the development of SNHL in "high risk" preterm infants of birthweight <1500 g.[102] Infants were classified as "high risk" on the basis of the occurrence of one or more complications which included among others: i) birth asphyxia; ii) need for assisted ventilation; iii) pneumothorax; iv) proven infection; and v) periventricular hemorrhage. These investigators observed that the duration of hyperbilirubinemia and the number of acidotic episodes during the period of hyperbilirubinemia were significantly greater in preterm infants with SNHL as compared to hearing intact controls. When they later adopted a more aggressive practice in the management of hyperbilirubinemia similar to that of Anagnostakis *et al.*, they observed no new cases of SNHL in very low birth weight infants.[102]

Subsequently, Bergman and co-workers reported that prolonged respirator care, hyperbilirubinemia and hyponatremia were associated with the development of SNHL in preterm infants <1500 g[103] suggesting for the first time that the general underlying severity of the infants clinical course was an index of risk for SNHL. Of note, the peak serum bilirubin level as an independent variable was not significantly different between affected infants and controls on univariable testing. An additional observation of interest from this study was the finding that hyponatremia was associated with SNHL. As stated by the authors, the use of furosemide (a known ototoxic agent[104]) could have served as a link between the development of both hyponatremia and SNHL, but on univariable testing no significant difference in the use of furosemide was found between the hearing impaired and control groups. The use of aminoglycoside and total dose of aminoglycoside, however, was significantly associated with SNHL; in fact all affected infants had received aminoglycoside treatment. This observation is important as it relates to the hyponatremia, given the known synergistic interaction between loop diuretics and aminoglycoside therapy in producing irreversible ototoxicity.[104–107] It may be that affected infants were exposed to concurrent aminoglycoside and furosemide treatment whereas non-affected infants were not. Whether such a phenomenon was operative in this study cohort cannot be determined from the published data but offers an alternative explanation for the development of SNHL in their affected infants; an explanation that is supported by more recent investigations.[11,12]

The aforementioned studies as a group suggest that bilirubin is a potential adjunct to the genesis of SNHL but do not provide overwhelming support for its role as an independent risk factor for SNHL in preterm infants. Moreover, these studies must be considered in the context of other investigations that do not support the claim that hyperbilirubinemia and SNHL are related in very-low-birth weight preterm infants. For example, the follow-up data from the NICHD Randomized Controlled Trial of Phototherapy for Neonatal Hyperbilirubinemia demonstrated that phototherapy and control groups had similar rates of SNHL (phototherapy: 1.8%; control: 1.9%[108]) and that the severity of hearing loss when detected was not related to maximum serum bilirubin levels.[108] These infants were managed using conservative exchange transfusion guidelines, e.g., serum bilirubin levels of 13 mg/dl or less for high risk < 1,500 g infants, thus limiting the scope of their conclusions to this restricted range of bilirubin levels. Nevertheless, these data do suggest that this degree of hyperbilirubinemia is not associated with ototoxic potential.

More recent studies are also not entirely consistent with the notion that hyperbilirubinemia is causally related to SNHL in the very-low-birth weight infant. It is ironic that one of these studies is that of van de Bor and colleagues published in 1989[83] that raised the specter that maximal serum bilirubin level and cerebral palsy were causally related [a conclusion not borne out by follow-up at 5 years of age].[84] In their 1989 publication, not only was there no difference between the various maximum serum bilirubin concentration groups with respect to SNHL, but none of the infants in the study cohort with maximum serum bilirubin levels of 14.7 mg/dl or greater (14.7–17.5 mg/dl: $n = 44$; >17.5 mg/dl: $n = 6$; Table 2, ref# 83) had SNHL on follow-up.[83]

Another recent study confirms Bergman's earlier suggestion that the severity of the premature infants clinical course is the primary factor associated with the genesis of SNHL[11] while still others demonstrate that repeated exposure to ototoxic medications[11,12] or combinations of ototoxic drugs may play an important role[11,12] in the development of SNHL. In neither of these studies, however, was marked hyperbilirubinemia observed, limiting their application to address the role of severe hyperbilirubinemia in the genesis of SNHL in preterm infants. Nevertheless, the results of these studies i) suggest that moderate levels of hyperbilirubinemia pose little threat to the central nervous system of the preterm neonate, and ii) underscore the important role that other factors play in the genesis of SNHL in this population. In this regard, it is of interest to note that a significant decrease in the prevalence of SNHL in low-birth-weight preterm infants was observed upon the discontinuation of benzyl alcohol use in the NICU,[12] a change in practice also associated with a significant decline in kernicterus in preterm infants.[80] Whether benzyl alcohol was a causative factor itself in the genesis of these clinical problems or simply a predisposing factor is unknown. Some speculate that benzyl alcohol exposure led directly to concomitant neuronal injury that enhanced the susceptibility of the neuron to bilirubin toxicity.[80,109] Others suggest that as a membrane fluidizer, benzyl alcohol may have increased the permeability of the blood–brain barrier, leading to greater CNS bilirubin infux and risk for bilirubin associated neuronal injury. These remain unanswered questions. These data, however, should give us pause in assigning causation of SNHL to individual factors within the complex array of treatments provided in the NICU setting.

Consistent with the general tenor of the aforementioned literature on SNHL in preterm infants, the Guidelines for Perinatal Care of the American Academy of Pediatrics (3rd Edition)[110] conclude that "although there is some evidence of an association between hyperbilirubinemia and neurodevelopmental handicaps less severe than those associated with classic bilirubin encephalopathy, a cause-and-effect relationship has not been established. Furthermore, there is no information presently available to suggest that treating mild jaundice will prevent such handicaps".[110] Further clinical investigation is necessary to provide additional insights on the neurotoxic potential of bilirubin in premature neonates.

HYPERBILIRUBINEMIA AND PULMONARY HEMORRHAGE

Descriptive studies from the late 1940's and early 1950's cite an association between pulmonary hemorrhage and kernicterus.[111–113] These reports are frequently referenced in neonatal and pediatric texts and, on this basis, some have inferred a direct causal linkage between marked hyperbilirubinemia and the genesis of pulmonary bleeding. On closer inspection, however, it is apparent that a causal role for hyperbilirubinemia per se in the pathogenesis of pulmonary hemorrhage is doubtful.[114–117]

First of all, the cited reports allegedly linking kernicterus with pulmonary hemorrhage are descriptive in nature[111–113] and essentially limited to severely affected and fatal cases of erythroblastosis fetalis.[111–113,118,119] Severely affected infants with erythroblastosis fetalis have anemia, marked hypoalbuminemia, extramedullary hematopoiesis, frequently thrombocytopenia and a disturbance of coagulation,[118] and occasionally hydrops fetalis. The resultant increased intravascular hydrostatic and decreased oncotic pressures increase pulmonary capillary filtration pressure, a condition that may be further exacerbated by asphyxia and attendant left ventricular failure – common findings in severely affected and fatal cases of erythroblastosis fetalis. This constellation of forces can readily lead to hemorrhagic pulmonary edema in these critically ill neonates. Thus, the compromised cardiopulmonary status of severely affected cases of erythroblastosis fetalis is itself sufficient to account for the occurrences of pulmonary hemorrhage observed, i.e., it is not necessary to invoke a causal role for hyperbilirubinemia in this process. Indeed, in infants without erythroblastosis fetalis no association exists between kernicterus and pulmonary hemorrhage, i.e., pulmonary hemorrhage is not more frequent in kernicteric infants as compared with their non-kernicteric counterparts,[114–117](William Silverman, M.D., personal communication).

Secondly, data from animal models on this question provide conflicting results. One study that explored the effects of a sustained intravenous bilirubin infusion on neonatal animals suggested that hyperbilirubinemia was associated with multiple visceral hemorrhages, including the lungs, in 25–40% of subjects.[120] The conclusions of this investigation, however, are limited by the observation that several of the study animals manifested an early circulatory collapse and anoxia in response to the bilirubin infusion,[120] conditions well known to generate pulmonary hemorrhage themselves. In marked contrast, data reported on jaundiced Gunn rats, a widely used animal model of hyperbilirubinemia and kernicterus, demonstrate a significantly lower prevalence of pulmonary hemorrhage in kernicteric (9 of 26 rats) as compared with non-kernicteric (7 of 9 rats) animals [$p < 0.05$ Fishers Exact test], despite significantly higher serum bilirubin levels in the kernicteric group [16.7 ± 0.9 vs. 10.7 ± 1.4 mg/dl, $P < 0.01$].[121] The data on Gunn rats are in direct conflict with the notion that kernicterus or hyperbilirubinemia contribute to the genesis of pulmonary hemorrhage.

Finally, we are not aware of any cases of pulmonary hemorrhage in more recent reports of non-erythroblastotic infants with marked hyperbilirubinemia alone. This group encompasses a large number of infants, which along with the aforementioned human studies and conflicting results in animal models, argues against hyperbilirubinemia or kernicterus per se as a causal agents or predisposing conditions for pulmonary hemorrhage in humans.

SUMMARY

The classic triad of choreoathetosis, sensorineural hearing deficits, and impaired ocular supraversion was recognized decades ago as pathognomonic for the diagnosis of hyperbilirubinemic encephalopathy. Today these adverse neurodevelopmental sequelae are seldom seen secondary to a marked decrease in the prevalence of Rh sensitized pregnancies and the intensive management of hyperbilirubinemia in infants with hemolytic disease. Nevertheless there continues to be debate and study regarding the level of hyperbilirubinemia at which neurotoxicity is manifest in healthy full term infants without hemolysis and in infants born prematurely (<37 completed weeks gestation). The realization that instances of extreme hyperbilirubinemia can develop in otherwise healthy breast fed term or near term infants has renewed interest in this clinical area. In the future, an enhanced understanding of the epidemiology and pathogenesis of extreme hyperbilirubinemia in term and near term infants will likely further reduce the incidence of chronic postkernicteric neurodevelopmental sequelae.

References

1. Evans., P.R. and Polani, P.E., The neurological sequelae of Rh sensitization, *Quart. J. Med.* 1950; **19**: 129–149.
2. Vaughan III, V.C., Allen F.H. and Diamond, L.K., Erythroblastosis fetalis. IV. Further observations on kernicterus, *Pediatrics* 1950; **6**: 706–716.
3. Byers, R.K., Paine, R.S. and Crothers, B., Extrapyramidal cerebral palsy with hearing loss following erythroblastosis, *Pediatrics* 1955; **15**: 248–254.
4. Craig, W.S., Convulsive movements occurring in the first 10 days of life, *Arch. Dis. Child.* 1960; **35**: 336–344.
5. Perlstein, M.A., The late clinical syndrome of posticteric encephalopathy, *Pediatr. Clin. North Am.* 1960; **7**: 665–687.
6. Van Praagh, R., Diagnosis of kernicterus in the neonatal period, *Pediatrics* 1961; **28**: 870–876.
7. Notter, M.F.D. and Kendig, J.W., Differential sensitivity of neural cells to bilirubin toxicity, *Exp. Neurol.* 1986; **94**: 670–682.
8. Ahdab-Barmada, M., Neonatal kernicterus: neuropathologic diagnosis. In: Levine, R.L. and Maisels, M.J., eds. Hyperbilirubinemia in the Newborn. Columbus, OH: Ross Laboratories, 1983; 2–10.
9. Ahdab-Barmada, M. and Moossy, J., The neuropathology of kernicterus in the premature neonate: diagnostic problems, *J. Neuropathol. Exp. Neurol.* 1984; **43**: 45–56.
10. Foley, J., Dyskinetic and dystonic cerebral palsy, *Acta. Paediatr.* 1992; **81**: 57–60.
11. Salamy, A., Eldredge, L. and Tooley, W.H., Neonatal status and hearing loss in high-risk infants, *J. Pediatr.* 1989; **114**: 847–852.
12. Brown, D.R., Watchko, J.F. and Sabo, D., Neonatal sensorineural hearing loss associated with furosemide: a case-control study, *Dev. Med. Child Neurol.* 1991; **33**: 816–823.
13. Hoyt, C.S., Billson, F.A. and Alpins, N., The supranuclear disturbances of gaze in kernicterus, *Ann. Opthamol.* 1978; **10**: 1487–1492.
14. Marcus, J.C., The clinical syndromes of kernicterus. In: Levine, R.L. and Maisels, M.J., eds. Hyperbilirubinemia in the Newborn. Columbus, OH: Ross Laboratories, 1983, pp. 18–26.
15. Palmer, C. and Smith, M.B., Assessing the risk of kernicterus using nuclear magnetic resonance, *Clin. Perinatol.* 1990; **17**: 307–329.
16. Inoue, E., Hori, S. and Narumi, Y., Portal-systemic encephalopathy: presence of basal ganglia lesions with high signal intensity on MR images, *Radiology* 1991; **179**: 551–555.
17. Penn, A.A., Enzmann, D.R., Hahn, J.S. and Stevenson, D.K., Kernicterus in a full term infant, *Pediatrics* 1994; **93**: 1003–1006.
18. Martich-Kriss, V., Kollias, S.S. and Ball, W.S., MR findings in kernicterus, *Am. J. Neuroradiol.* 1995; **16**: 819–821.
19. Yokochi, K., Magnetic resonance imaging in children with kernicterus, *Acta. Paediatr.* 1995; **84**: 937–939.
20. Grobler, J.M. and Mercer, M.J., Kernicterus associated with elevated predominately direct-reacting bilirubin, *S. Afr. Med. J.* 1997; **87**: 146.
21. Hoon, A.H., Reinhardt, E.M., Kelley, R.I., Breiter, S.N., Morton, D.H., Naidu, S. and Johnston, M.V., Brain magnetic resonance imaging in suspected extrapyramidal cerebral palsy: observations in distinguishing genetic-metabolic from acquired causes, *J. Pediatr.* 1997; **131**: 240–245.
22. Day, R. and Haines, M.S., Intelligence quotients of children recovered from erythroblastosis fetalis since the introduction of exchange transfusion, *Pediatrics* 1954; **13**: 333–337.
23. Johnston, W.H., Angara, V., Baumal, R., Hawke, W.A., Johnson, R.H., Keet, S. and Wood, M., Erythroblastosis fetalis and hyperbilirubinemia: A five year follow-up with neurological, psychological, and audiological evaluation, *Pediatrics* 1967; **39**: 88–92.

24. Ozmert, E., Erdem, G., Topcu, M., Yurdakok, M., Tekinalp, G., Genc, D. and Renda, Y., Long-term follow-up of indirect hyperbilirubinemia in full-term Turkish infants, *Acta. Paediatr.* 1996; **85**: 1440–1444.

25. Johnson, L. and Boggs, T.R., Bilirubin-dependent brain damage: incidence and indications for treatment. In: Odell, G.B., Schaffer, R. and Simopoulos, A.P., eds. Phototherapy in the Newborn: An Overview. Washington, D.C., National Academy of Sciences, 1974, pp. 122–149.

26. Beutler, E., G6PD deficiency, *Blood* 1994; **84**: 3613–3636.

27. MacDonald, M.G., Hidden risks: early discharge and bilirubin toxicity due to glucose-6-phosphate dehydrogenase deficiency, *Pediatrics* 1995; **96**: 734–738.

28. Valaes, T., Severe neonatal jaundice associated with glucose-6-phosphate dehydrogenase deficiency: pathogenesis and global epidemiology, *Acta. Paediatr.* Suppl. 1994; **394**: 58–76.

29. Mores, A., Fargasova, I. and Minarikova, E., The relation of hyperbilirubinemia in newborns without isoimmunization to kernicterus, *Acta. Paediatr.* 1959; **48**: 590–602.

30. Killander, A., Michaelsson, M., Muller-Eberhard, U. and Sjolin, S., Hyperbilirubinemia in full term newborn infants: A follow-up study, *Acta. Paediatr. Scand.* 1963; **52**: 481–484.

31. Killander, A., Muller-Eberhard, U. and Sjolin, S., Indications for exchange transfusion in newborn infants with hyperbilirubinemia not due to Rh immunization, *Acta. Paediatr. Scand.* 1960; **49**: 377–390.

32. Newman, T.B. and Maisels, M.J., Does hyperbilirubinemia damage the brain of healthy full-term infants? *Clin. Perinatol.* 1990; **17**: 331–358.

33. Newman, T.B. and Maisels, M.J., Evaluation and treatment of jaundice in the term newborn: a kinder, gentler approach, *Pediatrics* 1992; **89**: 809–818.

34. Hardy, J.B. and Peeples, M.O., Serum bilirubin levels in newborn infants: distributions and associations with neurologic abnormalities during the first year of life, *Johns Hopkins Med. J.* 1971; **128**: 265–272.

35. Fohl, E. and Lombos, O., The prognosis of neonatal hemolysis due to A-B-O incompatibility, without exchange transfusion, *Ann. Pediatr.* 1964; **203**: 279–287.

36. Holmes, G.E., Miller, J.B. and Smith, E.E., Neonatal hyperbilirubinemia in production of long-term neurological deficits, *A.J.D.C.* 1968; **116**: 37–43.

37. Culley, P., Powell, J. and Waterhouse, J., Sequelae of neonatal jaundice, *Br. Med. J.* 1970; **3**: 383–386.

38. Bengtsson, B. and Verneholt, J., A follow-up study of hyperbilirubinemia in healthy, full term infants without isoimmunization, *Acta. Paediatr. Scand.* 1974; **63**: 70–80.

39. Newman, T.B. and Klebanoff, M.A., Neonatal hyperbilirubinemia and long-term outcome: another look at the Collaborative Perinatal Project, *Pediatrics* 1993; **92**: 651–657.

40. Newman, T.B., Escobar, G.J., Branch, P.T., Armstrong, M.A., Folck B.F. and Gardner, M.N., Incidence of extreme hyperbilirubinemia in a large HMO, *Ambulatory Child Health* 1997; **3**: 203.

41. Seidman, D.S., Paz, I., Stevenson D.K., Laor, A., Danon, Y.L. and Gale, R., Neonatal hyperbilirubinemia and physical and cognitive performance at 17 years of age, *Pediatrics* 1991; **88**: 828–833.

42. Maisels, M.J. and Newman, T.B., Kernicterus in otherwise healthy, breast-fed term newborns, *Pediatrics* 1995; **96**: 730–733.

43. Bancroft, J.D., Kreamer, B. and Gourley, G.R., Gilbert syndrome accelerates development of neonatal jaundice, *J. Pediatr.* 1998; **132**: 656–660.

44. Kaplan, M., Renbaum, P., Levy-Lahad, E., Hammerman, C., Lahad, A. and Beutler, E., Gilbert syndrome and glucose-6-phosphate dehydrogenase deficiency: a dose-dependent genetic interaction crucial to neonatal hyperbilirubinemia, *Proc. Natl. Acad. Sci. USA* 1997; **94**: 12128–12132.

45. Brown, A.K. and Johnson, L., Loss of concern about jaundice and the reemergence of kernicterus in full-term infants in the era of managed care. In: Fanaroff, A.A. ed. The Year Book of Neonatal and Perinatal Medicine, St. Louis: Mosby, 1996, pp. xvii–xxviii.

46. Johnson, L., Hyperbilirubinemia in the term infant: when to worry, when to treat, *N.Y. State J. Med.* 1991; **91**: 483–489.

47. Maisels, M.J. and Newman, T.B., Jaundice in full term and near term babies who leave the hospital within 36 hours – the pediatrician's nemesis, *Clin. Perinatol.* 1998; **25**: 295–302.

48. Billing, B.H., Cole, P.G. and Lathe, G.H., Increased plasma bilirubin in newborn infants in relation to birth weight, *B.M.J.* 1954; **2**: 1263–1265.

49. Kemper, K., Forsyth, B. and McCarthy, P., Jaundice, terminating breast feeding, and the vulnerable child, *Pediatrics* 1982; **84**: 773–778.

50. Newman, T.B., Easterling, M.J. and Stevenson, D.K., Laboratory evaluation of jaundice in newborns. Frequency, cost, and yield, *A.J.D.C.* 1990; **144**: 364–368.

51. American Academy of Pediatrics, Provisional Committee for Quality Improvement and Subcommittee on Hyperbilirubinemia. Practice parameter: management of hyperbilirubinemia in the healthy term newborn, *Pediatrics* 1994; **94**: 558–562.
52. Erratum, *Pediatrics* 1995; **95**: 458–461, 1995.
53. Aiden, R., Corner, B. and Tovey, G., Kernicterus and prematurity, *Lancet* 1950; **1**: 1153–1154.
54. Zuelzer, W.W. and Mudgett, R.T., Kernicterus: etiologic study based on an analysis of 55 cases, *Pediatrics* 1950; **6**: 452–474.
55. Crosse V.M., Meyer, T.C. and Gerrard, J.W., Kernicterus and prematurity, *Arch. Dis. Child.* 1955; **30**: 501–508.
56. Meyer, T.C., A study of serum bilirubin levels in relation to kernicterus and prematurity, *Arch. Dis. Child.* 1956; **31**: 75–80.
57. Crosse, V.M., Wallis, P.G. and Walsh, A.M., Replacement transfusion as a means of preventing kernicterus of prematurity, *Arch. Dis. Child.* 1958; **33**: 403–408.
58. Crosse, V.M. and Obst, D., The incidence of kernicterus (not due to haemolytic disease) among premature babies. In: Sass-Korstak, A., ed. Kernicterus. Toronto, Canada: University of Toronto Press, 1961; 4–9.
59. Koch, C.A., Jones, D.V., Dine, M.S. and Wagner, E.A., Hyperbilirubinemia in premature infants: a follow-up study, *J. Pediatr.* 1959; **55**: 23–29.
60. Heimer, C.B., Braine, M.D., Kowlessar, M. *et al.*, The sequelae of neonatal hyperbilirubinemia of prematurity at age one year, *AJDC* 1960; **100**: 495–496.
61. Shiller, J.G. and Silverman, W.A., The lack of association between hyperbilirubinemia and brain damage of prematurity, *AJDC* 1960; **100**: 496–497.
62. Shiller, J.G. and Silverman, W.A., Uncomplicated hyperbilirubinemia of prematurity, *AJDC* 1961; **101**: 587–592.
63. Silverman, W.A. Discussion, *AJDC* 1960; **100**: 497–500.
64. Wishingrad, L., Cornblath, M., Takakuwa, T. *et al.*, Studies of non-hemolytic hyperbilirubinemia in premature infants, *Pediatrics* 1965; **36**: 162–172.
65. Grewar, D.A.I., Experiences with kernicterus in premature infants. In: Sass-Korstak, A., ed. Kernicterus. Toronto, Canada: University of Toronto Press, 1961; 13–19.
66. Koch, C.A., Hyperbilirubinemia in premature infants: a follow-up study, II; *Pediatr.* 1964; **65**: 1–11.
67. Vuchovich, D.M., Haimowitz, N., Bowers, N.D., Cosbey, J. and Hsia, D., The influence of serum bilirubin levels upon the ultimate development of low birthweight infants, *J. Ment. Defic. Res.* 1965; **9**: 51–60.
68. Harris, R.C., Lucey, J.F. and MacLean, J.R., Kernicterus in premature infants associated with low concentrations of bilirubin in the plasma, *Pediatrics* 1958; **21**: 875–883.
69. Stern, L. and Denton, R.L., Kernicterus in small premature infants, *Pediatrics* 1965; **35**: 483–485.
70. Gartner, L.M., Snyder, R.N., Chabon, R.S. and Bernstein, J., Kernicterus: high incidence in premature infants with low serum bilirubin concentrations, *Pediatrics* 1970; **45**: 906–917.
71. Ackerman, B.D., Dyer, G.Y. and Leydorf, M.M., Hyperbilirubinemia and kernicterus in small premature infants, *Pediatrics* 1970; **45**: 918–925.
72. Keenan, W.J., Perlstein, P.H., Light, I.J. and Sutherland, J.M., Kernicterus in small sick premature infants receiving phototherapy, *Pediatrics* 1972; **49**: 652–655.
73. National Institute of Child Health Human Development randomized, controlled trial of phototherapy for neonatal hyperbilirubinemia, *Pediatrics* 1985; **75**(suppl): 385–441.
74. Scheidt, P.C., Mellits, E.D., Hardy, J.B., Drage, J.S. and Boggs, T.R., Toxicity to bilirubin in neonates: infant development during first year in relation to maximum neonatal serum bilirubin concentration, *J. Pediatr.* 1977; **91**: 292–297.
75. Naeye, R.L., Amniotic fluid infections, neonatal hyperbilirubinemia, and psychomotor impairment, *Pediatrics* 1978; **62**: 497–503.
76. Turkel, S.B., Guttenberg, M.E., Moynes, D.R. and Hodgman, J.E., Lack of identifiable risk factors for kernicterus, *Pediatrics* 1980; **66**: 502–506.
77. Kim, M.H., Yoon, J.J., Sher, J. and Brown, A.K., Lack of predictive indices in kernicterus: a comparison of clinical and pathologic factors in infants with and without kernicterus, *Pediatrics* 1980; **66**: 852–858.
78. Maisels, M.J., Clinical studies of the sequelae of hyperbilirubinemia. In: Levine, R.L. and Maisels, M.J., eds. Hyperbilirubinemia in the Newborn. Columbus, OH: Ross Laboratories, 1983; 26–35.
79. Turkel, S.B., Miller, C.A., Guttenberg, M.E., Moynes, D.R. and Hodgman, J.E., A clinical pathologic reappraisal of kernicterus, *Pediatrics* 1982; **69**: 267–272.

80. Jardine, D.S. and Rogers, K., Relationship of benzyl alcohol to kernicterus, intraventricular hemorrhage, and mortality in preterm infants, *Pediatrics* 1989; **83**: 153–160.

81. Watchko, J.F. and Claassen, D., Kernicterus in premature infants: current prevalence and relationship to NICHD Phototherapy Study exchange criteria, *Pediatrics* 1994; **93**: 996–999.

82. Pearlman, M.A., Gartner, L.M., Lee, K., Morecki, R. and Horoupian, D.S., Absence of kernicterus in low-birth-weight infants from 1971- through 1976: comparison with findings in 1966 and 1967, *Pediatrics* 1978; **62**: 460–464.

83. van de Bor, M., Zeben-van der Aa, T.M., Verloove-Vanhorick, S.P., Brand, R. and Ruys, J.H., Hyperbilirubinemia in preterm infants and neurodevelopmental outcome at 2 years of age: Results of a National Collaborative Survey, *Pediatrics* 1989; **83**: 915–920.

84. van de Bor, M., Ens-Dokkum, M., Schreuder, A.M., Veen, S., Brand, R. and Verloove-Vanhorick, S.P., Hyperbilirubinemia in low birth weight infants and outcome at 5 years of age, *Pediatrics* 1992; **89**: 359–364.

85. O'Shea, T.M., Dillard, R.G., Klinepeter, K.L. and Goldstein, D.J., Serum bilirubin levels, intracranial hemorrhage, and the risks of developmental problems in very low birth weight neonates, *Pediatrics* 1992; **90**: 888–892.

86. Graziani, L.J., Mitchell, D.G., Kornhauser, M., Pidcock, F.S., Merton, D.A., Stanley, C. and McKee, L., Neurodevelopment of preterm infants: neonatal neurosonographic and serum bilirubin studies, *Pediatrics* 1992; **89**: 229–234.

87. Ikonen, R.S., Kuusinen, E.J., Janas, M.O., Koivikko, M.J. and Sorto, A.E., Possible etiologic factors in extensive periventricular leukomalacia of preterm infants, *Acta Paeditr. Scand.* 1988; **77**: 489–495.

88. Trounce, J.Q., Shaw, D.E., Levine, M.I. and Rutter, N., Clinical risk factors and periventricular leucomalacia, *Arch. Dis. Child.* 1988; **63**: 17–22.

89. Ikonen, R.S., Koivkko, M.J., Laippala and Kuusinen, E.J., Hyperbilirubinemia, hypocarbia and periventricular leukomalacia in preterm infants: relationship to cerebral palsy, *Acta. Paediatr.* 1992; **81**: 802–807.

90. Banker, B.Q. and Larroche, J.C., Periventricular leukomalacia of infancy. a form of neonatal anoxic encephalopathy, *Arch. Neurol.* 1962; **7**: 386–410.

91. Friis-Hansen, B., Perinatal brain injury and cerebral blood flow in newborn infants, *Acta. Paediatr. Scand.* 1985; **74**: 323–331.

92. Young, R.S.K., Hernandez, M.J. and Yagel, S.K., Selective reduction of blood flow to white matter during hypotension in newborn dogs: a possible mechanism of periventricular leukomalacia, *Ann. Neurol.* 1982; **12**: 445–448.

93. Calvert, S.A., Hoskins, E.M., Fong, K.W. and Forsyth, S.C., Etiological factors associated with the development of periventricular leukomalacia, *Acta. Paediatr. Scand.* 1987; **76**: 254–259.

94. Crabtree, N. and Gerard, J., Perceptive deafness associated with severe neonatal jaundice. A report of sixteen cases, *J. Laryngol.* 1950; **64**: 482–506.

95. Dublin, W.B., Neurologic lesions of erythroblastosis fetalis in relation to nuclear deafness, *Am. J. Clin. Pathol.* 1951; **21**: 935–939.

96. Chisin, R., Perlman, M. and Sohmer, H., Cochlear and brain stem responses in hearing loss following neonatal hyperbilirubinemia, *Ann. Otol. Rhinol. Laryngol.* 1979; **88**: 352–357.

97. Crichton, J.U., Dunn, H.G., McBurney, A.K., Robertson, A.M. and Tredger, E., Long term effects of neonatal jaundice on brain function in children of low birth weight, *Pediatrics* 1972; **49**: 656–670.

98. Douek, E., Bannister, L.H., Dodson, H.C., Ashcroft, P. and Humphries, K.N., Effects of incubator noise on the cochlea of the newborn, *Lancet* 1976; **2**: 1110–1113.

99. McDonald, A.D., Deafness in children of very low birth weight, *Arch. Dis. Child.* 1964; **39**: 272–277.

100. Abramovich, S.J., Gregory, S., Slemick, M. and Stewart, A., Hearing loss in very low birthweight infants treated with neonatal intensive care, *Arch. Dis. Child.* 1979; **54**: 421–426.

101. Anagnostakis, D., Petmezakis, J., Papazissis, G., Messaritakis, J. and Matsaniotis, N., Hearing loss in low-birth-weight infants, *AJDC* 1982; **136**: 602–604.

102. de Vries, L.S., Lary, S. and Dubowitz, L.M.S., Relationship of serum bilirubin levels to ototoxicity and deafness in high-risk low-birth-weight infants, *Pediatrics* 1985; **76**: 351–354.

103. Bergman, I., Hirsch R.P., Fria, T.J., Shapiro, S.M., Holzman, I. and Painter, M.J., Cause of hearing loss in the high-risk premature infant, *J. Pediatr.* 1985; **106**: 95–101.

104. Rybak, L.P., Furosemide ototoxicity: clinical and experimental aspects, *Laryngoscope 95*: Suppl. 1985; **38**: 1–14.

105. Brummett, R.E., Effects of antibiotic–diuretic interactions in the guinea pig model of ototoxicity, *Reviews of Infectious Diseases* Suppl. 1981; **3**: S216–S223.

106. Brummett, R.E. and Fox, K.E., Studies of aminoglycoside ototoxicity in animal models. In: Welton, A., Neu, H.C., eds. The Aminoglycosides. Microbiology, Clinical Use and Toxicology. New York: Marcel Dekker, 1982.

107. Brummett, R.E., Traynor, J., Brown, R. and Himes, D., Cochlear damage resulting from kanamycin and furosemide, *Acta. Otolaryngol.* 1975; **80**: 86–92.

108. Scheidt, P.C., Bryla, D.A., Nelson, K.B. Hirtz, D.G. and Hoffman, H.J., Phototherapy for neonatal hyperbilirubinemia: six-year follow-up of the National Institute of Child Health and Human Development clinical trial, *Pediatrics* 1990; **85**: 455–463.

109. Volpe, J.J., Bilirubin and brain injury. In: Volpe, J.J., Neurology of the Newborn. 3rd ed. Philadelphia: W.B. Saunders, 1995, pp. 490–514.

110. Guidelines for Perinatal Care. 3rd ed. Elk Grove Village, IL, American Academy of Pediatrics, 1992, 204–210.

111. Ahvenainen, E.K. and Call, J.D., Pulmonary hemorrhage in infants. A descriptive study, *Am. J. Path.* 1952; **28**: 1–18.

112. Zuelzer, W.W. and Mudgett, R.T., Kernicterus. Etiologic study based on an analysis of 55 cases, *Pediatrics* 1950; **6**: 452–474.

113. Vaughan, V.C., Kernicterus in erythroblastosis fetalis, *J. Pediatr.* 1946; **29**: 462–473.

114. Silverman, W.A., Andersen, D.H., Blanc, W.A. and Crozier, D.N., A difference in mortality rate and incidence of kernicterus among premature infants allotted to two prophylactic antibacterial regimens, *Pediatrics* 1956; **18**: 614–625.

115. Silverman, W.A., Neonatal Bilirubinemia. In: Silverman, W.A., Dunham's Premature Infants. 3rd ed. New York: Paul B. Hoeber, Inc., 1961, pp. 199–223.

116. Silverman, W.A., Other Noninfectious Pulmonary Conditions. In: Silverman, W.A., Dunham's Premature Infants. 3rd ed. New York: Paul B. Hoeber, Inc., 1961, pp. 251–258.

117. Van Praagh, R., Causes of death in infants with hemolytic disease of the newborn (erythroblastosis fetalis), *Pediatrics* 1961; **28**: 223–233.

118. Diamond, L.K., Allen, F.H., Vann, D.D. and Powers, J.R., Round table discussion: erythroblastosis fetalis, *Pediatrics* 1952; **10**: 337–347.

119. Chessells, J.M. and Wigglesworth, J.S., Haemostatic failure in babies with Rhesus isoimmunization, *Arch. Dis. Child.* 1971; **46**: 38–45.

120. Rozdilsky, B. and Olszewski, J., Experimental study of the toxicity of bilirubin in newborn animals, *J. Neuropath. Exper. Neurol.* 1961; **20**: 193–205.

121. Johnson, L., Sarmiento, F., Blanc, W.A. and Day, R., Kernicterus in rats with an inherited deficiency of glucuronyl transferase, *A.M.A. Am. J. Dis. Child.* 1959; **97**: 591–608.

Clinical Management

10 The Clinical Approach to the Jaundiced Newborn

M. Jeffrey Maisels

Department of Pediatrics, William Beaumont Hospital, Royal Oak, Michigan, USA

NORMAL SERUM BILIRUBIN LEVELS AND THE NATURAL HISTORY OF NEONATAL JAUNDICE

In spite of multiple studies of normal newborn populations, the definition of what represents a "normal bilirubin level" has proven elusive. The main reason for this is that total serum bilirubin (TSB) levels vary considerably depending on the racial composition of the population, the incidence of breast-feeding, other genetic and epidemiologic factors and the laboratory methods used for measuring bilirubin levels (see Figure 10.1 and Chapter 3). Mean TSB bilirubin levels in cord blood range from 1.4–1.9 mg/dl (24–32 μmol)[1,2] and elevated cord TSB levels are associated with an increased risk of hyperbilirubinemia.[2–5] For years textbooks have described the natural history of neonatal jaundice as a serum bilirubin level that rises after birth, reaches its apex on about the 3rd day and then declines by about a week – a description consistent with the infants reported by Gartner *et al*.[6] These infants were all formula fed, half were black and half white and reference to Figure 10.1 shows that their TSB levels are quite different from those of a predominantly breast fed population. In populations where 60–70% or more of the infants have been fully or partially breast-fed, the TSB levels are substantially higher, do not reach their peak until the 4th or 5th day and, when followed for long enough, show no clinically important decline even by the 6th or 7th day. In a study of 312 breast-fed English infants, the mean TSB level on day 6 was 8.4 mg/dl (144 μmol/l).[7] Thus, TSB levels obtained from newborns prior to hospital discharge (unless they remain in hospital for 5–7 days) are quite misleading,[8] because they will miss the peak bilirubin levels in a large portion of the population.

For many years we have used population norms derived from the data of the National Collaborative Perinatal Project (CPP).[9] This study was conducted from 1955–1961 when 30% or fewer mothers breast-fed their infants in hospital. Serum bilirubin levels were measured at about 48 hours on every one of 34,049 infants, with

Address for correspondence: M. Jeffrey Maisels, M.D., 3535 W. 13 Mile Road, Royal Oak, MI 48073, Phone: (248) 551-0412, Fax: (248) 551-5998, E-mail: jmaisels@beaumont.edu

Total Serum Bilirubin

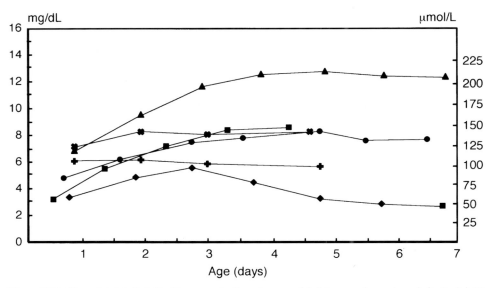

Figure 10.1. Mean total daily bilirubin concentrations in normal full term and near-term infants. (▲) 50 healthy Japanese newborn infants, 37–42 weeks of gestation, all breast-fed. Excludes Rh and ABO incompatibility.[112] (✖) 176 term breast-fed Canadian infants. Excludes Rh hemolytic disease, but includes 9 ABO incompatible infants with positive Coombs tests. 17 infants received phototherapy[1] (✚) 164 Canadian term formula-fed infants, 7 ABO incompatible with positive Coombs tests and 3 received phototherapy.[1] (■) 1087 term Israeli infants, 78% fully or partially breast-fed[16] (●) 56 Nigerian term AGA infants. Excludes ABO or Rh incompatibility and G6PD deficiency. Infants were "largely breast-fed".[113] (◆) 29 full-term American infants, all formula fed, about 50% African-American and 50% Caucasian.[6] From Maisels.[114]

birth weights >2500 gm, and repeated daily if the initial level was ≥10 mg/dl (171 μmol/l) until the value decreased to <10 mg/dl (171 μmol/l). Although this population included sick infants and those with hemolytic disease, 95% of all infants had TSB concentrations that did not exceed 12.9 mg/dl (215 μmol/l), and this (95th percentile) became the accepted upper limit of "physiologic jaundice". In a hospitalized population of 2,297 consecutive infants who weighed more than 2500 gm and were admitted to a well baby nursery between 1976 and 1980, we found that bilirubin levels of 13 mg/dl (222 μmol/l) or greater occurred in 6% of the population[8] virtually identical with the incidence (6.2%) in the CPP. More recent data[10–12] suggest that, at least in the US, we now see many more jaundiced babies and the bilirubin levels found in the normal population are significantly higher than previously reported. Thus, in Bhutani's population, (≥35 weeks gestation, 43% white, 41% black, 4% Asian, 59% fully or partially breast fed) the 95th percentile was a TSB of about 17.5 mg/dl (300 μmol/l).[11] In an international multicenter study of 261 well babies ≥36 weeks gestation from nurseries in the US, Hong Kong, and Israel (42% white, 14% black, 29% East Asian or Pacific Islander, 72% fully or partially breast fed) the 50th percentile for a TSB level at 96 ± 6.0 hr was 8.7 mg/dl (149 μmol/l) and the 95th

Total Serum Bilirubin

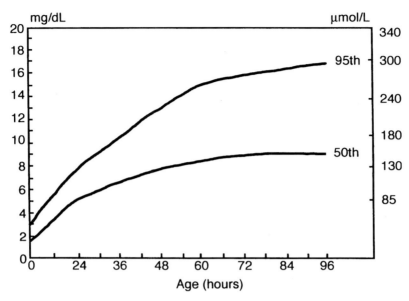

Figure 10.2. Smoothed curves from studies in diverse populations illustrating the expected velocity of total serum bilirubin (TSB) levels and approximate values for the 50th and 95th percentiles. Data for cord blood values come from the studies of Davidson,[3] and Saigal,[1] values in the first 12 hours from Frishberg[15] and subsequent values from Bhutani,[11] Seidman,[16] Maisels,[12] and Wood.[7] Data for the 95th percentile are primarily obtained from the data of Bhutani,[11] but also from the studies of Newman[10] and Maisels.[12] These data represent values that might be expected in a predominantly breast-fed (60–70%) population. In view of the significant variations in different populations (see Figure 10.1) as well as the variations found in laboratory measurement,[14] the values provided should be used only as rough guidelines. Nevertheless, this graph can be useful in plotting the course of neonatal jaundice because it will demonstrate when the velocity of the TSB increase deviates significantly from the curves shown. *Note that the values must be plotted according to the infant's age in hours, not days.* Infants who have values that exceed the 95th percentile deserve an evaluation to determine a potential cause for the jaundice and they require careful surveillance and follow-up to prevent the development of extreme hyperbilirubinemia. Infants whose TSB values approach the upper percentiles, should also receive closer scrutiny. On the other hand, those whose values fall well below the 50th percentile probably require minimal surveillance and follow-up for jaundice.[11] From Maisels.[114]

percentile 15.1 mg/dl (258 µmol/l).[12] In 11 Kaiser Permanente Northern California hospitals the 95th percentile was a TSB of 17.4 mg/dl (298 µmol/l).[10] Thus, it is clear that we need to revise our criteria for the normal range of TSB levels in the newborn. The upper limit of "normal" (see below for a discussion of what this term means) in predominantly breast fed populations is a TSB of 15–17.5 mg/dl (291 µmol/l). This implies that 5–6 day old breast-fed infants with TSB levels below about 17 mg/dl (291 µmol/l) do not require any laboratory investigation to find out *why* they are jaundiced. They may well require careful follow-up, however. The normal mean bilirubin level for this type of population on day 5–7 is about 8–10 mg/dl (137–171 µmol/l).

Another important factor accounting for the variation in TSB levels is the difficulty in obtaining accurate and consistent laboratory measurements, a problem that has been recognized for 4 decades[13] and shows no sign of resolution. In a recent study of 14 university hospital laboratories, a sample with a TSB concentration of 14.8 mg/dl (253 μmol/l) produced TSB measurements ranging from 11.5 to 20.9 mg/dl (197–357 μmol/l).[14]

Using data from 8 different studies[1,3,7,10–12,15,16] of populations in which 60–70% of the infants were breast fed, we have constructed smoothed curves that provide a guide to the expected course of bilirubin levels in this type of population. (Figure 10.2) Although these data cannot be applied to all populations, they should be useful for plotting the course of jaundice in newborns. The velocity of the increase in TSB can be used to make decisions about evaluation, follow-up, and potential intervention.

"Physiologic Jaundice" and the Concept of a Normal Serum Bilirubin

Because at some point during the first week of life essentially every newborn has a TSB level that exceeds 1 mg/dl (17 μmol/l), the upper limit of normal for an adult, and about 2/3 or more will appear clinically jaundiced, this type of transient hyperbilirubinemia has been called "physiologic jaundice". Nevertheless, there is good reason to consider abandoning this term. First, as discussed above, because of the significant differences in bilirubin levels in different populations (Figure 10.1), it is difficult, if not impossible, to define what is normal or abnormal, physiologic or nonphysiologic. Second, defining the term "normal" is in itself a difficult task.[17] A *diagnostic* definition of normal implies that if a result falls outside of a defined range then there is a known probability of a specific disease being present. For example, a 2 day old term newborn infant who has a thyroxine (T4) level of 4 μg/dl (51 nmol/l) almost certainly has congenital hypothyroidism and this diagnosis can be confirmed by means of additional laboratory studies (TSH, etc.). On the other hand, in an infant with a TSB level of 18–20 mg/dl (308–340 μmol/l, and above the 95th percentile) on day 5, the likelihood of finding a specific etiology is less than 5%.[18,19] Hour-specific TSB levels, however, can be very informative.[11] A TSB of 10 mg/dl (171 μmol/l) at age 12 hours is almost certainly due to a hemolytic process even if the precise cause of the increased bilirubin production is not yet known.

Another definition of normal utilizes the "*risk factor approach*". This is based on the relationship of bilirubin levels in the newborn to the development of kernicterus or the later development of more subtle manifestations of bilirubin encephalopathy (cognitive or neurological). As discussed in detail in Chapter 9, we have been unable, so far, to associate a specific risk of damage with a particular TSB level. Perhaps the most useful definition of normal for hyperbilirubinemia is the *therapeutic* definition. Here a normal range defines the bilirubin level beyond which a specific therapy *will likely do more good than harm*. Although the ranges are only approximate, the recommendations contained in the American Academy of Pediatrics' (AAP) guidelines for the use of phototherapy in term newborns are examples of the application of this principle.[20] For example, the AAP recommends using phototherapy in any infant whose bilirubin level reaches 15 mg/dl (257 μmol/l) between 25 and 48 hours of life. While a level of 15 mg/dl (257 µmol/l) at that age poses no imminent threat to the infant's well-being, it is well above the 95th percentile,[11] is most likely due to an increase in bilirubin production and, if untreated, might increase to a level that is dangerous to the infant. The suggested intervention, phototherapy, is both safe and effective and, under these circumstances, is much more likely to do good than harm.

With the exception of an early, or rapidly rising bilirubin level that suggests hemolysis, the *diagnostic* definition of normal for indirect hyperbilirubinemia (or so-called physiologic jaundice) is of very limited value. The *risk factor* definition may have some utility, and the *therapeutic* definition is probably the most useful.

There are even stronger reasons for abandoning the use of the term "physiologic jaundice" when we deal with the premature infant. If untreated, low birth weight infants have exaggerated and prolonged hyperbilirubinemia with peak TSB levels that exceed those of fullterm infants and are slower to return to baseline values. While this may be considered "physiologic" because it occurs in all preterm infants, in very low birth weight infants TSB levels well within the "physiologic" range are considered potentially hazardous and are treated with phototherapy. Thus, the natural history of hyperbilirubinemia in the very low birth weight infant is never observed and defining certain bilirubin levels as "physiologic" in this population is both misleading and potentially dangerous. Using a diagnostic definition of normal, a TSB level of 10 mg/dl (171 µmol/l) on day 4 in a 750 g neonate is considered completely "physiologic" and no investigation need be done to identify a *cause* for this jaundice. Nevertheless, almost all neonatologists would *treat* this infant with phototherapy implying that this value exceeds the therapeutic definition of normal and that treatment is more likely to do good than harm. Thus, in neonatal intensive care units today, the term "physiologic" jaundice has no meaning and no utility, and should be abandoned.

Direct Bilirubin Levels

Increased direct bilirubin levels, by themselves, generally do not represent a threat to the infant so that neither the risk factor nor the therapeutic definitions of normal are useful. As with TSB levels, there are multiple causes for elevations of direct bilirubin. Nevertheless, any elevation of direct bilirubin beyond the age of 2–3 weeks mandates consideration of the known causes of cholestatic jaundice because identification of a treatable cause such as a choledochal cyst or extrahepatic biliary atresia and appropriate surgical intervention will decrease the likelihood of cirrhosis. In biliary atresia, a delay in performing a portoenterostomy or Kasai procedure significantly worsens the prognosis.[21]

THE APPROACH TO A JAUNDICED INFANT

In October 1994 the Provisional Committee for Quality Improvement and Sub-Committee on Hyperbilirubinemia of the American Academy of Pediatrics (AAP) published a "Practice Parameter" dealing with the management of hyperbilirubinemia in the healthy term newborn.[20] Although the subject of some discussion[22,23] the practice parameter has proven to be a very useful guide in the management of the jaundiced infant[24] and is discussed in detail below (see Treatment of Hyperbilirubinemia).

Clinical Evaluation

Identifying clinically significant jaundice

The AAP algorithm (see Figure 10.3) begins with the evaluation of a term newborn with jaundice, and subsequently recommends measurement of the infant's total serum bilirubin level if the jaundice appears to be "clinically significant by medical judgment". The problem with this recommendation is that the ability of clinicians to diagnose "clinically significant" jaundice varies widely.[3,25–27] Some studies suggest that the ability of physicians and nurses to estimate serum bilirubin levels clinically is no better than guess-work,[27] while others have shown that newborns whose bilirubin levels exceed 12 mg/dl (205 µmol/l) will, at least, always be identified as "jaundiced".[3,25] Noninvasive (transcutaneous) devices for estimating serum bilirubin provide substantially greater accuracy than visual assessment. (See section on non-invasive bilirubin measurement).[26,28,29]

The cephalocaudal progression of jaundice

In newborns, jaundice is detected by blanching the skin with digital pressure, thus revealing the underlying color of the skin and subcutaneous tissue. This dermal icterus is seen first in the face and then progresses in a cordad manner to the trunk and extremities so that for a given bilirubin level, the skin of the face will appear more yellow than that of the foot. First observed over 100 years ago, and confirmed by several investigators using both visual observation as well as transcutaneous bilirubinometry, the cephalocaudal progression of dermal icterus is a useful clinical tool,[25,30–35] but is probably unreliable once the bilirubin level exceeds 12 mg/dl (139 µmol/l).[25] Knudsen suggests that the cephalocaudal color difference in newborns is best explained by conformational change in the bilirubin–albumin complex. Following its formation, bilirubin is bound tightly to albumin and the initial binding process is extremely rapid (within 10 msec). This is followed by a train of slower changes in the conformation of the bilirubin–albumin complex commencing within 1 to 30 seconds, final conformation being reached 8 minutes after the initial binding.[36] This time course suggests that, initially, there is a lower bilirubin-binding affinity to albumin (until the final stage of conformation has occurred) and thus less effective bilirubin–albumin binding in the blood immediately after it has left the reticuloendothelial system. The affinity increases after the blood reaches the distal portions of the body and the conformational changes in the bilirubin–albumin complex are completed. Knudsen suggests that some of the yellow color of the skin is the result of precipitated bilirubin acid and, in the presence of reduced bilirubin binding affinity to albumin, there is an increased precipitation of bilirubin acid and thus an increase in the yellow color of the skin. This is more likely to occur in the proximal parts of the body because of the conformational changes in the young bilirubin–albumin complexes. Consistent with this hypothesis, Knudsen found that there was a significant and linear correlation between the cephalocaudal color difference, the plasma bilirubin concentration and the square of the hydrogen ion concentration.[34] The cephalocaudal color difference was inversely related to the reserve albumin concentration thus suggesting that the conformational change in the young bilirubin–albumin complex enhances the precipitation of bilirubin acid in the skin of the proximal parts of the body. If this is the mechanism, then objective measurement of the yellow color of the skin using transcutaneous bilirubinometry could be a better predictor of potential bilirubin encephalopathy than a serum bilirubin measurement.

Noninvasive measurements of bilirubin

In 1960, Gosset[37] described the use of the Ingram Icterometer (Cascade Healthcare Products, Salem, OR). A piece of transparent plastic is pressed against the nose and the yellow color of the blanched skin is matched with the appropriate yellow stripe painted on the plastic. As a screening tool, the Icterometer performs as effectively as a much more sophisticated instrument, the Minolta Air Shields Jaundice Meter.[29,38] The Jaundice Meter was the first handheld instrument to use the principles of reflectance spectrophotometry to measure the yellow color of the skin and subcutaneous tissues, and it has been shown to be a very useful screening device in homogenous populations.[29,38,39] Routine use of the Jaundice Meter in our nursery produced a 36% reduction in the number of serum bilirubin measurements obtained[39] but because of the difficulty in using this instrument in heterogeneous populations, it has not been widely accepted in the United States.

Newer devices might overcome these disadvantages. The TLcBiliTest (Chromatic Color Sciences International, Inc., New York, NY) has an algorithm incorporated into the device that has been designed to examine the luminosity of the skin and incorporate the underlying color of normal skin. The changes in the yellow component of the spectrum are observed separately and are used as a bilirubin estimate. In a study of 900 infants, an excellent correlation was found between the transcutaneous bilirubin and the TSB concentrations ($r = 0.956$).[26] These measurements were made in a mixed population of white, African-American, Hispanic, and Asian infants. Preliminary data are also available for an instrument known as the BiliCheck[TM] (Respironics, Pittsburgh, PA) that suggest that it too is capable of performing transcutaneous bilirubin measurements in a mixed population.[40] If these results are confirmed in additional studies, the use of these instruments will prove of enormous benefits to infants and healthcare workers and should obviate the need for serum bilirubin determinations in many circumstances.

Laboratory Evaluation – Seeking a Cause for the Jaundice

Tables 10.1 and 10.2 provide an approach to the clinical and laboratory evaluation of the jaundiced newborn. For many years, standard texts have recommended a battery

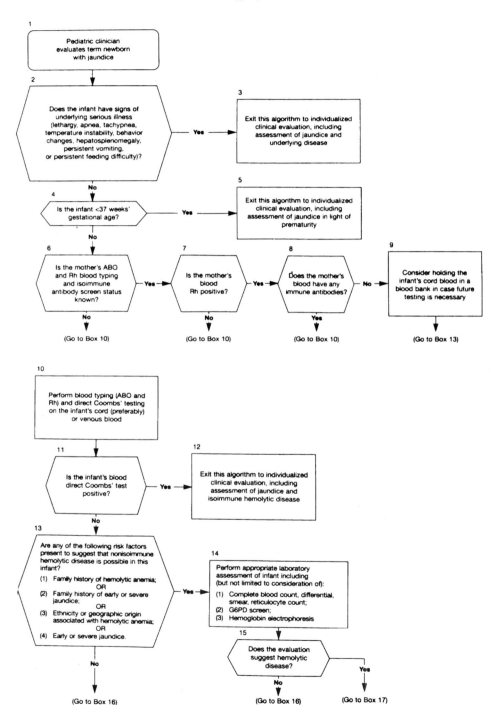

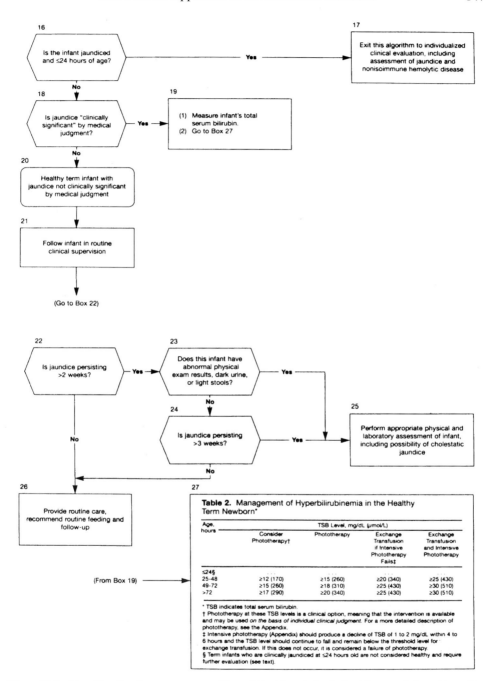

16

Is the infant jaundiced and ≤24 hours of age?

Yes →

17

Exit this algorithm to individualized clinical evaluation, including assessment of jaundice and nonisoimmune hemolytic disease

No ↓

18

Is jaundice "clinically significant" by medical judgment?

Yes →

19

(1) Measure infant's total serum bilirubin.
(2) Go to Box 27

No ↓

20

Healthy term infant with jaundice not clinically significant by medical judgment

↓

21

Follow infant in routine clinical supervision

↓

(Go to Box 22)

22

Is jaundice persisting >2 weeks?

Yes →

23

Does this infant have abnormal physical exam results, dark urine, or light stools?

Yes →

No ↓

24

Is jaundice persisting >3 weeks?

Yes →

25

Perform appropriate physical and laboratory assessment of infant, including possibility of cholestatic jaundice

No ↓

No ←

26

Provide routine care, recommend routine feeding and follow-up

27

Table 2. Management of Hyperbilirubinemia in the Healthy Term Newborn*

(From Box 19) →

Age, hours	TSB Level, mg/dL (μmol/L)			
	Consider Phototherapy†	Phototherapy	Exchange Transfusion if Intensive Phototherapy Fails‡	Exchange Transfusion and Intensive Phototherapy
≤24§	...	...	...	...
25-48	≥12 (170)	≥15 (260)	≥20 (340)	≥25 (430)
49-72	≥15 (260)	≥18 (310)	≥25 (430)	≥30 (510)
>72	≥17 (290)	≥20 (340)	≥25 (430)	≥30 (510)

* TSB indicates total serum bilirubin.
† Phototherapy at these TSB levels is a clinical option, meaning that the intervention is available and may be used on the basis of individual clinical judgment. For a more detailed description of phototherapy, see the Appendix.
‡ Intensive phototherapy (Appendix) should produce a decline of TSB of 1 to 2 mg/dL within 4 to 6 hours and the TSB level should continue to fall and remain below the threshold level for exchange transfusion. If this does not occur, it is considered a failure of phototherapy.
§ Term infants who are clinically jaundiced at ≤24 hours old are not considered healthy and require further evaluation (see text).

Figure 10.3. Algorithm for the management of hyperbilirubinemia in the healthy term infant. From *The American Academy of Pediatrics*.[20]

Table 10.1. Guidelines for initial evaluation and follow up of jaundice in apparently healthy term and near-term infants.[1]

Clinical observation	Initial actions	Other evaluations	Follow-up
Onset of jaundice in first 24 hours[2]	Clinical evaluation[3] Measure TSB and TcB[4]	Blood group (ABO, Rh) Direct Coombs Test CBC, smear for red cell morphology, reticulocyte count[6]	Repeat TSB in 4–24 hours[5]
Onset of jaundice 24–72 hours	Clinical evaluation Assess cephalocaudal distribution[7] TcB	TSB if indicated by TcB or clinical evaluation	Clinical evaluation and/or TcB or TSB within 24–72 hours and repeat as necessary

[1] These guidelines apply to the evaluation and follow-up of the majority of jaundiced newborns who are cared for in well baby nurseries and are ≥35 weeks gestation. They cannot take into account all possible situations. The term "apparently healthy" refers to an infant who has no clinical signs suggesting the possibility of other diseases such as respiratory distress, poor feeding, lethargy, temperature instability, etc.
[2] 24 hours is a long time in the life of a newborn infant. Jaundice at age 4 hours is essentially always due to a hemolytic process whereas jaundice at age 23 hours may be normal.
[3] Clinical evaluation refers to a review of the obstetric history, events of labor and delivery and physical examination of the newborn which should include an evaluation for cephalhematomas, bruising, and hepatosplenomegaly.
[4] In some nurseries a TcB measurement (using the Minolta/Air Shields Jaundice Meter) is used as a screening device and a decision to measure the TSB is based on the TcB level. If a TSB is done, the simultaneous measurement of a TcB allows subsequent TcB measurements to be used to follow the baby and to determine the necessity for additional bilirubin measurements. Recently developed TcB devices could largely replace TSB measurements.
[5] The frequency of obtaining repeated TSB measurements depends on the initial TSB level and the age at which it occurred. A TSB of 5 mg/dl at age 4 hours must be repeated within 4 hours whereas the same level at 23 hours could be repeated in 12–24 hours.
[6] These investigations lack both sensitivity and specificity, but may be helpful in confirming the diagnosis of ABO hemolytic disease or other rarer courses of hemolysis.
[7] Jaundice is first seen in the face. As the TSB increases, jaundice appears in the trunk, abdomen and extremities.
TSB, total serum bilirubin; TcB, transcutaneous bilirubin.
From Maisels.[114]

of tests for any infant whose TSB level at any time exceeds 12–13 mg/dl (205–222 μmol/l) because of a belief that such levels represent potentially "pathologic" jaundice. But as mentioned above, not only are there significant differences in TSB levels in different populations but recent data show that the 95th percentile is about 15–17.5 mg/dl (290–308 μmol/l).[10–12] Furthermore, the usual laboratory tests used (hematocrit, CBC, reticulocyte count, smear, blood type and Coombs test) are neither specific nor sensitive. These tests were performed on almost 5,000 jaundiced infants who weighed >2500 gm and whose TSB levels had exceeded the "physiologic" range. A diagnosis was suggested in fewer than 20% of infants.[41,42] Even in infants who are readmitted to hospital in the first 2 weeks of life with clearly abnormal TSB levels of 18–20 mg/dl (308–340 μmol/l) or higher, these investigations are usually unrewarding.[19] As can be seen in Table 10.3, in about 95% of term or near term very jaundiced newborns, no pathologic cause of jaundice can be identified. Perhaps the

Table 10.2. Additional laboratory evaluation of the jaundiced term and near term infant.

Indications	Maneuvers
Suspicion of hemolytic disease or anemia (e.g., pallor, early jaundice or TSB > 8 mg/dl [137 μmol/l] by 24 hours or > 13 mg/dl [222 μmol/l] by 48 h of life)	Blood type, group, and Coombs test, if not obtained with cord blood. Complete blood count and smear Reticulocyte count
East Asian, Mediterranean or Nigerian infants with TSB > 15 mg/dl (257 μmol/l). Any infant with late-onset jaundice or TSB ≥18 mg/dl (308 μmol/l)	Measure glucose-6-phosphate dehydrogenase
Jaundice beyond 3 weeks of age	Direct bilirubin level, urine dipstick for bilirubin, inspect stools for color. Check results of newborn thyroid screen, evaluate infant for signs or symptoms of hypothyroidism
Infant ill	Direct bilirubin level, check urine for reducing substances, check results of newborn screen for galactosemia and other inborn errors, and evaluate for sepsis

TSB, total serum bilirubin concentration.
From Maisels.[114]

Table 10.3. Discharge diagnosis in 306 infants admitted with severe hyper-bilirubinemia.*

Diagnosis	Number	Percentage
Hyperbilirubinemia of unknown cause or breast-milk jaundice	290	94.8
Cephalhematoma or bruising	3	1.0
ABO hemolytic disease†	11	3.6
Anti-E hemolytic disease	1	0.3
Galactosemia	1	0.3
Sepsis	0	

*Infants were readmitted after discharge as newborns. Mean age at admission was 5 days (range, 2–17 days), and mean bilirubin level was 18.5 ± 2.8 mg/dl (range 12.7–29.1 mg/dl).
† Mother was type O, infant was type A or B, direct Coombs test was positive.
From Maisels, M.J. and Kring, E.[19]

ability to measure end-tidal carbon monoxide concentrations in these infants will identify some who are producing large quantities of bilirubin even though they have no obvious cause for hemolysis.[43]

It makes no sense to attempt to interpret bilirubin levels without considering the infant's precise age in hours.[11] Figure 10.1 illustrates the natural history of neonatal jaundice in different populations and Figure 10.2 an approximation of the range of bilirubin levels to be expected in a mixed race population in which 60–70% of infants are breast fed. Any infant whose bilirubin level exceeds the 95th percentile or in whom the rate of rise appears to be crossing percentiles, deserves evaluation and careful follow-up. Nevertheless, in most cases it is unlikely that a precise cause of the aberrant trend will be found.

Screening for isoimmunization

All mothers should be tested for ABO and Rh (D) typing and a serum screen performed for unusual isoimmune antibodies.[44] If such perinatal testing has not been performed, then a direct Coombs test, a blood type and an Rh (D) type on the infant's (cord) blood should be done and this should always be done if the mother is Rh negative. In addition to identification of potentially Rh sensitized infants, this testing is obligatory because it identifies Rh negative mothers who require anti-D gammaglobulin to prevent Rh (D) sensitization.

The diagnosis of ABO hemolytic disease

It is difficult to be confident about a diagnosis of ABO hemolytic disease. (see Chapter 4). About 45% of Americans of western European descent have type O blood and a similar percentage are type A. Types B and AB make up the balance. The equivalent percentages for African-Americans are 50% type O, 29% type A, 17% type B and 4% AB.[45] As a result, OA incompatibility is by far the most common form of ABO incompatibility encountered in the US. ABO incompatibility tends to run in families. One study found an 88% risk of recurrence of ABO hemolytic disease in infants at risk of the disease who were born to parents whose first born child was similarly affected.[46]

Ozolek, *et al.*[47] prospectively analyzed cord blood samples of 4,996 consecutive live born infants for their blood type, hematocrit and the results of the direct antiglobulin test (DAT or Coombs test) and the indirect Coombs test. The direct Coombs test detects antibodies attached to the red cell while the indirect Coombs test detects IgG antibody in the serum. Only 0.29% of type A, B or AB infants who were incompatible with their type A or B mothers had a positive DAT result, whereas 32% of type A or B infants born to type O mothers had positive DATs. A positive DAT was the best predictor of an elevated bilirubin level, but only 20% of infants with a positive DAT developed TSB levels $\geq$12.8 mg/dl (224 µmol/l). (Table 10.4) In a

Table 10.4. Bilirubin levels in ABO incompatible infants according to Coombs test.

Coombs test result	Peak serum bilirubin $\geq$ 12.8 mg/dl (224 µmol/L)
Direct antiglobulin (Coombs) test positive	46/225 (20.4%)
Indirect Coombs test positive	29/309 (9.4%)
Both tests negative	38/488 (7.8%)

From Ozolek *et al.*[47]

Norwegian study of 2,463 infants, 19.6% of DAT positive OA or OB incompatible infants required phototherapy.[48] These large prospective studies confirm what has been found in other smaller studies: although about 1/3 of group A or B infants born to group O mothers have anti-A or anti-B antibodies attached to their red cells, only 1 in 5 of those with a positive DAT have a *modest to significant degree* of hyperbilirubinemia and severe jaundice in these infants is quite uncommon.[47,49–52] Thus, although it can on occasion, be severe, ABO hemolytic disease *is not a common cause of severe hyperbilirubinemia* (Table 10.3) and while there is certainly a wide spectrum of hemolysis in ABO hemolytic disease, this diagnosis should generally not be made unless there is a positive DAT and clinical jaundice within the first 12–24 hours. Reticulocytosis and the presence of microspherocytes on the smear help to confirm the diagnosis. Nevertheless, most clinicians have seen the occasional infant in whom all of the above criteria for the diagnosis of ABO hemolytic disease were present yet the direct Coombs test was negative. Presumably such cases reflect the technical vicissitudes of Coombs testing in the laboratory.

In these days of cost containment, a question that is commonly asked is: should a blood type and direct Coombs test be performed on the cord blood of all infants of group O mothers? A recent survey found that 58% of hospital blood banks in the US were routinely performing Coombs tests and blood typing on newborn cord bloods. About 36% of hospitals tested all cord bloods routinely and 35% tested those of type O or Rh negative mothers.[53] When such testing is done, however, the results are frequently ignored by the responsible pediatrician[53,54] and it is unlikely that routine screening, except in infants of Rh negative mothers, is warranted[47,53] provided appropriate surveillance and follow-up are assured.

Infants with severe jaundice

In those infants with severe jaundice (TSB levels >17–18 mg/dl [291–308 µmol/l]) it is worth looking for ABO immunization and other causes of hemolysis (Table 4.1, Chapter 4). If ABO incompatibility or some other cause of hemolytic disease is strongly suspected, these infants generally deserve more aggressive therapy than those with nonhemolytic jaundice. In the absence of hemolysis and any abnormal historical or physical findings, jaundice *by itself* is almost never a sign of serious illness and, although some reports have suggested that unexplained indirect hyperbilirubinemia may be the only manifestation of sepsis in otherwise healthy-appearing newborns,[55–57] this is certainly a rare occurrence. Of 306 newborns admitted to our pediatric ward within 21 days of birth because of severe indirect hyperbilirubinemia (peak TSB levels 18.5 ± 2.8; range 12.7–29.1 mg/dl, [316 ± 4.8, 217–498 µmol/l]) not one case of sepsis was identified (upper 95% confidence limits for the risk of sepsis = 1%) (see Table 10.3).[19] However, infants who exhibit some of the signs or symptoms listed in Table 10.5 deserve careful evaluation, particularly those who have late onset jaundice after physiologic icterus has resolved, those with direct hyperbilirubinemia and those with something in the history, physical examination or laboratory investigation that is out of the ordinary.

Table 10.5. Danger signs in jaundiced infants.

Family history of significant hemolytic disease
Onset of jaundice in first 24 hours of life
Onset of jaundice after day 3 of life
Vomiting
Lethargy
Poor feeding
Fever
High-pitched cry
Dark urine
Light stools

From Maisels.[114]

Changing Times and Jaundiced Newborns

A possible resurgence of kernicterus

There is some anecdotal evidence that kernicterus has reemerged from a status of near extinction to one that is of concern to pediatricians.[58-63] However, it is difficult to compare the incidence of kernicterus in the population today with the incidence in the last 30 years, because there has been no uniform surveillance for the reporting of such cases over the last 3–4 decades, no uniform case definition for kernicterus and, most important, no denominators for the case reports listed. Short hospital stays following delivery seem to have played a role in many of these cases[58,59] and an additional contributing factor could be the belief that hyperbilirubinemia, no matter how extreme, is harmless if it occurs in an otherwise healthy breast-fed infant. Reports of kernicterus in such infants indicate that this is not the case.[63]

Early discharge and the risk of jaundice

There is a world-wide trend towards shortening the length of hospital stay for newborns and there is some evidence that early discharge itself seems to be associated with an increased risk of significant hyperbilirubinemia[18,59,64-66] and even kernicterus.[58] In 20 of 21 cases of kernicterus collected by Brown and Johnson[58] and in all 4 cases reported by MacDonald[59] there were short postpartum hospital stays. Although the AAP has recommended only that infants discharged at less than 48 hours be seen within 2–3 days after discharge,[20,67] our data and those of Soskolne, *et al.* show that the risk of readmission for hyperbilirubinemia is increased and is of similar magnitude *whether the infant was discharged at less than 48 hours or between 48 and 72 hours.*[18,65]

Why babies discharged early should be at a greater risk for developing significant hyperbilirubinemia is not clear. Perhaps mothers who have had more time to receive counseling from nursing staff and, in particular, lactation counseling during their hospital stay will nurse their babies more effectively. There is good evidence that more frequent and effective lactation[68,69] as well as improved caloric intake,[70] decreases the likelihood of hyperbilirubinemia. There is also evidence that early discharge affects the ability of mothers to assimilate and process the information that they receive regarding lactation and infant care.[71] As a result, they may nurse their infants less effectively. One thing is certain: *if babies leave hospital before they are 36 hours old, their peak bilirubin level will occur after they are discharged*. Thus, jaundice today is largely an outpatient problem and if we want to be able to identify and prevent the occurrence of extreme hyperbilirubinemia in the occasional baby, we need to develop a consistent approach to the monitoring and surveillance of these infants.

More jaundiced newborns

As discussed above, the incidence of neonatal jaundice is increasing. In the Collaborative Perinatal Project (CPP, 1959–1966), the 95th percentile was a TSB $\geq$ 13 mg/dl (222 µmol/l)[9] while in 3 recent studies, the 95th percentile was 15.0–17.5 mg/dl (265–308 µmol/l).[10–12] Newman[42] found that 10% of white babies born between 1980 and 1982 had peak TSB levels $\geq$13 mg/dl (222 µmol/l) but by 1986 to 1987 the proportion had increased to 14%.[72] In the CPP, which predated phototherapy, only 0.8% of infants had a peak TSB level of $\geq$20 mg/dl (342 µmol/l)[9] compared with 2% of infants in a recent study of 11 Kaiser Permanente Northern California hospitals.[10] Some of the factors that may be responsible for this increase in jaundice include an increase in the number of infants breast-fed on discharge from the hospital (30% in the 1960's, 60% in 1997),[73] an increase in the population of east Asian babies in the US, and short hospital stays.

A compressed time frame

The ever-shrinking hospital stay requires a readjustment in our thinking with regard to the meaning of specific bilirubin levels, but this has proved to be a difficult adjustment for pediatricians[54,74] who have become accustomed to using a specific bilirubin level (irrespective of the baby's age) as a cause for reassurance or concern. As illustrated in Figures 10.2 and 10.4, however, a serum bilirubin level of 8 mg/dl (137 µmol/l) in a baby on "day 2" could be on the 95th, 75th or 40th to 50th percentile depending on whether the baby was 24.1, 36, or 47.9 hours old respectively. A TSB of 8 mg/dl at 24.1 hours is on the 95th percentile and requires an evaluation for the presence of hemolysis (blood type, Coombs test, etc.) and close follow-up, while the same level at 47.9 hours requires no investigation or close follow-up.

A UNIFIED APPROACH TO PREVENTING KERNICTERUS

Epidemiologic Risk Factors

Assuming that most babies leave the hospital within 48 hours of delivery, how do we identify those who are (or are not) at risk for developing a bilirubin level that might be a threat to the infant's well-being? Clearly, only a very small number of the

154   *M. Jeffrey Maisels*

Table 10.6. Common obstetric and neonatal factors that significantly increase the risk of nonhemolytic hyperbilirubinemia in healthy term and near-term infants.

Previous jaundiced sibling	Male sex
East Asian race	Breast feeding
Oxytocin use in labor	Caloric deprivation and larger weight loss
Macrosomic infant of diabetic mother	Visible jaundice before discharge
Bruising cephalhematoma,	G6PD deficiency
vacuum extraction	Short Hospital Stay
Gestation 35–38 weeks	

4 million babies born every year in the US suffer bilirubin encephalopathy but, if we assume that this condition is almost always preventable, then it is worthwhile taking reasonable steps to prevent its occurrence. Table 10.6 lists those factors that are clinically significant and most consistently associated with an increase in the risk of severe nonhemolytic jaundice. Because these risk factors are common and the risk of severe hyperbilirubinemia is small, individually, they are of limited use as predictors of significant hyperbilirubinemia. Nevertheless, if no risk factors are present, the risk of severe hyperbilirubinemia is extremely low, but if several are present in the same infant, the risk of hyperbilirubinemia increases significantly. Some factors, such as breast-feeding and decreasing gestation seem to play a particularly important role in the rare reported cases of extreme hyperbilirubinemia and kernicterus. It is remarkable that essentially every recently described case of kernicterus has occurred in a breast fed infant[58–60,63] even when the infant had an underlying hemolytic process.[59,60] In addition, most cases have occurred in infants <40 weeks gestation.

The epidemiology of neonatal jaundice is discussed in detail in Chapter 3.

Universal newborn bilirubin screening

Infants who are clinically jaundiced in the first few days are much more likely to develop subsequent significant hyperbilirubinemia[18,65] and there is an association between bilirubin levels in cord blood and subsequent bilirubin concentrations.[2,3]

Bhutani and coworkers obtained TSB levels in 2,840 term and near-term healthy infants and established a bilirubin nomogram for the first week of life.[11] (Figure 10.4)* The population studied was 43% white, 41% African-American, 4% Hispanic, 4% Asian and 8% other and 59% of mothers attempted breast-feeding in the first week (49.5% exclusively breastfed). Infants with ABO incompatibility and positive Coombs tests were excluded as were Rh sensitized infants. Those who were ≥ 35 weeks gestation were included if their birth weight was ≥2500 gm and those who were ≥ 36 were included if their birth weights were ≥2000 gm. The investigators plotted bilirubin levels against the infant's age in hours and created percentiles that

---

* In this study, the TSB levels at the 40th percentile after about 72 hours are much higher than reported in any other study to date and are almost certainly biased as a result of patient selection. (See commentary by Maisels and Newman[75] for a discussion of this issue.)

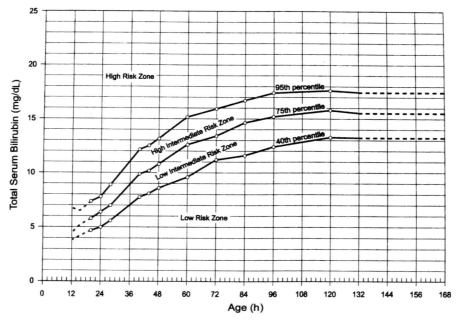

Figure 10.4. Risk designation of term and near-term well newborns based on their hour-specific serum bilirubin values. (Dotted extensions are based on <300 TSB values/epoch.) From Bhutani *et al.*[11]

Table 10.7. Predischarge bilirubin levels and risk of subsequent hyperbilirubinemia.

TSB before discharge		TSB after discharge
Percentile	*N*	*>95th percentile*
>95th	172 (6.1%)	68/172 (39.5%)
76th–95th	356 (12.5%)	46/356 (12.9%)
40th–75th	556 (19.6%)	12/556 (2.15%)
<40th	1756 (61.8%)*	0/1756
Total	2840	126 (4.4%)

*Newborn TSB were obtained between 18 and 72 hours and 61.8% of all values obtained were below the 40th percentile.
TSB, Total serum bilirubin level.
From Bhutani *et al.*[11]

defined a high risk (above the 95th percentile), a low risk (values below the 40th percentile) and an intermediate risk (40th–95th percentiles) zone. They used this nomogram to see if an initial TSB level obtained prior to discharge would predict the likelihood that a subsequent TSB level would exceed the 95th percentile. The results of the study are shown in Table 10.7. Of Coombs negative infants whose initial TSB levels fell in the intermediate zone 58/912 (6.4 %) subsequently had a TSB level above the 95th percentile, 39.5% (68/172) of those who were initially above the 95th percentile remained at that level, but no infant whose initial TSB level was in the low risk zone, had a subsequent TSB that exceeded the 95th percentile.

These data suggest that obtaining a single serum bilirubin level on every baby prior to discharge can be a very useful way of predicting the risk (or absence of risk) of subsequent significant hyperbilirubinemia and, if confirmed in other studies, suggests that there is a group of infants who, *at least as far as hyperbilirubinemia is concerned*, do not require early follow-up. This type of information should be very useful in populations where early follow-up is difficult or impossible. Similarly, infants whose bilirubin levels fall in the high risk zone require much more careful surveillance and follow-up until there is laboratory evidence supporting a declining TSB level. Because of the variability in the measurement of TSB and the desire of the investigators to achieve a negative predictive value that was close to certainty, the 40th percentile rather than the 50th percentile was selected as a demarcator for the minimal risk zone. Using this percentile, the negative predictive value was 100%. The authors did not indicate if there was any difference in the predictive value of the predischarge TSB level if it was taken early or later in the hospital course, but because of the natural history of neonatal hyperbilirubinemia, it is likely that the later the TSB is obtained prior to discharge, the closer it will correlate with the ultimate peak value. This may be important, particularly in infants of 35–36 weeks gestation.[76]

Measuring bilirubin production

When heme is catabolized, carbon monoxide (CO) is produced in equimolar quantities with bilirubin and a measurement of blood carboxyhemoglobin (COHb) concentration, CO production or CO excretion provides a measurement of bilirubin production.[43,77] The recent development of a simple, noninvasive method of measuring end tidal CO, corrected for ambient CO ($ETCO_c$)[43] provides for the first time, a noninvasive technique for quantifying hemolysis. Measurements of $ETCO_c$ prior to discharge should identify those infants with high or low rates of bilirubin production and can provide additional help in predicting the likelihood (or lack thereof) of severe hyperbilirubinemia.[78,79]

Preventing extreme hyperbilirubinemia

Jaundice is very common, but extreme hyperbilirubinemia is rare. Maximum bilirubin levels of more than 25 mg/dl (428 µmol/l) occur in about 1 in 750 infants[10] and levels of more than 30 mg/dl (513 µmol/l) in about 1–3 per 10,000 infants.[10,64] To make sure that we do not miss these rare babies, however, we need to follow and measure serum bilirubin levels on many more who will never develop severe hyperbilirubinemia. Recognizing the risks associated with short hospital stays, the AAP recommended that "follow-up should be provided to all neonates discharged less than 48 hours after birth by a health care professional in an office, clinic or at home within 2–3 days of discharge".[20] A subsequent AAP statement shortened the follow-up time to "within 48 hours of discharge".[67]

If every baby, irrespective of risk factors, were seen within 72–96 hours of birth, significantly jaundiced infants should be identified and appropriate follow-up and intervention (where necessary) instituted. Those few infants with a Coombs positive hemolytic anemia are almost always jaundiced before they are 24 hours old. Thus, in a perfect world, most risk assessment prior to discharge would be superfluous. In the real world, however, it is not possible to see every baby in follow-up, particularly in rural areas where distances may be vast, and weather conditions may preclude travel at certain times of the year. In addition, mothers do not always comply with a request to return and pediatricians in the US have not yet demonstrated that they are convinced of the necessity for this type of follow-up. Many infants discharged at less than 48 hours are not being seen earlier than 1–2 weeks after discharge.[54] Finally, although the AAP recommends this type of early follow-up only for babies discharged before 48 hours, 2 studies have shown that infants discharged between 48 and 72 hours are at as great a risk for readmission with significant jaundice as those discharged before 48 hours.[18,65] Thus, we recommend that any infant discharged at less than 72 hours should be seen by a health care professional within 1–3 days of discharge. A suggested approach to the management and follow-up of these babies is shown in Tables 10.1 and 10.2.

TREATING NEONATAL JAUNDICE

Term and Near Term Newborns

Recommendations for treatment of full-term and near-term infants are given in Table 10.8. These guidelines were developed by the AAP under the original heading "Management of Hyperbilirubinemia in the Healthy Term Newborn".[20] This has

Table 10.8. Management of hyperbilirubinemia in the apparently healthy term and near term newborn.

Age(h)	TSB* Level, mg/dl (μmol/l)			
	Consider phototherapy[†]	*phototherapy*	*Exchange transfusion if intensive phototherapy fails*[‡]	*Exchange transfusion and intensive phototherapy*
≤24[§]	–	–	–	–
25–48	≥12 (205)	≥15 (260)	≥20 (340)	≥25 (430)
49–72	≥15 (260)	≥18 (310)	≥25 (430)	≥30 (510)
>72	≥17 (290)	≥20 (340)	≥25 (430)	≥30 (510)

* TSB indicates total serum bilirubin.
  [†] Phototherapy at these TSB levels is a clinical option, meaning that the intervention is available and may be used on the basis of individual clinical judgment.
  [‡] Intensive phototherapy should produce a decline of TSB of 1 to 2 mg/dl within 4–6 hours, and the TSB level should continue to fall and remain below the threshold level for exchange transfusion. If this does not occur, it is considered a failure of phototherapy.
  [§] Term infants who are clinically jaundiced at ≤ 24 hours old are not considered healthy and require further evaluation.
From *Pediatrics*, 1994; **94**: 560.

M. Jeffrey Maisels

been modified to read "... in the *Apparently Healthy Term and Near Term Newborn*". The AAP's recommendations refer to newborns of ≥37 weeks gestation, but there are many infants at 34–36 weeks gestation who are cared for in well baby nurseries and managed no differently from those ≥37 weeks. Some clinicians may prefer to use slightly lower TSB levels for intervention with phototherapy and/or exchange transfusions for infants who are 35–36 weeks gestation and this is a matter of individual judgment.

No formal review of the compliance with, or efficacy of, the AAP guidelines has been carried out, but there seems little doubt that if all significantly jaundiced infants were identified and these guidelines followed, essentially no cases of kernicterus would occur. One of the key differences between the AAP's practice parameter and previous guidelines is that the practice parameter contemplates exchange transfusion *only when intensive phototherapy fails* (see Chapter 12) unless the first TSB obtained is in excess of 30 mg/dl (513 μmol/l). Even in the face of such extreme hyperbilirubinemia, by the time a blood sample has been obtained, typed and cross-matched for an exchange transfusion, intensive phototherapy may well have reduced the TSB by as much as 10 mg/dl (171 μmol/l),[80] in which case a decision might be made to withhold the exchange transfusion. In virtually every case of kernicterus reported over the last decade[58–60,63] the bilirubin level has far exceeded those at which the AAP guidelines call for intervention (Table 10.8). Dr. William Robertson, who chaired the subcommittee responsible for producing the AAP's practice parameter, has recently reflected on these guidelines and writes:

> How does the 1994 practice parameter on management of hyperbilirubinemia in the healthy term newborn appear through the retrospectoscope in 1998? Naturally, I am biased, but it looks good, given its purpose of providing guidance, *not certainty*. A guideline is similar to the white lines on both sides of the highway, we all try to stay between those white lines, except when unusual circumstances such as a flat tire make us pull off the road and outside the lines to attend to the crisis.[24]

One criticism of the AAP practice parameter is that although it is intended to provide guidelines for intervention in healthy infants, the bilirubin levels chosen for phototherapy suggest that the infants may not, in fact, be healthy. This is particularly so for bilirubin levels in the early portion of the time periods 25–48 hours and 49–72 hours. For example, the guidelines recommend phototherapy when the bilirubin level is ≥15 mg/dl (260 μmol/l) in a 25–48 hour old infant (Table 10.8). But a TSB of ≥15 mg/dl (260 μmol/l) at 26 hours is far above the 95th percentile and is even >95th percentile for a 48 hour old infant (see Figure 10.4).[11] The same can be said for a TSB of 18 mg/dl (310 μmol/l) at 49–72 hours and 20 mg/dl (340 μmol/l) at >72 hours. Thus, although these treatment levels are quite appropriate, by definition, infants who qualify for treatment may not be "healthy" and may have an underlying component of increased bilirubin production, or inadequate bilirubin clearance, or both, and such infants merit investigation for the cause of their hyperbilirubinemia.

Intervention in the Breastfed Infant

Of infants who develop bilirubin levels high enough to require phototherapy and who do not have evidence of isoimmunization or other obvious hemolytic disease, 80–90% are fully or partially breast-fed.[8,19] Table 10.9 suggests an approach to the prevention and treatment of jaundice associated with breast-feeding. Observational studies show that increasing the frequency of breast-feeding during the first few days after birth decreases TSB levels.[68,69,81] We performed a controlled trial in which mothers were randomly assigned to a frequent or demand breast-feeding schedule and we found no significant difference between the TSB levels measured in the 2 groups at an average age of 55 hours.[82] Given the natural history of jaundice in breast feeding infants, it is very likely that maximum bilirubin levels had not yet been achieved in these infants. On the other hand, the observational data of Yamauchi *et al.* show a very strong inverse and linear relationship between the frequency of nursing in the first 24 hours and the probability of hyperbilirubinemia on day 6.[69]

In many hospitals it is a common practice to provide supplemental feedings of water or dextrose water to breast-fed infants in the mistaken belief that this will lower their TSB levels. On the contrary, this practice consistently increases TSB levels[83,84] and should be abandoned. Furthermore, an increase in dextrose water intake in the first 3 days of life was significantly related to a decrease in breast milk intake on the 4th day,[85] and water supplementation decreases the number of infants who are exclusively breast-fed at age 3 months.[86]

When the TSB in a breast-fed infant reaches a level at which intervention is being considered, a number of options exist and are listed in Table 10.9. Two randomized controlled trials have evaluated some of these interventions. When TSB levels reached 15 mg/dl (257 μmol/l), Amato *et al.* compared the effect of interrupting breast-feeding versus phototherapy.[87] There was no difference between the groups in the amount of time needed to reduce the TSB to <12 mg/dl (205 μmol/l). In a controlled clinical trial, Martinez and colleagues compared the effect of 4 different interventions on hyperbilirubinemia in 125 full term breast-fed infants[88] who were enrolled when their TSB levels reached 17 mg/dl (291 μmol/l). The primary outcome

Table 10.9. Approaches to the prevention and treatment of jaundice associated with breast-feeding.

Prevention
1. Encourage frequent nursing (i.e., at least eight times per day)
2. Do not supplement with water or dextrose water

Treatment options
1. Observe
2. Discontinue nursing, substitute formula
3. Alternate feedings of breast milk and formula
4. Discontinue nursing, administer phototherapy
5. Continue nursing, administer phototherapy*

* Author's preferred intervention.
From Maisels.[114]

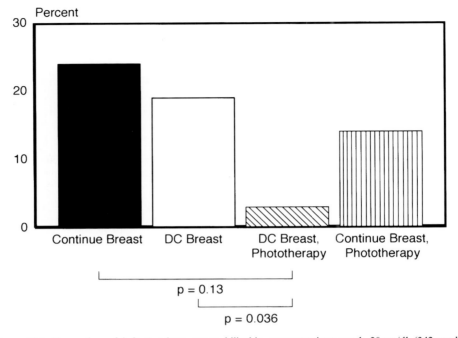

Figure 10.5. Proportion of infants whose serum bilirubin concentrations reach 20 mg/dl (342 μmol/l) following 1 of 4 interventions. Infants were enrolled when their TSB levels reached 17 mg/dl (291 μmol/l). They were randomly assigned for groups: (A) Continue breast feeding. (B) Discontinue breast feeding and substitute formula. (C) Discontinue breast feeding and receive phototherapy. (D) Continue breast feeding and receive phototherapy. Note that infants received standard (not intensive) phototherapy (see text). From Martinez *et al.*[88]

variable was the proportion of infants whose TSB concentrations reached 20 mg/dl (342 μmol/l) and the results are shown in Figure 10.5. In neither of these studies was intensive phototherapy used.[89] Although it seems reasonable to offer the mother a choice of the interventions listed in Table 10.9, we believe that any interruption of nursing is undesirable and, unless extreme hyperbilirubinemia is present (TSB levels in excess of 25 mg/dl [428 μmol/l]), it is our practice to recommend that breast-feeding be continued while the infant is treated with intensive phototherapy (see Chapter 12).[89]

Low Birth Weight Infants

Table 10.10 provides suggested guidelines for the management of hyperbilirubinemia in low birth weight infants. Over the last decade, there has been a remarkable decrease in the incidence of kernicterus found in autopsied infants who died in NICU's and some of this may be due to the liberal use of phototherapy. Certainly, phototherapy has dramatically decreased the necessity for exchange transfusion which, in low birth weight infants, is now almost exclusively carried out in the occasional infant with

Table 10.10. Approaches to the use of phototherapy and exchange transfusion in low birth-weight infants.[a]

Birth weight (g)	Total bilirubin level (mg/dl [μmol/l][b])	
	Phototherapy[c]	Exchange Transfusion[d]
<1500	5–8 (85–140)	13–16 (220–275)
1500–1999	8–12 (140–200)	16–18 (275–300)
2000–2499	11–14 (190–240)	18–20 (300–340)

[a] Note that these guidelines reflect ranges used in neonatal intensive care unites. They cannot take into account all possible situations. In some units, prophylactic phototherapy is used for all infants who weigh <1500 g. Higher intervention levels may be used for small-for-gestational-age infants, based on gestational age rather than birth weight.
[b] Consider initiating therapy at these levels. Range allows discretion based on clinical conditions or other circumstances (see Table 10.11).
[c] Used at these levels and in therapeutic doses, phototherapy should, with few exceptions, eliminate the need for exchange transfusions.
[d] Levels for exchange transfusion assume that bilirubin continues to rise or remains at these levels despite intensive phototherapy (see Chapter 12).
From Maisels.[114]

severe Rh hemolytic disease or extensive bruising. In a cohort of 833 infants with birth weights between 500 and 1500 gm born in North Carolina between 1985 and 1989, only 2 infants (0.24%) underwent exchange transfusion.[90] We have not performed a single exchange transfusion in our population of newborns with birthweights <1500 g in the last 10 years.[91] As pointed out in Chapter 11, previously used criteria for exchange transfusion in the low birth weight population have been questioned[92] and the use of more effective phototherapy[89] has rendered moot much of the debate regarding exchange transfusion in this population. Furthermore, exchange transfusion at low bilirubin levels is very inefficient and is less effective than phototherapy in achieving a prolonged reduction of bilirubin levels in infants with nonhemolytic jaundice.[93]

As shown in Table 10.10, phototherapy is generally used according to a sliding scale – the lower the birth weight, the lower the TSB level at which phototherapy is instituted. Although this practice is followed widely, there is little evidence to support it and, in view of the known antioxdant properties of bilirubin, some have raised the possibility that maintaining very low TSB levels by the aggressive use of phototherapy might be associated with an increase in severe retinopathy of prematurity.[94] On the other hand, in a study of 157 surviving infants of 23–26 weeks gestation, DeJonge *et al.* found no association between bilirubin levels, severe ROP, or any stage of ROP.[95]

Special Circumstances

For term, near-term and very low-birth-weight infants, special circumstances may exist that require a more aggressive approach to treatment than provided in Tables 10.8 and 10.10. Table 10.11 lists some of the conditions that may modify intervention for hyperbilirubinemia.

Table 10.11. Conditions that may modify intervention for hyperbilirubinemia.

Immediate exchange transfusion
  Clinical signs of bilirubin encephalopathy

Earlier or prophylactic phototherapy due to increased procedural risk of morbidity and mortality or technical difficulty in performing exchange transfusion
  Serious complication with previous exchange transfusion
  Serious cardiovascular, coagulation, or other disease
  Potential graft-versus-host reaction (e.g., abdominal surgery, omphalocele)

Earlier phototherapy or exchange transfusion due to possible increased risk of bilirubin toxicity
  Serum bilirubin rising more than 1 mg/dl (17 μmol/l) per hour
  Serum albumin <2.5 mg/dl
  Reduced bilirubin-binding capacity, if measured
  Persistent, severe, metabolic or respiratory acidosis[a]
  Persistent, severe hypercapnia[a]
  Persistent, severe hypoxia[a]
  Sepsis
  Very sick low birth-weight infants

[a] Attempt to correct blood gas abnormality.
From Maisels.[114]

Elevated Direct Reacting or Conjugated Bilirubin levels

There are no helpful data and, as a result, little guidance on how we should deal with the occasional infant who has a high TSB as well as a significant elevation of direct reacting bilirubin. Because direct reacting bilirubin is not toxic to the central nervous system, some authors have suggested guidelines for exchange transfusion based on the level of indirect serum bilirubin level only. More recently, however, most guidelines have either ignored the subject or have referred to total bilirubin levels as the criteria for treatment. Kernicterus has been described in a full term infant with the bronze baby syndrome in which the maximum TSB level was 18 mg/dl (308 μmol/l) and the direct reacting bilirubin was 4.1 mg/dl (17 μmol/l).[96] I have reviewed at least 3 medical records of term or near term infants who developed clinical kernicterus and whose TSB levels were >20 mg/dl (340 μmol/l) but, because of significant elevations in the direct bilirubin levels, the indirect bilirubin levels were well below 20 mg/dl and no exchange transfusions were done. Grobler and Mercer reported classical kernicterus in an infant with Rh erythroblastosis fetalis who developed a TSB of 45.2 mg/dl (773 μmol/l) of which 31.6 mg/dl (540 μmol/l) was direct reacting.[97] These are, of course, anecdotal observations, but they raise the question of how elevated direct bilirubin levels should be addressed. It is possible that direct-reacting bilirubin causes competitive displacement of indirect bilirubin from its binding site to albumin. Ebbesen found that infants with elevated direct bilirubin levels of 6.4–9.9 mg/dl (109–169 μmol/l) and the bronze baby syndrome, had a decrease in reserve albumin binding capacity.[98] On the other hand, some infants with extremely high, but predominantly direct reacting, serum bilirubin levels have come to no harm. A common recommendation is that direct bilirubin concentrations should not be subtracted from the total bilirubin level unless they exceed 1/2 of the TSB concentration. Clearly, this approach would not have benefited the infant described above.[97]

Hemolytic Disease

As discussed in Chapter 9 infants with hemolytic disease are generally at a greater risk for the development of bilirubin encephalopathy than are non hemolyzing infants with similar bilirubin levels. The reasons for this are not clear. In the early studies of Rh disease, almost all infants were delivered prematurely (to prevent stillbirth) and many were asphyxiated and severely ill. It is highly unlikely that the risk of kernicterus in infants with Rh disease, treated in today's intensive care environment and with similar TSB levels would be nearly as great. Although it has been suggested that infants with hemolytic disease may have a decrease in their bilirubin-binding capacity, when measured, this has not been found to be the case.[99] Similarly, we have no obvious explanation for the increased risk of bilirubin encephalopathy in infants with G6PD deficiency.

In almost all cases of Rh hemolytic disease, phototherapy should be used quite early, as soon as there is evidence for a rapidly rising serum bilirubin level. In ABO hemolytic disease, on the other hand, early rising serum bilirubin levels frequently level off and decline spontaneously and phototherapy is often unnecessary.[50] Nevertheless, a reasonable rule of thumb for ABO hemolytic disease is to institute phototherapy at TSB levels 1–2 mg/dl (17–34 µmol/l) below those given in Table 10.8. If, in spite of intensive phototherapy, serum bilirubin levels approach 18–20 mg/dl (308–342 µmol/l) in any infant with hemolytic disease, exchange transfusion should be considered.

Intravenous gammaglobulin (IVIG) has been used successfully in Rh and ABO hemolytic disease and, in controlled trials, has been shown to reduce the need for exchange transfusions.[100,101] The use of metalloporphyrins has decreased TSB levels in infants with Coombs positive ABO incompatibility and G6PD deficiency[102,103] (see Chapter 13 on pharmacologic treatment). Early studies of the natural history of Rh and ABO hemolytic disease provided useful predictions of whether or not the serum bili-rubin concentration would reach 20 mg/dl (342 µmol/l). As a result, rules of thumb were developed for exchange transfusion based on cord blood TSB levels and on rising TSB levels at different ages. The use of intensive phototherapy and IVIG has rendered these guidelines largely irrelevant. Nevertheless, if intensive phototherapy and the use of IVIG do not control a rising serum bilirubin level, or if the TSB rapidly approaches 18–20 mg/dl (308–242 µmol/l), then an exchange transfusion is indicated.

Repeat Exchange Transfusions

In general, the criteria for repeat exchange transfusions are similar to those used for the initial exchange.

Hydrops Fetalis

The pathogenesis of hydrops fetalis with its attendant edema and serous effusions is not clear. It commonly occurs when the fetal hemoglobin drops below 6–7 gm/dl. The rapid production of severe anemia in fetal sheep produced hydrops associated with an increased central venous pressure and placental edema whereas the same degree of anemia produced over a longer period did not produce hydrops, placental edema or an increased central venous pressure.[104] In Rh isoimmunization, fetal edema may result from the extensive erythropoiesis that takes place in the fetal liver. This can disrupt the portal circulation and impair albumin synthesis.[105,106] Fetuses with severe hydrops also have elevated atrial natriuretic factor concentrations.[107] Hypoxia produces myocardial dysfunction with increased umbilical venous pressure that leads to the release of atrial natriuretic factor.[108] Severely affected infants die from progressive cardiorespiratory failure in which asphyxia and hyaline membrane disease play a major role. In one hydropic fetus with erythroblastosis fetalis, pulsed Doppler studies of left and right ventricular outputs were obtained over time. Despite severe anemia, cardiac outputs were normal and remained normal after *in utero* percutaneous intravascular transfusions, which reversed the hydrops.[109] These measurements of normal cardiac output *in utero* suggest that high output failure due to anemia is not the mechanism for hydrops in these infants and supports the hypothesis that portal hypertension and disruption of normal liver function from extra medullary hematopoiesis is the primary mechanism for the development of hydrops in isoimmune hemolytic disease of the fetus.[109]

Hydropic infants generally suffer significant hypoxia *in utero* and women who are to deliver such infants should be managed exclusively in perinatal centers capable of the full range of obstetric and neonatal intensive care. Hydropic infants and those who are severely anemic (hematocrit <35%) and asphyxiated, demand immediate treatment. Exchange transfusion of about 50 ml/kg of packed cells soon after birth raises the hematocrit to about 40%. Phlebotomy should be not be performed routinely on these infants because they are usually normovolemic and may even be hypovolemic.[109–111] No manipulations of blood volume should be performed without appropriate measurements of central venous and arterial blood pressures. For accurate monitoring of central venous pressure, however, the umbilical venous catheter must enter the inferior vena cava by way of the ductus venosus. If the catheter is in a portal vein or the umbilical vein, the pressures so measured are meaningless and preclude interpretation of the infant's circulatory status. In addition, before making therapeutic decisions based on measurements of central venous pressure, the physician must also correct acidosis, hypercarbia, hypoxia and anemia. Serum glucose levels should be monitored carefully, because hypoglycemia is common.

References

1. Saigal, S., Lunyk, O., Bennett, K.J. and Patterson, M.C., Serum bilirubin levels in breast- and formula-fed infants in the first 5 days of life, *Can. Med. Assoc. J.* 1982; **127**: 985–989.
2. Knudsen, A., Prediction of the development of neonatal jaundice by increased umbilical cord blood bilirubin, *Acta. Pediatr. Scand.* 1989; **78**: 217–221.
3. Davidson, L.T., Merritt, K.K. and Weech, A.A., Hyperbilirubinemia in the newborn, *Am. J. Dis. Child* 1941; **61**: 958–980.
4. Rosenfeld, J., Umbilical cord bilirubin levels as a predictor of subsequent hyperbilirubinemia, *J. Fam. Pract.* 1986; **23**: 556–558.

5. Risemberg, H.M., Mazzi, E., MacDonald, M.G. *et al.*, Correlation of cord bilirubin levels with hyperbilirubinemia in ABO incompatibility, *Arch. Dis. Child.* 1977; **52**: 219–222.
6. Gartner, L.M., Lee, K.-S., Vaisman, S. *et al.*, Development of bilirubin transport and metabolism in the newborn rhesus monkey, *J. Pediatr.* 1977; **90**: 513–513.
7. Wood, B., Culley, P., Roginski, C., Powell, J. and Waterhouse, J., Factors affecting neonatal jaundice, *Arch. Dis. Child.* 1979; **54**: 111–115.
8. Maisels, M.J., Gifford, K., Antle, C.E. *et al.*, Normal serum bilirubin levels in the newborn and the effect of breast feeding, *Pediatrics* 1986; **78**: 837–843.
9. Hardy, J.B., Drage, J.S. and Jackson, E.C., The First Year of Life: The Collaborative Perinatal Project of the National Institutes of Neurological and Communicative Disorders and Stroke. Baltimore, MD: Johns Hopkins University Press, 1979.
10. Newman, T.B., Escobar, G.J., Branch, P.T. *et al.*, Incidence of extreme hyperbilirubinemia in a large HMO, *Amb. Child Health* 1997; **3**: 203 (abstract).
11. Bhutani, V.K., Johnson, L. and Sivieri, E.M., Predictive ability of a predischarge hour-specific serum bilirubin for subsequent significant hyperbilirubinemia in healthy-term and near-term newborns, *Pediatrics* 1999; **103**: 6–14.
12. Maisels, M.J., Fanaroff, A.A., Stevenson, D.K. *et al.*, Serum bilirubin levels in an international, multiracial newborn population, *Pediatr. Res.* 1999; **45**: 167A.
13. Mather, A., Reliability of bilirubin determinations in icterus of the newborn infant, *Pediatrics* 1960; **26**: 350–350.
14. Vreman, H.J., Verter, J., Oh, W. *et al.*, Interlaboratory variability of bilirubin measurements, *Clin. Chem.* 1996; **42**: 869–873.
15. Frishberg, Y., Zelicovic, I., Merlob, P. and Reisner, S.H., Hyperbilirubinemia and influencing factors in term infants, *Isr. J. Med. Sci.* 1989; **25**: 28–31.
16. Seidman, D., Personal Communication, 1998.
17. Sackett, B.L., Haynes, R.B. and Tugwell, P., Clinical epidemiology. A Basic Science for Clinical Medicine. Boston: Little, Brown and Company, 1985.
18. Maisels, M.J. and Kring, E.A., Length of stay, jaundice and hospital readmission, *Pediatrics* 1998; **101**: 995–998.
19. Maisels, M.J. and Kring, E., Risk of sepsis in newborns with severe hyperbilirubinemia, *Pediatrics* 1992; **90**: 741–743.
20. American Academy of Pediatrics, Provisional committee for Quality Improvement and Subcommittee on Hyperbilirubinemia, Practice parameter: Management of hyperbilirubinemia in the healthy term newborn, *Pediatrics* 1994; **94**: 558–562.
21. Davenport, M., Kerkar, N., Mieli-Vergani, G. *et al.*, Biliary atresia: The King's College Hospital experience (1974–1995), *J. Pediatr. Surg.* 1997; **32**: 479–485.
22. Seidman, D. and Stevenson, D., The issues of hyperbilirubinemia, *Pediatrics* 1995; **96**: 543.
23. Newman, T.B., Klebanoff, M.A. and Maisels, M.J., Bilirubin problem – The debate continues, *Pediatrics* 1996; **98**: 165–166.
24. Robertson, W.O., Personal reflections on the AAP practice parameter on management of hyperbilirubinemia in the healthy term newborn, *Pediatrics in Review* 1998; **19**: 75–77.
25. Madlon-Kay, D.J., Recognition of the presence and severity of newborn jaundice by parents, nurses, physicians, and icterometer, *Pediatrics* 1997; **100 E3**:
26. Tayaba, R., Gribetz, D., Gribetz, I. and Holzman, I.R., Noninvasive estimation of serum bilirubin, *Pediatrics* 1998; **102 E3**:
27. Moyer, V.A., Ahn, C. and Sneed, S., Accuracy of clinical judgment in neonatal jaundice. Program and abstracts. Ambulatory Pediatric Association, 38th Annual Meeting, New Orleans, 1998.
28. Maisels, M.J. and Kring, E., Trancutaneous bilirubinometry decreases the need for serum bilirubin measurements and saves money, *Pediatrics* 1997; **99**: 599–601.
29. Schumacher, R.E., Non-invasive measurements of bilirubin in the newborn, *Clin. Perinatol*, 1990; **17**: 417.
30. Ebbesen, F., The relationship between the cephalo-pedal progress of clinical icterus and the serum bilirubin concentration in newborn infants without blood type sensitization, *Acta. Obstet. Gynaecol. Scand.* 1975; **54**: 329–332.
31. Kramer, L.I., Advancement of dermal icterus in the jaundiced newborn, *Am. J. Dis. Child.* 1969; **118**: 454–454.
32. Hegyi, T., Hiatt, M., Gertner, I. *et al.*, Transcutaneous bilirubinometry: the cephalocaudal progression of dermal icterus, *Am. J. Dis. Child.* 1981; **135**: 547.
33. Knudsen, A., The cephalocaudal progression of jaundice in newborns in relation to the transfer of bilirubin from plasma to skin, *Early Hum. Dev.* 1990; **22**: 23.

34. Knudsen, A., The influence of the reserve albumin concentration and pH on the cephalocaudal progression of jaundice in newborns, *Early Hum. Dev.* 1991; **25**:

35. Knudsen, A. and Broderson R., Skin colour and bilirubin in neonates, *Arch. Dis. Child.* 1989; **64**: 605.

36. Jacobsen, J. and Brodersen R., Albumin-bilirubin binding mechanism: kinetic and spectroscopic studies of binding of albumin and xanthobilirubic acid to human serum albumin, *J. Biol. Chem.* 1983; **10**: 6319.

37. Gossett, I.H., A Perspex icterometer for neonates. *Lancet* 1960; **1**: 87–88.

38. Schumacher, R.E., Thornbery, J. and Gutcher, G.R., Transcutaneous bilirubinometry: A comparison of old and new methods, *Pediatrics* 1985; **76**: 10–14.

39. Maisels, M.J. and Kring, E., Transcutaneous bilirubinometry decreases the need for serum bilirubin measurements and saves money, *Pediatrics* 1997; **99**: 599.

40. Bhutani, V, Johnson, L.H., Gourley, G. and Adler S., Transcutaneous measurement of total serum bilirubin by multi-wavelength spectral reflectance (Bilicheck™): Accuracy and precision in newborn babies, *Ped. Res.* 1999; **45**: 186A.

41. Maisels, M.J., Gifford, K.L., Antle, C.E. *et al.*, Jaundice in the healthy newborn infant: A new approach to an old problem, *Pediatrics* 1988; **81**: 505–511.

42. Newman, T.B., Easterling, M.J., Goldman, E.S. and Stevenson, D.K., Laboratory evaluation of jaundiced newborns: Frequency, cost and yield, *Am. J. Dis. Child.* 1990; **144**: 364–368.

43. Stevenson, D.K. and Vreman, H.J., Carbon monoxide production in neonates, *Pediatrics* 1997; **100**: 252–254.

44. American Academy of Pediatrics, College of Obstetrics and Gynecology. Guidelines for Perinatal Care. 4th ed. Elk Grove Village, ILL: American Academy of Pediatrics, 1997.

45. Giblet, E.R., Blood groups and blood transfusion. In: Braunwald, E., Isselbacher, K.J., Petersdordf, R.G., Wilson, J.D., Martin, J.B., Fauci, A.S., eds. 11th ed. New York: Harrison's Principles of Internal Medicine, 1987: 1483–1489.

46. Katz, M.A., Kanto, W.P. and Korotkin, J.H., Recurrence rate of ABO hemolytic disease of the newborn, *Obstet. Gynecol.* 1982; **59**: 611–614.

47. Ozolek, J., Watchko, J. and Mimouni, F., Prevalence and lack of clinical significance of blood group incompatibility in mothers with blood type A or B, *J. Pediatr.* 1994; **125**: 87–91.

48. Meberg, A. and Johansen, K.B., Screening for neonatal hyperbilirubinaemia and ABO alloimmunization at the time of testing for phenylketonuria and congenital hypothyreosis, *Acta. Paediatr.* 1998; **87**: 1269–1274.

49. Kanto, W.P., Marino, B., Godwin, A.S. and Bunyapen, C., ABO hemolytic disease: A comparative study of clinical severity and delayed anemia, *Am. J. Dis. Child.* 1978; **62**: 365–369.

50. Osborn, L.M., Lenarsky, C., Oakes, R.C. and Reiff M.I., Phototherapy in full-term infants with hemolytic disease secondary to ABO incompatibility, *Pediatrics* 1984; **74**: 371–374.

51. Quinn, M.W., Weindling, A.M. and Davidson, D.C., Does ABO incompatibility matter? *Arch. Dis. Child.* 1988; **63**: 1258–1260.

52. Serrao, P.A. and Modanlou, H.D., Significance of anti-A and anti-B isohemagglutinins in cord blood of ABO incompatible newborn infants: Correlation with hyperbilirubinemia, *J. Perinatol*, 1989; **9**: 154–158.

53. Leistikow, E.A., Collin, M.F., Savastano, G.D. *et al.*, Wasted health care dollars. Routine cord blood type and Coombs' testing, *Arch. Pediatr. Adolesc. Med.* 1995; **149**: 1147–1151.

54. Maisels, M.J. and Kring, E.A., Early discharge from the newborn nursery: Effect on scheduling of follow-up visits by pediatricians, *Pediatrics* 1997; **100**: 72–74.

55. Chavalitdhamrong, P.-O., Escobedo, M.B., Barton, L.L. *et al.*, Hyperbilirubinemia and bacterial infection in the newborn, *Arch. Dis. Child.* 1975; **50**: 652–652.

56. Linder, N., Yatsiv, I., Tsur, M. *et al.*, Unexplained neonatal jaundice as an early diagnostic sign of septicemia in the newborn, *J. Perinatol*, 1988; **8**: 325–327.

57. Rooney, J.C., Hill, D.J. and Danks, D.M., Jaundice associated with bacterial infection in the newborn, *Am. J. Dis. Child.* 1971; **122**: 39–41.

58. Brown, A.K. and Johnson, L., Loss of concern about jaundice and the reemergence of kernicterus in full term infants in the era of managed care. Yearbook of Neonatal and Perinatal Medicine. St. Louis, MO. Mosby, 1996; xvii–xxviii.

59. MacDonald, M., Hidden risks: early discharge and bilirubin toxicity due to glucose-6-phosphate dehydrogenase deficiency, *Pediatrics* 1995; **96**: 734–738.

60. Penn, A.A., Enzman, D.R., Hahn, J.S. *et al.*, Kernicterus in a full term infant, *Pediatrics* 1994; **93**: 1003–1006.

61. Sola, A. and Kitterman, J.A., Changes in clinical practice and bilirubin encephalopathy in "healthy term newborns", *Pediatr. Res.* 1995; **37**: 145A.

62. Washington, E.C., Ector, W., Abboud, M., *et al.*, Hemolytic jaundice due to G6PD deficiency causing kernicterus in a female newborn, *South Med.* 1995; **88**: 776–779.

63. Maisels, M.J. and Newman, T.B., Kernicterus in otherwise healthy, breast-fed term newborns, *Pediatrics* 1995; **96**: 730–733.

64. Lee, K.-S., Perlman, M. and Ballantyne, M., Association between duration of neonatal hospital stay and readmission rate, *J. Pediatr.* 1995; **127**: 758–766.

65. Soskolne, E.L., Schumacher, R., Fyock, C. *et al.*, The effect of early discharge and other factors on readmission rates of newborns, *Arch. Pediatr. Adolesc. Med.* 1996; **150**: 373–379.

66. Liu, L.L., Clemens, C.J., Shay, D.K., Davis, R.L. and Novack, A.H., The safety of newborn discharge. The Washington State experience, *JAMA* 1997; **278**: 293–298.

67. American Academy of Pediatrics, Committee on the Fetus and Newborn. Hospital stay for healthy term newborns, *Pediatrics* 1995; **96**: 788–790.

68. De Carvalho, M., Klaus, M.H. and Merkatz, R.B., Frequency of breastfeeding and serum bilirubin concentration, *Am. J. Dis. Child.* 1982; **136**: 737–738.

69. Yamauchi, Y. and Yamanouchi, I., Breast-feeding frequency during the first 24 hours after birth in full-term neonates, *Pediatrics* 1990; **86**: 171–175.

70. Fevery, J., Fasting hyperbilirubinemia: Unraveling the mechanism involved, *Gastroenterology* 1997; **113**: 1707–1313.

71. Eidelman, A.L., Hoffman, M.W. and Kaitz, M., Cognitive deficits in women after childbirth, *Obstet. Gynecol*, 1993; **81**: 764–767.

72. Newman, T.B., Unpublished data, 1999.

73. Ryan, A.S., The resurgence of breastfeeding in the United States, *Pediatrics* 1997; **99**(4): E12.

74. Maisels, M.J. and Newman, T.B., Jaundice in full term and near-term babies who leave the hospital within 36 hours. The pediatrician's nemesis, *Clin. Perinatol.* 1998; **25**: 295–302.

75. Maisels, M.J. and Newman, T.B., Predicting hyperbilirubinemia in newborns: The importance of timing, *Pediatrics* 1999; **103**: 493–495.

76. Johnson, L. and Bhutani, V.K., Guidelines for management of the jaundiced term and near-term infant, *Clin. Perinatol.* 1998; **25**: 555–574.

77. Maisels, M.J., Pathak, A., Nelson, N.M. *et al.*, Endogenous production of carbon monoxide in normal and erythroblastotic newborn infants, *J. Clin. Invest.* 1971; **50**: 1–1.

78. Chan, M.-L., Ho, H.-T., Ip, K.-S. *et al.*, Prediction of hyperbilirubinemia in healthy term-and near-term Chinese newborns, *Pediatr. Res.* 1999; **45**: 188A.

79. Stevenson, D.K., Young, B.W., Maisels, M.J. *et al.*, The incidence of increased bilirubin production in hyperbilirubinemic neonates as indexed by breath carbon monoxide (CO), *Pediatr. Res.* 1999; **45**: 227A.

80. Hansen, T.W.R., Acute management of extreme neonatal jaundice – the potential benefits of intensified phototherapy and interruption of enterohepatic bilirubin circulation, *Acta. Paediatr.* 1997; **86**: 843–846.

81. Varimo, P., Simil, S., Wendt, L. and Kolvisto, M., Frequency of breast feeding and hyperbilirubinemia, *Clin. Pediatr.* 1986; **25**: 112.

82. Maisels, M.J., Vain, N., Acquavita, A.M. *et al.*, The effect of breast-feeding frequency on serum bilirubin levels – a randomized controlled trial, *Am. J. Obstet. Gynecol.* 1994; **170**: 880–883.

83. De Carvalho, M., Holl, M. and Harvey, D., Effects of water supplementation on physiological jaundice in breast fed babies, *Arch. Dis. Child.* 1981; **56**: 568–569.

84. Nicoll, A., Ginsburg, R. and Tripp, J.H., Supplementary feeding and jaundice in newborns, *Acta. Pediatr. Scand.* 1982; **71**: 759–761.

85. Kuhr, M. and Paneth, N., Feeding practices and early neonatal jaundice, *J. Pediatr. Gastr. Nutr.* 1982; **1**: 485–488.

86. Herrera, A.J., Supplemented versus unsupplemented breast feeding, *Perinatology-Neonatology* 1984; 70–71.

87. Amato, M., Howald, H. and von Muralt, G., Interruption of breast-feeding vs. phototherapy as treatment of hyperbilirubinemia in full term infants, *Helv. Paediatr. Acta.* 1985; **40**: 127–131.

88. Martinez, J.C., Maisels, M.J., Otheguy, L. *et al.*, Hyperbilirubinemia in the breast-fed newborn: a controlled trial of four interventions, *Pediatrics* 1993; **91**: 470

89. Maisels, M.J., Why use homeopathic doses of phototherapy? *Pediatrics* 1996; **98**: 283–287.

90. O'Shea, T.M., Dillard, R.G., Klinepeter, K.D. *et al.*, Serum bilirubin levels, intracranial hemorrhage, and the risk of developmental problems in very low birth weight infants, *Pediatrics* 1992; **90**: 888–892.

91. Maisels, M.J., Is exchange transfusion for hyperbilirubinemia in danger of becoming extinct? *Pediatr. Res.* 1999; **45**: 210A.

92. Watchko, J. and Claassen, D., Kernicterus in premature infants: current prevalence and relationship to NICHD phototherapy study exchange criteria, *Pediatrics* 1994; **93**: 996–999.

93. Tan, K.L., Comparison of the effectiveness of phototherapy and exchange transfusion in the management of nonhemolytic neonatal hyperbilirubinemia, *J. Pediatr.* 1975; **87**: 609–609.

94. Yeo, K.L., Perlman, M., Hao, Y. and Mullaney, P., Outcomes of extremely premature infants related to their peak serum bilirubin concentrations and exposure to phototherapy, *Pediatrics* 1998; **102**: 1426–1431.

95. DeJonge, M.H., Khuntia, A., Maisels, M.J. and Bandagi, A., Bilirubin levels and severe retinopathy of prematurity in 23–26 week estimated gestational age infants, *J. Pediatr.* 1999; **135**: 102–104.

96. Clark, C.F., Torii, S., Hamamoto, Y. and Kaito, H., The "bronze baby" syndrome: postmortem data, *J. Pediatr.* 1976; **88**: 461–464.

97. Grobler, J.M. and Mercer, M.J., Kernicterus associated with elevated predominately direct-reacting bilirubin, *S. Afr. Med. J.* 1997; **87**: 146.

98. Ebbesen, F., Low reserve albumin for binding of bilirubin in neonates with deficiency of bilirubin excretion and bronze baby syndrome, *Acta. Paediatr. Scand.* 1982; **71**: 415–410.

99. Catterton, Z., Carp, W., Bunyaten, C. *et al.*, Bilirubin binding capacity in ABO hemolytic disease of the newborn, *Clin. Res.* 1979; **27**: 817A.

100. Sato, K., Hara, T., Kondo, T., Iwao, H., Honda, S. and Ueda, K., High-dose intravenous gamma-globulin therapy for neonatal immune haemolytic jaundice due to blood group incompatibility, *Acta. Paediatr. Scand.* 1991; **80**: 163–166.

101. Rubo, J., Albrecht, K., Lasch, P. *et al.*, High-dose intravenous immune globulin therapy for hyperbilirubinemia caused by Rh hemolytic disease, *J. Pediatr.* 1992; **121**: 93–97.

102. Kappas, A., Drummond, G.S., Manola, T. *et al.*, Sn-protoporphyrin use in the management of hyperbilirubinemia in term newborns with direct Coombs'-positive ABO incompatibility, *Pediatrics* 1988; **81**: 485–497.

103. Valaes, T., Drummond, G.S. and Kappas, A., Control of hyperbilirubinemia in glucose-6-phosphate dehydrogenase-deficient newborns using an inhibitor of bilirubin production, Sn-meso-porphyrin, *Pediatrics* 1998; **101** (5):5 URL: http://www.pediatrics.org/cgi/content/full/101/5/el

104. Blair, D.K., Vander Straten, M.C. and Gest, A.L., Hydrops fetalis in sheep from rapid induction of anemia, *Pediatr. Res.* 1994; **35**: 560–564.

105. Nicolaides, K.H., Warenski, J.C. and Rodeck, C.H., The relationship of fetal plasma protein concentration and hemoglobin level to the development of hydrops in rhesus isoimmunization, *Am. J. Obstet. Gynecol.* 1985; **152**: 341–344.

106. Grannum, P.A., Copel, J.A., Moya, F.R. *et al.*, The reversal of hydrops fetalis by intravascular intrauterine transfusion in severe isoimmune fetal anemia, *Am. J. Obstet. Gynecol.* 1988; **158**: 914–919.

107. Moya, F.R., Grannum, P.A., Riddick, L. *et al.*, Atrial natriuretic factor in hydrops fetalis caused by Rh isoimmunization, *Arch. Dis. Child.* 1990; **65**: 683–686.

108. Weiner, C., Nonhematologic effects of intravascular transfusion on the human fetus, *Semin. Perinatol.* 1989; **13**: 338–341.

109. Barss, V.A., Doubilet, P.M., St.John-Sutton, M., Cartier, M.D. and Frigoletto, F.D., Cardiac output in a fetus with erythroblastosis fetalis: assessment using pulsed Doppler, *Obstet. Gynecol.* 1987; **70**: 442–444.

110. Phibbs, R.H., Johnson, P. and Tooley, W.H., Cardiorespiratory status of erythroblastotic newborn infants. II. Blood volume, hematocrit, and serum albumin concentration in relation to hydrops fetalis, *Pediatrics* 1974; **53**: 13–23.

111. Nicolaides, K.H., Clewell, W.H. and Rodeck, C.H., Measurement of human fetoplacental blood volume in erythroblastosis fetalis, *Am. J. Obstet. Gynecol.* 1987; **157**: 50–53.

112. Yamauchi, Y. and Yamanouchi, I., Transcutaneous bilirubinometry in normal Japanese infants, *Acta. Paediatr. Jpn.* 1989; **31**: 65–72.

113. Okolo, A.A., Omene, J.A. and Scott-Emaukpor, A.B., Physiologic jaundice in the Nigerian neonate, *Biol. Neonate* 1988; **53**: 132–137.

114. Maisels, M.J., Neonatal jaundice, In: Avery, G.B., Fletcher, M.A. and MacDonald, M.G., Neonatology: pathophysiology and management of the newborn. J.B.Lippincott Co., 5th ed. Philadelphia, 1999; 765–820.

11 Exchange Transfusion in the Management of Neonatal Hyperbilirubinemia

Jon F. Watchko

Division of Neonatology and Developmental Biology, Department of Pediatrics, University of Pittsburgh School of Medicine, Pittsburgh, Pennsylvania, USA

HISTORICAL ASPECTS

Phototherapy and exchange transfusion are the mainstays of treatment for infants with hyperbilirubinemia. Exchange transfusion occupies a unique place in the history of neonatal jaundice because it was the first intervention to permit effective control of hyperbilirubinemia and thus, prevent kernicterus in infants with Rh isoimmunization.[1-3] The original description of exchange transfusion in the management of an infant with icterus gravis neonatorum actually predated by two decades an understanding of the pathophysiology of this disease. This remarkably prescient account by Hart, published in 1925,[4] detailed the clinical course of an infant born on December 18, 1924 to a family that had lost 6 previous newborns to icterus gravis neonatorum. Their sole surviving child had also experienced severe jaundice as a neonate and subsequently suffered from chorea. Thus, trouble with their current newborn had been anticipated. When jaundice intensified on day 3 of life a colleague of Hart's, J.L. MacDonald, M.D., also from the Hospital for Sick Children in Toronto, performed an exchange transfusion on the approximately 8 lb male neonate. The rationale for using an exchange transfusion was the belief by Hart that the infant's life was at risk because of an unknown toxin circulating in the blood and the hope that removing sufficient toxin might prevent the progress of the disease.[4] He stated that "as both parents and I felt that if something drastic was not done at once the child was certainly going to die as the six other previous males had done, it was decided to do an exsanguination transfusion".[4] Hart described the procedure as follows:

> Dr J.L. MacDonald ... exsanguinated three hundred cc. of blood from the anterior fontanelle at the same time transfusing 335 cc. of blood into the internal saphenous vein at the left ankle. The transfusion was commenced after 20 cc. of blood had been removed and **the transfusion and exsanguination went on synchronously until the required quantity had been used**, and we ended by giving the baby 35 cc. more than had been removed. ... By the following morning the jaundice was much less intense.[4]

169

The infant survived the procedure, was spared the effects of hyperbilirubinemic encephalopathy and thrived.[4,5] The paper by Hart provided a detailed description of familial icterus gravis neonatorum, evinced an in depth understanding of this disease, and set the stage for therapeutic refinements in exchange transfusion two decades later by Wallerstein,[6] following the discovery of the Rh factor by Landsteiner in 1940.[7] Harry Wallerstein, a hematologist by training, recognized that many infants with erythroblastosis fetalis (hemolytic disease of the newborn) died of the disease in the absence of severe anemia and postulated (analogous to Hart) that a "factor of toxemia, possibly arising from the stromal substance of the lysed red blood cells, undoubtedly plays an important role in the fatal outcome in these cases".[6] Moreover, he felt that the administration of Rh negative blood alone would not ameliorate the problem in all cases, a fact borne out in subsequent study.[8] Wallerstein postulated that it was "desirable to remove the known Rh positive blood of the infant and to replace it with Rh negative blood. Such a procedure would either minimize or entirely prevent the action of the hemolytic end products upon the ... brain ganglia".[6] Wallerstein used the sagittal sinus to withdraw the Rh positive blood from the affected infants ($n = 3$) and administered the Rh negative blood via a cannulated peripheral vein and calculated that at the completion of the exchange transfusion (250 cc [∼ *single volume exchange*]) only 25% of the original Rh positive red cells would remain in the infants circulation.[6] These early exsanguination-transfusion procedures, however, were complicated by the fact that sagittal vein puncture was a dangerous procedure particularly in newborn infants where anatomical relations were often distorted as a result of cranial molding during labor and delivery. Further important refinements in the technique of exchange transfusion were made by Wiener and colleagues[9] who utilized the radial artery for blood removal and the saphenous vein for blood infusion and by Diamond and co-workers who were the first to utilize special plastic catheters placed in the umbilical vein,[10,11] thus making it possible for the average practitioner to perform this procedure.

THERAPEUTIC GOALS OF EXCHANGE TRANSFUSION

Exchange transfusion in infants with erythroblastosis fetalis accomplishes four desirable goals in addition to the immediate control of hyperbilirubinemia: these are 1) the removal of antibody-coated red blood cells [a source of "potential" bilirubin], 2) the correction of anemia [if present], 3) the removal of maternal antibody and 4) the removal of other potential toxic byproducts of the hemolytic process. The efficiency of red cell exchange is dependent on the fraction of blood volume exchanged (Figure 11.1).[12] Approximately 85% of the infant's red blood cells are removed by a double volume exchange (Figure 11.1).[12]

A newborn's blood volume is ∼85 ml/kg and a "double volume" exchange refers to an exchange of twice the blood volume or ∼170 ml/kg. The exchange transfusion is much less efficient in the removal of total body bilirubin because the majority of the infant's bilirubin is in the extravascular compartment.[13] In fact, although a double volume exchange transfusion removes 110% of circulating bilirubin (extravascular

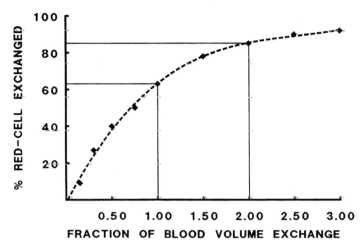

**EFFICIENCY OF RED-CELL EXCHANGE
VS. FRACTION OF BLOOD VOLUME EXCHANGED**

Figure 11.1. Efficiency of exchange transfusion as a fraction of blood volume exchanged. Derived from Veall and Mollison[12] and based on intermittent substitution "push-pull" method of exchange.

bilirubin enters the blood during the exchange), only 25% of total body bilirubin is removed. Post-exchange bilirubin levels are ~60% of pre-exchange levels, but the re-equilibration of bilirubin between the vascular and extravascular compartments produces a rebound of serum bilirubin levels to 70–80% pre-exchange levels.[14] The equilibration of intra- and extravascular bilirubin is rapid (~30 min), a finding that prompted Valaes to trial a "two-stage" exchange transfusion.[13] In this approach, the double volume exchange was interrupted midway for 30 minutes to allow time for the passage of bilirubin from the tissues into the circulation and potentially enhance the efficacy of the exchange.[13] Although increased bilirubin removal was demonstrated using this technique,[13] it has never attained widespread use. The paper by Valaes describing these findings is an excellent source of information on bilirubin tissue distribution and the dynamics of bilirubin removal by exchange transfusion.[13] The clinical indications for exchange transfusion are detailed in Chapter 10.

TECHNIQUES AND PROCEDURES

Exchange transfusions are most readily performed via the umbilical vein using a 5 or 8 Fr umbilical catheter inserted just far enough to obtain free flow of blood (usually no more than the distance between the xiphoid process and umbilicus). The "push-pull" method with a single syringe and special four way stopcock assembly permits a single operator to complete the procedure (Figure 11.2).

Alternatively, the exchange transfusion may be performed by simultaneous infusion through an umbilical venous catheter placed in the inferior vena cava and

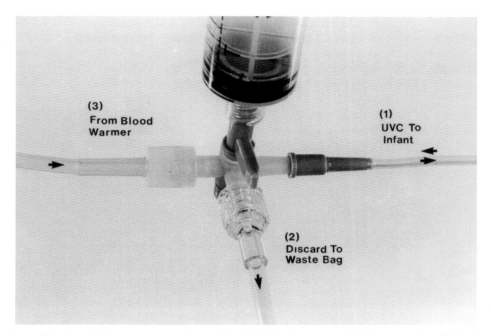

Figure 11.2. Special four-way stop cock assembly. (1) Male adapter to umbilical venous line; (2) female adapter to waste container; and (3) attachment to blood bag and warmer. The stop cock handle points to the port that is open to the syringe and stop cock handle is rotated in a clockwise fashion when correctly assembled (e.g., first, withdraw aliquot from infant; second, discard to waste container; third, draw fresh blood from bag, and then forth, infuse into infant to complete one cycle).

withdrawal from an umbilical arterial catheter. Infusion through the umbilical arterial catheter should be avoided, if possible, because of the theoretical risk of aortic retrograde flow that may perfuse the central nervous system with hypoxic/acidotic exchange blood. Fresh citrate-phosphate-dextrose blood (<72 hours old; and devoid of the offending antigen in the case of immune mediated hemolytic disease) cross-matched to the infant should be used. Although the risk for graft-versus-host disease following an exchange transfusion is extremely rare, blood for exchange transfusion should be irradiated if possible, particularly in the infant who is premature. The blood should be warmed to body temperature by a blood/fluid warmer. The actual exchange should be performed slowly in aliquots of 5 (to 10) cc/kg body weight with each withdrawal-infusion cycle approximating 3-min duration.[15] Using this approach, a double volume exchange should take ~1.5 ± 0.5 hours. This rate of exchange has been demonstrated to be both safe and efficient.[16] Although some clinicians have not attributed importance to the speed of exchange.[17,18] a slower exchange rate avoids deleterious hemodynamic changes which can be quite profound as demonstrated by Aranda and Sweet (Figure 11.3).[15] The wide fluctuations in blood pressure observed during rapid exchange may adversely affect cerebral[19] and/ or gastrointestinal blood flow.[20]

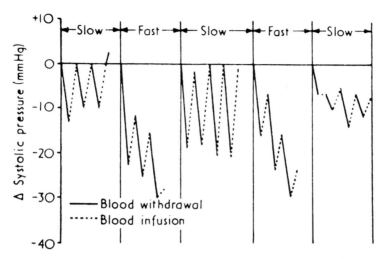

Figure 11.3. Aortic systolic blood pressure changes during slow (10 ml/3 min) and fast (10 ml/45−60 s) periods of blood withdrawal (solid line) and infusion (hatched line) in a preterm infant (2270 grams birthweight; 36 weeks gestation) undergoing an exchange transfusion. From Aranda and Sweet;[15] reprinted with permission from the BMJ Publishing Group.

During the exchange, the infants vital signs should be monitored closely, including ECG, respiration, oxygen saturation, temperature, and blood pressure. Symptomatic hypocalcemia will develop in 5% of healthy infants but supplemental calcium gluconate administration during the exchange transfusion has little effect on serum ionized calcium,[21–23] and too rapid infusion of calcium may cause bradyarrythmias or cardiac arrest. If symptomatic hypocalcemia develops, temporary cessation of the procedure will allow recovery toward normal calcium levels as the citrate (which binds calcium) is metabolized by the liver. Albumin need not be administered routinely before or during the exchange transfusion as this practice does not consistently increase the amount of bilirubin removed.[24,25] Post exchange studies should include: bilirubin, hemoglobin, platelet count, ionized calcium and serum glucose.

POTENTIAL HAZARDS OF EXCHANGE TRANSFUSION

The unintended consequences of exchange transfusion are potentially numerous and defined in Table 11.1. They include cardiovascular, hematologic, gastrointestinal, biochemical and infectious hazards among others.

Previously reported overall mortality rates associated with exchange transfusion ranged from 0.3 to 0.95 per 100 procedures,[26,27] and significant morbidity (apnea, bradycardia, cyanosis, vasospasm, thrombosis) was observed in 6.7% of infants who received exchange transfusion in the NICHD collaborative phototherapy study.[26] These rates, however, may not be generalizable to the current era if, like most procedures, frequency of performance is an important determinant of risk[28] and

Table 11.1. Potential complications of exchange transfusion.

Cardiovascular	Arrhythmias
	Cardiac arrest
	Volume overload
	Embolization with air or clots
	Thrombosis
	Vasospasm
Hematologic	Sickling (donor blood)
	Thrombocytopenia
	Bleeding (overheparinization of donor blood)
	Graft versus host disease
	Mechanical of thermal injury to donor cells
Gastrointestinal	Necrotizing enterocolitis
	Bowel perforation
Biochemical	Hyperkalemia
	Hypernatremia
	Hypocalcemia
	Hypomagnesemia
	Acidosis
	Hypoglycemia
Infectious	Bacteremia
	Virus infection (hepatitis, CMV)
	Malaria
Miscellaneous	Hypothermia
	Perforation of umbilical vein
	Drug loss
	Apnea

experience with exchange transfusion is decreasing.[29] It is quite possible that the mortality (and morbidity) for this now infrequently performed procedure might be considerably higher than previously reported. On the other hand, none of the reports prior to 1986 included contemporary monitoring capabilities such as pulse oximetry. Jackson recently reported a 2 percent overall mortality rate (2/106) associated with exchange transfusions between 1980 and 1995.[30] There was a 12 percent risk of serious complications attributable to exchange transfusion in ill infants.[30] Moreover, in infants classified as ill with medical problems in addition to hyperbilirubinemia, the incidence of exchange transfusion related complications leading to death was 8 percent.[30] There were no procedure related deaths in 81 healthy infants.[30] Symptomatic hypocalcemia, bleeding related to thrombocytopenia, catheter-related complications, and apnea-bradycardia requiring resuscitation were common serious morbidities observed in this study suggesting that exchange transfusion should be performed only in nurseries prepared to respond to these adverse events.[30]

One of the most serious associated complications of exchange transfusion is necrotizing enterocolitis.[30-35] The etiology of this complication remains unclear but may result from bowel ischemia related to portal venous congestion during the injection phase of the withdrawal-infusion exchange cycle,[20] and/or a sustained fall in arterial blood pressure when the exchange transfusion is performed too rapidly.[15]

Although, this and the other complications detailed in Table 11.1 are not altogether avoidable, they will occur less frequently if exchange transfusions are performed by experienced individuals in a neonatal intensive care unit with continuous monitoring (including pulse oximetry) and close attention to detail. Finally, although the risk is now very low, transfusion always carries some risk of acquired immunodeficiency syndrome and hepatitis.[36] The risk estimates (risk per tested unit) for transfusion transmitted viruses in the United States for the period 1991 through 1993 were as follows: for the human immunodeficiency virus (HIV), 1:493,000 (95% confidence interval, 202,000 to 2,778,000); for the human T-cell lymphotropic virus (HTLV), 1:641,000 (256,000 to 2,000,000); for the hepatitis C virus (HCV), 1:103,000 (28,000 to 288,000); and for the hepatitis B virus (HBV), 1:63,000 (31,000 to 147,000).[36]

References

1. Allen, F.H. Jr., Diamond, L.K. and Vaughan, V.C., III. Erythroblastosis fetalis. VI. Prevention of kernicterus, *Am. J. Dis. Child.* 1950; **80**: 779–791.
2. Hsia, D.Y., Allen, F.H., Gellis, S.S. and Diamond, L.K., Erythroblastosis fetalis VII. Studies of serum bilirubin in relation to kernicterus, *N. Engl. J. Med.* 1952; **247**: 668–671.
3. Mollison, P.L. and Cutbush, M., Haemolytic disease of the newborn. In: Gairdner, D. ed. Recent Advances in Pediatrics. New York, N.Y.: P. Blakiston and Son 1954; 110.
4. Hart, A.P., Familial icterus gravis of the newborn and its treatment, *Can. Med. Assoc. J.* 1925; **15**: 1008–1011.
5. Hart, A.P., Exsanguination transfusion in a newborn infant in 1925, *J. Pediatr.* 1948; **32**: 760.
6. Wallerstein, H., Treatment of severe erythroblastosis by simultaneous removal and replacement of the blood of the newborn infant, *Science* 1946; **103**: 583–584.
7. Landsteiner, K. and Weiner, A.S., An agglutinable factor in human blood recognizable by immune sera for Rhesus blood, *Proc. Soc. Exper. Biol. Med.* 1940; **43**: 223.
8. Vaughan, V.C., Allen, F.H. and Diamond, L.K., Erythroblastosis fetalis. I. Problems in the interpretation of changing mortality in erythroblastosis fetalis, *Pediatrics* 1950; **6**: 173–182.
9. Wiener, A.S., Wexler, I.B. and Grundfast, G.H., Therapy of erythroblastosis with exchange transfusion, *Bull, N.Y. Acad. Med.* 1947; **23**: 207–220.
10. Diamond, L.K., Erythroblastosis foetalis or haemolytic disease of the newborn, *Proc. Royal Soc. Med.* 1947; **40**: 546–550.
11. Diamond, L.K., Allen, F.H. and Thomas, W.O., Erythroblastosis fetalis. VII. Treatment with exchange transfusion, *N. Engl. J. Med.* 1951; **244**: 39–49.
12. Veall, N. and Mollison, P.L., The rate of red cell exchange in replacement transfusion, *Lancet* 1950; **2**: 792–797.
13. Valaes, T., Bilirubin distribution and dynamics of bilirubin removal by exchange transfusion, *Acta. Paediatr.* 1963; **52** (suppl 149): 1–115.
14. Brown, A.K., Zuelzer, W.W. and Robinson, A.R., Studies in hyperbilirubinemia. II. Clearance of bilirubin from plasma and extra vascular space in newborn infants during exchange transfusion, *Am. J. Dis. Child.* 1957; **93**: 274–286.
15. Aranda, J.V. and Sweet, A.Y., Alterations in blood pressure during exchange transfusion, *Arch. Dis. Child.* 1977; **52**: 545–548.
16. Forfar, J.O., Keay, A.J., Elliott, W.D. and Cumming, R.A., Exchange transfusion in neonatal hyperbilirubinemia, *Lancet* 1958; **2**: 1131–1137.
17. Boggs, T.R. and Westphal, M.C., Mortality of exchange transfusion, *Pediatrics* 1960; **26**: 745–755.
18. Boggs, T.R., Rapidity of Exchange, in Techniques of Exchange Transfusion, Supplement No. 1. to Reports of Ross Conferences on Pediatric Research, Thompson, S.G. ed. Columbus, OH: Ross Laboratories, 1962, pp. 46–47.
19. Bada, H.S., Chua, C., Salmon, J.H. and Hajjar, W., Changes in intracranial pressure during exchange transfusion, *J. Pediatr.* 1979; **94**: 129–132.
20. Touloukian, R.J., Kadar, A. and Spencer, R.P., The gastrointestinal complications of neonatal umbilical venous exchange transfusion. A clinical and experimental study, *Pediatrics* 1973; **51**: 36–43.

21. Ellis, M,I., Hey, E.N. and Walker, W., Neonatal death in babies with rhesus isoimmunization, *Q. J. Med.* 1979; **48**: 211–225.
22. Maisels, M.J., Li, T.K., Piechocki, J.T. and Werthman, M.W., The effect of exchange transfusion on serum ionized calcium, *Pediatrics* 1974; **53**: 683–686.
23. Wieland, P., Duc, G., Binswanger, U. and Fischer, J.A., Parathyroid hormone response in newborn infants during exchange transfusion with blood supplemented with citrate and phosphate: Effects of IV calcium, *Pediatr. Res.* 1979; **13**: 963–968.
24. Ruys, J.H. and van Gelderen, H.H., Administration of albumin in exchange transfusion, *J. Pediatr.* 1962; **61**: 413–417.
25. Chan, G. and Schiff, D., Variance in albumin loading in exchange transfusions, *J. Pediatr.* 1976; **88**: 609–613.
26. Keenan, W.J., Novak, K.K., Sutherland, J.M., Bryla, D.A. and Fetterly, K.L. Morbidity and mortality associated with exchange transfusion, *Pediatrics* (suppl) 1985; **75**: 417–421.
27. Hovi, L. and Siimes, M.A., Exchange transfusion with fresh heparinized blood is a safe procedure. *Acta. Paediatr. Scand.* 1985; **74**: 360–365.
28. Watchko, J.F. and Oski, F.A., Kernicterus in preterm newborns: past, present, and future, *Pediatrics* 1992; **90**: 707–715.
29. Newman, T.B. and Maisels, M.J., Evaluation and treatment of jaundice in the term newborn: A kinder gentler approach, *Pediatrics* 1992; **89**: 809–818.
30. Jackson, J.C., Adverse events associated with exchange transfusion in healthy and ill newborns. Pediatrics electronic pages [Online], e7, Available: http://www.pediatrics.org [May, 1997].
31. Castor, W.R., Spontaneous perforation of bowel in newborn following exchange transfusion, *Can. Med. Assoc. J.* 1968; **99**: 934–939.
32. Corkery, J.J., Dubowitz, V., Lister, J. and Moosa, A., Colonic perforation after exchange transfusion, *Br. Med. J.* 1968; **4**: 345–349.
33. Hilgartner, M.W., Lanzkowsky, P. and Lipsitz, P., Perforation of small and large intestine following exchange transfusion, *Am. J. Dis. Child.* 1970; **120**: 79–81.
34. Livaditis, A., Wallgren, G. and Faxelieus, G., Necrotizing enterocolitis after catheterization of the umbilical vessels, *Acta Paediatr. Scand.* 1974; **63**: 277–281.
35. Orme, R.L. and Eades, S.M., Perforation of the bowel in the newborn as a complication of exchange transfusion, *Br. Med. J.* 1968; **4**: 349–351.
36. Schreiber, G.B., Busch, M.P., Kleinman, S.H. and Korelitz, J.J., The risk of transfusion-transmitted viral infections, *N. Engl. J. Med.* 1996; **334**: 1685–1690.

12 Phototherapy

M. Jeffrey Maisels

Department of Pediatrics, William Beaumont Hospital, Royal Oak, Michigan, USA

We owe the development of phototherapy to an astute observation, made 40 years ago, by Sister J. Ward, the nurse in charge of the premature baby unit at the Rochford General Hospital in Essex, England. As described by Dr. R.H. Dobbs, consultant pediatrician, Sister Ward recognized the value of sunshine and fresh air to all, including premature babies, and she would take the "more delicate infants out into the courtyard, sincerely convinced that the combination of fresh air and sunshine would do them much more good than the stuffy, overheated atmosphere of the incubator".[1] During a ward round in 1956, Sister Ward showed the pediatricians a jaundiced, premature infant who appeared pale yellow except for a triangle of skin that was much yellower than the rest of the body. Apparently, a corner of the sheet had covered this part of the baby, and the Sister recognized that the rest of the baby had been "bleached" by the sun.*

A few weeks later, in the same nursery, a tube of blood was inadvertently exposed to sunlight for several hours and it was noted that the bilirubin level had fallen by 170 µmol/l (10 mg/dl). This confirmed the idea that visible light could affect serum bilirubin levels and the concept of using phototherapy as a clinical tool was born.[2] R.J. Cremer, et al. then showed that exposing jaundiced premature infants either to sunlight or to blue fluorescent lights effectively lowered their bilirubin levels.[2] At the time, Cremer was a pediatric resident (or registrar) in Dr. Dobbs' ward, and he went on to a career in family practice. Although Cremer's observations were published in 1958 and confirmed by Obes-Polleri and Hill in 1964,[3] it was not until Lucey and coworkers published their findings in 1968 that this simple, safe and effective treatment for hyperbilirubinemia achieved widespread acceptance in the United States.[4]

Phototherapy is now used worldwide for the treatment of hyperbilirubinemia; it is safe and it works. Although there exists a vast body of literature of human, animal

Address for correspondence: M. Jeffrey Maisels, M.D., 3535 W. 13 Mile Road, Royal Oak, Michigan 48073, Phone: (248) 551-0412, Fax: (248) 551-5998, E-mail: jmaisels@beaumont.edu
* It was only recognized more than a decade later that the mechanism for the bleaching of yellow serum – photooxidation – probably plays little role in the reduction of the serum bilirubin concentration in newborns treated with phototherapy.

and laboratory investigation dealing with the mechanisms of action, biological effects, complications, and clinical use of phototherapy, there is considerable misunderstanding about how phototherapy works, how it's dose is measured, and how it should be administered. The most comprehensive reference source for phototherapy is the 1993 monograph by Jährig *et al.*[5] to which the reader is referred for more detailed information and additional references not provided in this chapter.

TERMINOLOGY

Because few are familiar with the biology and photochemistry of light, it is helpful to consider light as an infusion of discrete photons of energy that correspond to the individual molecules of a drug in a conventional medication. Absorption of these photons by bilirubin molecules in the skin leads to the therapeutic effect in much the same way as binding of drug molecules to a receptor has a desired effect. Whereas drug dosages are conveniently measured in units of weight, photon dosages are more difficult to measure and are expressed in rather less familiar terms. To complicate matters further, there is no standardized method for reporting phototherapy dosages in the clinical literature; investigators have used different instruments with varying spectral responses, different filters and different units for expressing the results.[6] Clinical studies have shown that there are 3 major factors that influence the dose and, therefore, the efficacy of phototherapy. These are listed in Table 12.1 and Table 12.2 defines the radiometric quantities used in assessing the dose.

Table 12.1. Factors that determine the dose of phototherapy.

Spectrum of light emitted
Irradiance of light source
Design of phototherapy unit
Surface area of infant exposed to the light
Distance of infant from light source

From Maisels.[98]

Table 12.2. Radiometric quantities used.

Quantity	Dimensions	Usual units of measure
Irradiance (radiant power incident on a surface per unit area of the surface)	W/m^2	W/cm^2
Spectral irradiance (irradiance in a certain wavelength band)	W/m^2 per nm (or W/m^2)	$\mu/W/cm^2$ per nm
Spectral power (average spectral irradiance across a surface area)	W/m	mW/nm

From Maisels.[99]

Light Spectrum

The spectrum of light delivered by the phototherapy unit is determined by the type of light source and any filters used. Because of the optical properties of bilirubin and skin, the most effective lights are those with wavelengths that are predominantly in the blue-green spectrum.[7] Although commercially available fluorescent daylight and cool white tubes are commonly used, these tubes emit light at wavelengths of 300–700 nm but do not have a high output in the blue spectrum (425–475 nm).

Halogen (quartz halide) phototherapy lamps emit significant energy in the blue spectrum and are smaller, more portable and often more convenient to use than standard fluorescent tubes. However, halogen phototherapy lamps cannot be positioned closer to the infant than recommended by the manufacturer without incurring the risk of a burn, whereas fluorescent tubes can be brought very close to the infant in order to increase the irradiance.

A third type of light in common use is the fiberoptic light system. Here light is delivered from a high intensity lamp and transmitted down a fiberoptic bundle to a pad that can be placed directly in contact with the infant's skin.

There is a common misconception that ultraviolet light is used for phototherapy. None of the light systems described emit any significant amount of UV radiation. The small amount of UV light that is emitted by fluorescent tubes is in longer wavelengths (>320 nm) than those which cause erythema and, in any case, almost all UV light produced is absorbed by the glass wall of the fluorescent tube and by the plexiglass cover of the phototherapy unit.

Irradiance

There is a direct relationship between the efficacy of phototherapy and the *irradiance* used[8] (Figure 12.1) and irradiance is directly related to the distance between the light and the infant (Figure 12.2). Irradiance decreases rapidly with increasing distance and cannot be reliably estimated by eye. It is measured in watts per square centimeter or microwatts per square centimeter. The irradiance in a certain wavelength band is called the *spectral irradiance* and is expressed as $\mu W/cm^2/nm$. In the laboratory, spectral irradiance is measured with a precision instrument known as a spectroradiometer, which measures the flux of light over a series of discrete wavelengths. Clinicians and the manufacturers of phototherapy units usually use standard radiometers to measure the light output. These radiometers are relatively inexpensive and easy to operate but, unlike spectroradiometers, they take only a single measurement across a band of wavelengths – typically 425–475 or 400–480 nm. These bands of wavelengths are chosen because they represent the wavelengths at which bilirubin absorbs light maximally and will therefore undergo photochemical reactions to form excretable isomers and breakdown products.

Commercial radiometers measure the irradiance in a predetermined band but display the results as the spectral irradiance ($\mu W/cm^2/nm$). To do this, they simply divide the irradiance by the width of the wavelength band. Thus, a radiometer placed

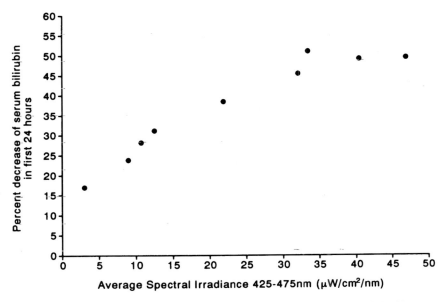

Figure 12.1. Relationship between average spectral irradiance and decrease in serum bilirubin concentration. Full-term infants with nonhemolytic hyperbilirubinemia were exposed to special blue light (Phillips TL 52/20 W) of different intensities. Spectral irradiance was measured as the average of readings at the head, trunk, and knees. Drawn from the data of Tan.[8]

30 cm below a phototherapy unit might measure an irradiance of $400\,\mu W/cm^2$ in the 400–480 nm band (a width of 80 nm) and will provide a readout of the spectral irradiance of $400/80 = 5\,\mu W/cm^2/nm$. Note, however, that under identical circumstances, a different radiometer that provided its measurement in the 425–475 nm band (a width of 50 nm) would display a spectral irradiance of 400/50 or $8\,\mu W/cm^2/nm$. Thus, published data on spectral irradiance using different radiometers and different phototherapy systems cannot be compared and commercial radiometers provide "at best an estimate of the effective irradiance."[6] The only measurements that can be compared are those taken using the same radiometer and similar light sources. Furthermore, expressing spectral irradiance as $\mu W/cm^2/nm$ (by dividing the irradiance by the band width) may not be appropriate because it is unlikely that the energy spectrum of the light source and the filter characteristics behave in a linear fashion over a range of 50–100 nm.[5] Thus it may be more appropriate to provide measurements in $\mu W/cm^2$ (rather than $\mu W/cm^2/nm$) and to document the spectral region in which the measurements were taken.

Radiometers are probably not essential pieces of equipment for every nursery, but they are useful for the purposes of quality control – to check the irradiance levels of phototherapy units and compare them with previous measurements. A sudden drop in irradiance might alert staff to a problem such as a damaged bulb or dirty reflectors in a phototherapy unit (for a more detailed discussion of radiometers see the study by ECRI).[6]

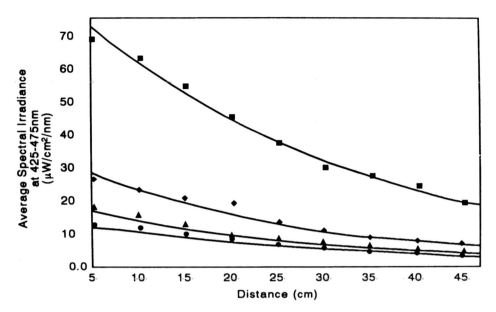

Figure 12.2. Effect of light source and distance from the light source to the infant on average spectral irradiance. Measurements were made across the 425 to 475 nm band using a commercial radiometer (Olympic Bilimeter Mark II). The phototherapy unit was fitted with eight 24-in fluorescent tubes. ■ indicates special blue, General Electric 20-W F20T12/BB tube; ◆ blue, General Electric 20-W F20T12/B tube; ▲ daylight blue, four General Electric 20-W F20T12/B blue tubes and four Sylvania 20-W F20T12/D daylight tubes; and ● daylight, Sylvania 20-W F20T12/D daylight tube. Curves were plotted using linear curve fitting (True Epistat; Epistat Services, Richardson, TX). The best fit is described by the equation $y = Ae^{Bx}$. From Maisels.[99]

The relationship between irradiance and the distance between the infant and the light source

Figure 12.2 shows that the light intensity (measured as spectral irradiance) is inversely related to the distance from the source. The relationship between intensity and distance is almost (but not quite) linear, indicating that these data do not obey the law of inverse squares, which states that the light intensity will decrease with the square of the distance. This law applies only to a point source of light and photo-therapy units do not provide a point source of light – the light source has some features of both a cylindrical and a planar source. Thus, the light intensity is a function of the distance but does not vary with the square of the distance.

Spectral Power

The *spectral power* is the product of the skin surface irradiance and the spectral irradiance across this surface area. Because both the irradiance and the surface area of the infant exposed to phototherapy are key elements in determining the efficacy of phototherapy, if we are to compare the dose of phototherapy received by 2 infants under different phototherapy systems, this can only be done by expressing the dose of phototherapy in terms of the spectral power delivered to the infant. The calculation of spectral power involves a measurement of the surface area of the infant exposed to phototherapy and the spectral irradiance delivered by the phototherapy system. For example, with fiberoptic phototherapy systems, the exposed surface area is assumed to be equal to the illuminated area of the fiberoptic pad. Assuming that the pad has an area of $134 \, cm^2$ and a maximum average spectral irradiance (400–480 nm) of $22 \, \mu W/cm^2/nm$, the spectral power can be calculated as $134 \times 22 = 2948 \, \mu W/nm$ or $2.9 \, mW/nm$. When a standard overhead bank of fluorescent phototherapy tubes is used, the whole surface of the infant facing the light is assumed to be the surface area exposed. Surface area can be obtained from standard nomograms.[9] The surface area of a normal term newborn (length 50 cm, weight 3.5 kg) is approximately $0.22 \, m^2$ or $2200 \, cm^2$. For a baby lying prone or supine under a bank of phototherapy lights, one can assume that the anterior (or posterior) surface of the infant is approximately equal to one-fourth of the total surface area or $550 \, cm^2$. Special blue tubes 15 cm above the infant provide an average spectral irradiance of $54 \, \mu W/cm^2/nm$ and therefore a spectral power of $550 \times 54 = 29700 \, \mu W/nm$ or $29.7 \, mW/nm$. But infants are not flat, so all of these calculations are approximations at best.

MECHANISM OF ACTION

Phototherapy is a mechanism for detoxifying bilirubin and it does this by converting bilirubin to photoproducts that are less lipophilic than bilirubin and can bypass the liver conjugating system and be excreted without further metabolism.[10,11] Bilirubin is one of the few substances in the body that absorbs light and light can produce a biologic response only if it is absorbed by a photoreceptor molecule. The presence of a photoreceptor at a location accessible to light is a prerequisite for the action of phototherapy.[11] Exactly where the process of phototherapy takes place in the skin is unknown. In the blood, bilirubin is found in the unbound ("free") form or bound to albumin and red cells . It is also present in extravascular tissue. Christensen and Kinn observed that when they incubated cultured cells with bilirubin (allowing the bilirubin to be bound to the cells) and then irradiated these cells with visible light, no photoisomers were formed whereas the expected photoisomers were found in irradiated samples of bilirubin/albumin mixtures.[12] These findings suggest that the conversion of bilirubin to photoisomers during phototherapy does not take place in skin cells but most likely in bilirubin bound to albumin in the vessels or in the interstitial space.

When a photoreceptor absorbs light, it may undergo a change in molecular structure (isomerization) and the efficiency of this photochemical process is defined by the value of π, the *quantum yield*. Photoreceptors have to absorb photons in order to change their energy state to an unstable electronic configuration and produce a change in molecular structure (isomerization). This process occurs in *picoseconds* and the rate of formation of the new isomer depends on the *quantum yield* (π) for the reaction, the absorption coefficient of the material (in this case bilirubin) at that wavelength, and the intensity of the light.[11]

The effectiveness of different light wavelengths is expressed *in vitro* and *in vivo* as an *action spectrum*. When applying an *in vitro* action spectrum to phototherapy, however, corrections have to be made for the optical properties of skin and the fact that skin blocks shorter wavelengths of visible light more than longer wavelengths. Thus, although a blue light (450 nm) might produce twice as much photoproduct as a green light (520 nm) of similar spectral power, it might only be 1.5 times as effective *in vivo* because skin transmits green light better than blue. Agati and coworkers have studied the quantum yields for photochemical reactions of bilirubin over the spectral range of bilirubin absorption. From their data and the optical properties of the skin, it appears that the most effective light source for phototherapy is one that emits in the blue-green spectral region between 490–510 nm.[7,13] Because of the combined effects of the quantum yield of the photoreaction converting bilirubin to the photoproduct lumirubin (see below), and the effect of the light spectrum on skin transmission, the most effective spectral band for the formation of lumirubin is probably towards a longer wavelength than those currently employed for phototherapy.

BILIRUBIN PHOTOCHEMISTRY

When bilirubin absorbs light, photochemical reactions occur. Although many such reactions have been observed *in vitro*, only 3 have been shown to occur *in vivo* during phototherapy.

Configurational (*Z, E*) Isomerization

Isomers are substances that have the same molecular formula, but different physico-chemical properties. *Configurational isomerization* occurs with compounds containing double bonds. Bilirubin contains 2 unsymmetrically substituted double bonds, one starting at carbon atom C4 and the other at C15 (Figure 12.3). Therefore, there are 4 possible configurational isomers of bilirubin. Pairs of configurational isomers are denoted by the letters *Z* or *E* and, therefore, the four bilirubin isomers are designated as: 4*Z*,15*Z*; 4*Z*,15*E*; 4*E*,15*Z*; 4*E*,15*E*. (Figure 12.4) Albumin-bound bilirubin, however, shows about a 100-fold preference for configurational isomerization at the double bond between C15 and C16 over the double bond between C4 and C5.[14] Thus, in infants receiving phototherapy, the stable 4*Z*,15*Z* isomer, (i.e., the one produced *in vivo* by the breakdown of hemoglobin) is converted predominantly to only 1 of the 3 other isomers – the 4*Z*,15*E* isomer (Figures 12.3 and 12.4). In this reaction, one of the end rings undergoes a 180 degree rotation around the double bond at C15. When this occurs, the polar N and O groups are exposed, making one end of the molecule polar and allowing it to be excreted in bile without conjugation. The formation of 4*Z*,15*E*-bilirubin is spontaneously reversible in the

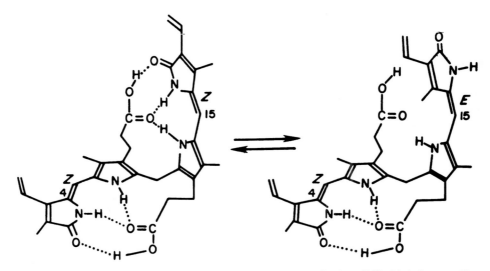

Figure 12.3. *Z–E* carbon–carbon double bond configurational isomerization of bilirubin in humans. From McDonagh, A.F. and Lightner, D.A.[10]

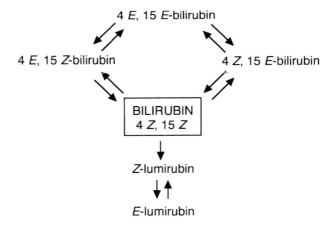

Figure 12.4. Configurational and structural isomers of 4Z,15Z bilirubin in infants undergoing photo-therapy. From Maisels.[98]

dark, unlike photo-oxidation or lumirubin formation (see below). This reverse re-action is slow when the pigment is bound to serum albumin but occurs rapidly in bile. Thus the 4Z,15E-bilirubin formed in the skin and excreted by the liver is readily converted back to ordinary unconjugated bilirubin. Furthermore, photochemical conversion of the normal Z,Z isomer to the less stable 4Z,15E isomer is reversible by light and irradiation of either isomer with visible light leads to rapid formation of the other.

The process by which bilirubin isomers are formed during phototherapy and then transported from the skin and excreted in the bile appears to be exceptionally efficient, at least in rats. When Gunn rats are exposed to phototherapy, virtually instantaneous changes occur in bile composition[15] and clearance of the 4Z,15E-bilirubin isomer is rapid. In infants, however, clearance of the light-generated 4Z,15E isomer is very slow[16] and a steady state concentration of the 2 isomers is achieved within 3 to 4 hours after the initiation of phototherapy. The steady state amount of the 4Z,15E isomer is dependent on the wavelength of the light used but is independent of intensity. Greater intensity leads to more rapid achievement of the steady-state concentrations but not the amounts.[14] Thus, although configurational isomerization is extremely rapid and accounts for the bulk of the photochemical outcomes, it probably plays only a minor role in lowering the serum bilirubin concentration because "although it is formed fastest, it has nowhere to go".[14]

Structural Isomerization

In this reaction (Figure 12.5), intramolecular cyclization of bilirubin (an irreversible process) occurs in the presence of light to form a substance known as *lumirubin* (also sometimes referred to as (*EZ*) cyclobilirubin) that can be excreted in bile (without the need for conjugation)[17] and in urine (but at a much lower rate than in bile).[18]

During phototherapy, the serum concentration of lumirubin is about 2–6% of the total serum bilirubin – considerably lower than the concentration of the configurational isomers which form about 20% of the total bilirubin, But lumirubin is cleared from the serum much more rapidly than the 4Z,15E isomer, the mean serum half life of lumirubin being less than 2 hours compared with 15 hours for the 4Z,15E isomer.[16] Costarino and colleagues showed that increasing the irradiance increased the amount of lumirubin present in the serum of premature infants but produced no

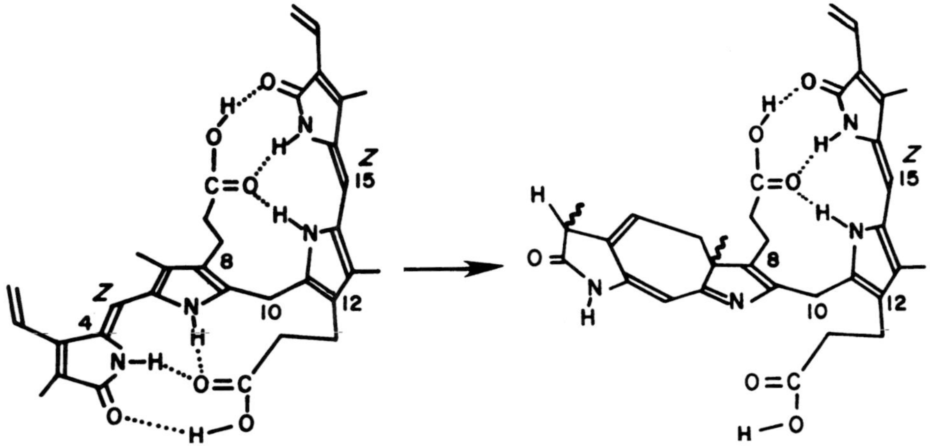

Figure 12.5. Intramolecular cyclization of bilirubin in presence of light to form lumirubin. From McDonagh, A.F. and Lightner, D.A.[10]

increase in the percentage of the configurational isomer[17] suggesting that lumirubin is responsible for the observed dose-response relation of phototherapy to the decrement in serum bilirubin. The formation of lumirubin is not reversible so that once formed it is excreted unchanged in the bile and urine. Quantitative data on the relative importance of urinary and biliary excretion are limited, but it is likely that the major route of bilirubin clearance during phototherapy is biliary excretion.[14]

It seems likely that lumirubin formation is mainly responsible for the phototherapy induced decline in serum bilirubin in the human infant, although it must be acknowledged that the evidence in support of this mechanism is relatively sparse. The contribution of $4E, 15E, 4E15Z$ and E-lumirubin have not been elucidated, nor has the relative contribution of photooxidation.[19] Although the half-life of the configurational isomers is long, increased concentrations of $4Z,15Z$-bilirubin have been found in bile during phototherapy.[20] As this $4Z,15Z$-bilirubin is almost certainly the result of reversion of the photoisomers to native bilirubin in the (dark) bile, it suggests that configurational isomerization makes more than a trivial contribution to the clearance of bilirubin. The general mechanisms of phototherapy are illustrated in Figure 12.6.

Note that although the same photochemical reactions occur in humans as in Gunn rats, because of species differences between the bilirubin–albumin complexes and the structure of albumin (or other binding proteins), there are differences in the

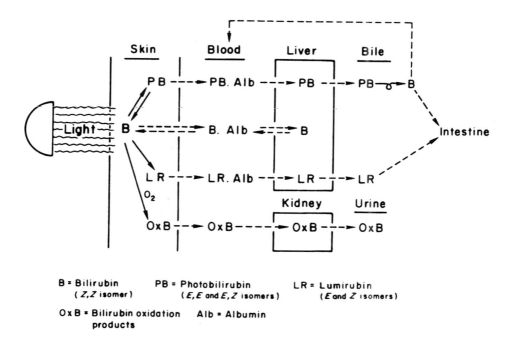

Figure 12.6. General mechanisms of phototherapy for neonatal jaundice. Chemical reactions (solid arrows) and transport processes (broken arrows) are indicated. Pigments may be bound to proteins in compartments other than blood. Some excretion of photoisomers, particularly lumirubin, in urine also occurs. From McDonagh, A.F. and Lightner, D.A.[10]

quantum yield in the 3 main photochemical pathways as well as rates of excretion of the photo products between the 2 species. Therefore the Gunn rat is a qualitative but not quantitative model of phototherapy in humans.

In the most detailed studies reported to date, we measured the pigment composition of plasma, duodenal bile and urine in a child with a clinical diagnosis of type I Crigler–Najjar syndrome before, during and after phototherapy.[19] Phototherapy converted about 20% of the bilirubin in the patient's circulation to 4Z,15E-bilirubin. Relatively small amounts of 4E,15Z bilirubin were also detectable along with traces of Z-lumirubin. The proportion of 4Z,15E-bilirubin declined slowly when phototherapy was suspended for 8 hours, but rapidly increased back to about 20% when the treatment was resumed. Bile samples collected during phototherapy contained Z-lumirubin, 4Z,15Z-bilirubin and, in 2 samples, both of the 4Z,15E and 4E,15Z-bilirubin photoisomers. Pigments were undetectable in 2 bile samples collected during the break in phototherapy. Urine samples collected during phototherapy contained all of the photoisomers with the exception of 4E,15E-bilirubin. Control experiments with synthetic photoisomers showed that 4Z,15E and 4E,15Z-bilirubin revert rapidly to natural bilirubin in bile and urine.

These studies demonstrate the collective importance of all of the isomerization reactions in enhancing the excretion of bilirubin during phototherapy and they show that calculating the relative contribution of individual compounds is difficult because of the rapid reversion of E-isomers to Z-isomers. They confirm previous observations that plasma clearance of 4Z,15E-bilirubin is slow and that Z-lumirubin is readily excreted in bile and urine, but indicate that the contribution of other isomers may not be negligible. In addition, they show that phototherapy swiftly converts a substantial fraction of the bilirubin in the circulation to a more polar, and presumably less toxic form.[19]

Finally, it is important to recognize that detoxification of bilirubin occurs

> ... with the flick of the light switch, although it may be hours before a decline in the plasma bilirubin concentration becomes evident. Just as the tip of an iceberg represents only a small proportion of its mass, the plasma bilirubin represents only about $\frac{1}{3}$ of the bilirubin in the body. It's disappearance in response to phototherapy is a secondary effect. Consequently, it is an insensitive, tardy, and possibly misleading parameter of the effectiveness of phototherapy. When a baby looks jaundiced, it is because pigment molecules and superficial tissues are absorbing blue light. What can be seen by eye is also accessible to the phototherapy lamp... Phototherapy is bound to accelerate the detoxification and elimination of bilirubin, irrespective of what the plasma concentration may show.[10]

Photo-oxidation

If a sample of serum containing bilirubin is left exposed to sunlight, the bilirubin gradually disappears (this is one of the observations that lead to the discovery of phototherapy). This bleaching phenomenon is the result of the photo-oxidation of bilirubin to water soluble, colorless products.[21] Because these products are small and polar, they can be excreted in the urine. Photo-oxidation is a slow process, however, and it is probably only a minor contributor to the elimination of bilirubin during phototherapy.

CLINICAL USE AND EFFICACY

Over 30 years of experience worldwide has confirmed the safety and efficacy of phototherapy. In their original description, Cremer, Perryman and Richards[2] cautiously suggested that although it was unlikely that phototherapy would "prove a substitute for exchange transfusion in the erythroblastotic infant with active haemolysis. . . . the method may be turned to clinical advantage in controlling the level of serum bilirubin in cases of jaundice of prematurity." It would be no exaggeration to say that phototherapy has succeeded beyond their wildest dreams. There are more than 50 published controlled trials of the clinical use of phototherapy[22] (See Maisels[22] for a description and analysis of each of these studies). These trials confirm that phototherapy is effective in preventing and treating hyperbilirubinemia and dramatically reduces the need for exchange transfusion.[22] Notwithstanding the obvious benefits of the use of Rh immune globulin in the prevention of Rh erythroblastosis fetalis, some idea of the magnitude of phototherapy's effect can be gauged by the fact that there are many residents in pediatric training programs today who, by the end of their 3 years of training, have never seen an exchange transfusion, let alone performed one. There may come a time when even those trained in the subspecialty of neonatology have little exposure to this procedure.[23]

Dose–Response Relationship

As described above, there is a clear relationship between the dose of phototherapy and the measured decrement in the serum bilirubin level (Figure 12.1).[8] The factors that influence the dose are the spectrum of light delivered by the phototherapy unit, the irradiance incident on the infant and the surface area of the infant exposed to phototherapy. The other important factor that influences how rapidly the serum bilirubin falls is the initial bilirubin level, the rate of decline being proportional to the initial bilirubin concentration.[24] Light treatment has its greatest impact during the first 24–48 hours of therapy, after which efficacy decreases. This is probably due to the fact that configurational isomers formed during light treatment revert to natural unconjugated bilirubin in the intestine after hepatic excretion.[19,25] This natural bilirubin is then reabsorbed via the enterohepatic circulation and contributes to the bilirubin load to be cleared by the liver.

Types of Light

Fluorescent tubes

The most widely used fluorescent light sources are daylight or cool white fluorescent tubes. These tubes provide energy in the 300–700 nm range with little output in the blue spectrum (Figure 12.2). They are useful and effective in providing prophylactic phototherapy where the objective is to control a slowly rising serum bilirubin level in a preterm or term infant. Because of their limited output in the blue spectrum, however, they are much less effective than special blue tubes. "Special blue" fluorescent tubes provide much more irradiance in the blue spectrum than other commercially available tubes and are the most effective light source currently available in the United States for phototherapy (Figure 12.2). They are labeled F20 T12/BB (General Electric, Westinghouse) or TL52/20W (Phillips). Note that these are different from regular blue tubes (labeled F20T12/B). Nursing staff working near special blue lights have complained of headaches, dizziness and nausea. Placing a screen or skirt around the light will shield staff from the effects of the light.[26] Because special blue tubes give infants a bluish tinge, pediatricians may be reluctant to use them in sick infants as they may obscure cyanosis. Generally however, these tubes are used to treat healthy full term infants readmitted to the hospital because of severe hyperbilirubinemia. These infants are in no distress and the fact that they look blue while receiving phototherapy is of little concern. If necessary, switching off the lights for a few seconds will provide reassurance. In infants in the NICU, who may need intensive phototherapy (see below) monitoring by pulse oximetry will provide all of the necessary information to ensure adequate oxygenation.

As discussed above, because of the known photochemical reactions of bilirubin and the optical properties of the skin, it is likely that the most effective light source for phototherapy is one that emits in a longer wavelength in the blue-green spectrum between 490–510 nm than the special blue lights currently in use. Donzelli *et al.* found that phototherapy with an experimental blue-green light source reduced serum bilirubin concentrations in preterm infants in the first 24 hours by 46.4% compared with 22.6% in the infants receiving special blue phototherapy ($p < .0001$).[27] This decrement is quite remarkable considering that the initial bilirubin level in the infants being treated was only about 240 μmol/l (14 mg/dl).

Halogen lamps

These high-pressure mercury vapor halide lamps provide reasonably good output in the blue range and have the advantage of being much more compact than lamps containing standard fluorescent tubes. However, unlike fluorescent lamps, they *cannot be brought close to the infant (to increase the irradiance)without incurring the risk of a burn*. These lamps are also mounted on a moveable arm and medical and nursing staff may unintentionally move the arm thus increasing the distance between the light and the infant and decreasing the effective irradiance. Standard fluorescent phototherapy lamps can be brought within 10 cm of an infant significantly increasing the irradiance (Figure 12.2) but without causing any significant increase in temperature (see below). In addition, the surface area covered by most halogen lamps is relatively small and the spectral power will be less than that produced by a bank of fluorescent lights. Finally, the field of irradiance produced by the halide lamps is quite heterogeneous, with a high intensity in the center and a marked decrease toward the sides that might impair their efficacy in relation to the energy output.[28]

Fiberoptic systems

Introduced in the late 1980s, fiberoptic phototherapy systems consist of a light that is delivered from a tungsten-halogen bulb through a fiberoptic cable and emitted from the sides and ends of the fibers inside a plastic pad. Two devices most widely used in the US are the Wallaby Phototherapy System (Fiberoptic Medical Products, Inc., Allentown, PA) and the BiliBlanket Phototherapy System (Ohmeda, Columbia, MD). In the Wallaby wraparound pad, the fiberoptic fibers are contained in a cummerbund, which can be wrapped around the infant whereas with the neonatal pad, the infant lies on the pad. In the Ohmeda system, the infant may lie on the woven fiberoptic pad or it may be tucked under a shirt while the infant is held. One advantage of these systems over conventional phototherapy systems is that eye patches are unnecessary, which eliminates the possibility of nasal obstruction from eyepads and the negative psychological effect on the parents of seeing a "blindfolded" baby. The equipment is also less bulky than conventional phototherapy equipment and infants can be held and nursed while they receive phototherapy. Fiberoptic systems also provide a convenient way to deliver double phototherapy when it is necessary to expose more of the infant's surface area (see below).

Both systems provide low and high intensity settings. A detailed evaluation of these devices has been conducted by ECRI, an organization that tests health devices.[6] At the highest light intensity (irradiance) settings, the Wallaby Neonatal and the Ohmeda pads produced an average spectral irradiance of about $22-23 \mu W/cm^2/nm$ in the 420–480 nm band. The wraparound pad of the Wallaby II produced approximately $8-9 \mu W/cm^2/nm$. The spectral power of the 2 systems is similar – about 3 mW/nm. The Ohmeda pad provides a more uniform irradiance than does the Wallaby pad[6] and it is possible that this has some clinical benefit. One limitation of fiberoptic phototherapy pads is that there is an inverse relationship between surface area and irradiance. For a given light source, enlarging the pad means that the light must be distributed over a greater area, thus reducing the irradiance (when compared with a smaller pad and the same light source). To achieve high levels of spectral irradiance ($>20 \mu W/cm^2/nm$ in the 425–475 nm range), manufacturers must compromise by reducing the size of the pad, which exposes a relatively small surface area of the infant to the light.[6]

Light emitting diodes

A new method of delivering high intensity narrow band (30 nm) light has recently been described.[29,30] The use of high intensity gallium nitride light emitting diodes (LEDs) permits high irradiance in the spectrum of choice (blue, blue-green, etc.) with minimal heat generation. The device is low weight, low voltage, low power and portable and could be an effective means of providing intensive phototherapy in the hospital or at home. To date, only limited clinical trials have been performed.

Full Term and Near Term Infants – Using Phototherapy Effectively

Phototherapy was initially used in low birthweight and full term infants, primarily to prevent slowly rising serum bilirubin levels from reaching levels that might require an exchange transfusion. When full term babies remained in hospital for 3–5 days and hyperbilirubinemia was treated quite aggressively,[25,31] large numbers of infants who became modestly jaundiced (serum bilirubin levels of 171–222 μmol/l, 10–13 mg/dl) received phototherapy and remained in the nursery until their bilirubin levels declined. For this prophylactic type of phototherapy, a relatively modest dose of phototherapy was quite adequate and readily supplied by using daylight or cool white fluorescent tubes. Because most infants in the United States (and in some other countries) are now discharged by 36 hours after birth, these bilirubin levels are seldom encountered in the well baby nursery and this type of phototherapy use has declined dramatically. Today, full term and near term infants who need phototherapy are generally those who have left the hospital and are readmitted on days 4–7 for treatment of serum bilirubin levels of 342 μmol/l (20 mg/dl) or higher. Levels of more than 428 μmol/l (25 mg/dl) are not unusual and much higher levels have been seen.[32,33] These infants need a therapeutic dose of phototherapy (sometimes termed intensive phototherapy) in order to get the bilirubin level down as soon as possible. As discussed above, the light spectrum, the irradiance and the exposed surface area are the key elements in determining the bilirubin response to phototherapy.

The most effective light source currently commercially available for phototherapy is that provided by special blue fluorescent tubes and maximum irradiance is achieved by bringing these tubes as close to the infant as possible. In order to do this, a full term infant should be in a bassinet, not an incubator, because the top of the incubator prevents the light from being brought sufficiently close to the infant. When intensive phototherapy is necessary in low birthweight infants, we place our special blue fluorescent lights between the radiant warmer and the warmer bed. In a bassinet it is possible to bring the fluorescent lights within about 10 cm of the infant. At this distance, special blue tubes provide an average spectral irradiance of more than 50 μW/cm^2/nm (see Figure 12.2). We have not observed significant warming of naked full term infants treated in this way with daylight or blue tubes. If slight warming does occur, the lamps can be elevated slightly. *Note, however, that halogen phototherapy lamps cannot be positioned closer to the infant than recommended by the manufacturers without incurring the risk of a burn.* The effect of increasing irradiance and a clear dose response relationship was first demonstrated by Tan who showed that infants exposed to an irradiance of 34 μW/cm^2/nm in the 425–475 nm range achieved declines in serum bilirubin levels of approximately 50% in the first 24 hours (Figure 12.1).[8] With standard phototherapy systems, a decline of 6–15% of the initial bilirubin level can be expected in the first 24 hours.[25]

In addition to the light spectrum and irradiance incident on the infant, the surface area of the infant exposed to phototherapy is another crucial element in determining its efficacy. The availability of fiberoptic pads has made it easy to increase the surface area of the infant exposed to phototherapy. This type of "double phototherapy" is approximately twice as effective as single phototherapy in low birthweight infants[26,34] and almost 50% better in full term infants.[26] The explanation for this difference in response is likely due to the fact that, at similar irradiance levels, the fiberoptic pad covers more of a small than a large infant. A simple way of increasing the surface area of the infant exposed to light is to place a reflecting material (a white sheet or aluminum foil) within or around the bassinet or incubator so that light is reflected onto the infant's skin.[35]

The use of special blue lights brought close to the baby together with fiberoptic pads placed below the baby, or other systems capable of providing 360 degree or double phototherapy have been termed "intensive phototherapy." Examples of placing fluorescent units both above and below the infant have been described.[33,36,37] Using a combination of a standard phototherapy unit above and 4 special blue tubes directly underneath the bassinet, Garg was able to produce an average decline of 43% in hyperbilirubinemic infants in the first 24 hours.[37] The infant was placed on a waterbed, which permitted transmission of the light and dissipated any heat generated by the lights.

Hansen reported his experience with 4 infants admitted with serum bilirubin levels of >500 µmol/l (>30 mg/dl), one of whom had unrecognized Rh erythroblastosis.[33] He used a radiant warmer bed with attached phototherapy lights on either side, two additional fluorescent units at 45 degree angles on both sides of the infant and placed the baby on a fiberoptic mat (Wallaby neonatal model). Infants were also fed ad lib with formula. A decline in serum bilirubin level of 170–185 µmol/l (10–11 mg/dl) occurred within 2 hours in 3 infants and 5 hours in the fourth and was felt to be the result of the intensive phototherapy together with formula feeding which, presumably, reduced the enterohepatic circulation. A 360 degree phototherapy system with special blue tubes has been used in France and produced a 30% decline in bilirubin within 4 hours in nonhemolyzing infants (R. Caldera, M.D. and Médipréma, Tours France, Letter, 1995).

In terms of spectral power, fiberoptic systems are significantly inferior to standard overhead lamps (see above) because the skin surface area illuminated is so much greater when overhead lamps are used. On the other hand, the therapeutic response could be improved by using 2 or even 3 pads to cover almost the entire lower surface of the infant. Tan's data suggest that there is a saturation point beyond which an increase in irradiance produces no added efficacy.[8,38] We do not really know, however, that a saturation point exists. Given that the conversion of bilirubin to excretable photoproducts is partly irreversible and follows first order kinetics, there may not be a saturation point. Certainly *with existing equipment there is no such thing as an overdose of phototherapy*.

Although the spectral power of the 2 systems is virtually identical, the Ohmeda BiliBlanket was more effective than the Fiberoptic Medical Wrap system when used to provide home phototherapy.[39] In other small trials of home phototherapy, the Wallaby system was equivalent to a 4 bulb home fluorescent unit.[40] Tan compared the efficacy of fiberoptic phototherapy using the standard Ohmeda BiliBlanket, a larger version of the Ohmeda BiliBlanket, double standard BiliBlankets (with the infant sandwiched between 2 blankets), and conventional daylight fluorescent phototherapy in full term infants with nonhemolytic jaundice.[41] The efficacy of double fiberoptic phototherapy and conventional phototherapy were similar and significantly better than the single large or the single standard fiberoptic mat.[41]

Concern for the potential mutagenic effects of light with wavelengths of 350–450 nm has led to the suggestion that green light (525 nm) should be used, but in clinical trials the efficacy of green light phototherapy has been inferior to special blue phototherapy.[42] It is possible that lamps emitting in the blue-green spectral region between 490–510 nm will prove more effective than available special blue lights.[27]

Preterm Infants

Conventional phototherapy using daylight or cool white fluorescent light, halogen lamps or fiberoptic pads have all been effective in decreasing serum bilirubin levels and the number of exchange transfusions performed in low birthweight infants both with and without hemolytic disease. In most of these studies, phototherapy was initiated prophylactically or at relatively low serum bilirubin levels (85–171 μmol/l, 5–10 mg/dl).[22,25]

Donzelli and coworkers[43] studied infants with birthweights ranging from 600–2500 g (gestation 25–37 weeks) and found that fiberoptic phototherapy with the Ohmeda BiliBlanket was as effective as conventional daylight fluorescent tubes but less effective than special blue fluorescent tubes. Costello, *et al.*,[44] in their study of low birth weight infants also found that the Ohmeda BiliBlanket was as effective as conventional phototherapy (4 white and 4 standard blue fluorescent lamps). We have conducted a controlled trial of infants less than 2500 g and compared the use of the Fiberoptic Medical (Wallaby) and the Ohmeda Bili Blanket in this population. Twenty-four hours after initiation of phototherapy the serum bilirubin in the Wallaby group had declined by $1.6 \pm 15.2\%$ compared with $12.8 \pm 15.3\%$ in the Ohmeda Bili Blanket group ($p = .006$). This suggests that in the low birthweight population the Ohmeda fiberoptic system is somewhat more effective than the Wallaby system. However, the mean bilirubin levels in the 2 groups at 24 hours and on the second day after initiating phototherapy were not significantly different, nor was there any significant difference in the number of infants who failed fiberoptic phototherapy or in whom a significant rebound occurred (Maisels, M.J. and Kring, E.A., unpublished data).

Intermittent Versus Continuous Phototherapy

Clinical studies comparing intermittent with continuous phototherapy have produced conflicting results.[5,45–47] Because all light exposure increases bilirubin excretion (compared with darkness), continuous phototherapy should be more efficient than intermittent phototherapy. The issue is quite complicated, however, because the efficacy of phototherapy is related exponentially to the initial bilirubin concentration and efficacy will thus decrease as the bilirubin level falls.[5] Jährig *et al.* speculate that rebound into the skin probably takes place when there is an interruption of phototherapy and question whether or not this (brief elevation in skin bilirubin) might improve efficiency when light therapy is restarted. They conclude that optimal therapy is achieved by using one hour on and one hour off phototherapy together with a regular change of the infant's position (supine to prone).[5] In practice, however, on-off cycles complicate nursing care and are probably more trouble than they are worth. There is no doubt, however, that phototherapy does not *need* to be continuous in the majority of circumstances. Phototherapy can and certainly should be interrupted during feeding or brief parental visits. On the other hand, when bilirubin levels are very high, intensive phototherapy should be administered continuously until a satisfactory decline in bilirubin level occurs or exchange transfusion is initiated.

Hydration

There is no evidence that excess fluid administration affects the serum bilirubin concentration. It is common, however, to find that infants who are breast fed and readmitted to hospital with high bilirubin levels have excess weight loss due to a combination of mild dehydration and poor caloric intake. In these infants it makes sense to provide supplemental calories and fluids using a milk-based formula because formulas inhibit the enterohepatic circulation of bilirubin and help to lower the bilirubin level. Because the photoproducts responsible for the decline in serum bilirubin are excreted in both urine and bile, maintaining adequate hydration and good urine output helps to improve the efficacy of phototherapy.[48] Routine supplementation (with dextrose water) of all infants receiving phototherapy is not indicated.

Lamp Life

In the first several hours of operation, there is a fairly rapid decline in irradiance in the blue spectrum from fluorescent tubes. There are no accepted recommendations regarding when these tubes should be changed although some recommend that they be changed after 600–800 hours of operation.[5] Measurements with a radiometer will help to confirm that phototherapy units are emitting adequate irradiance.

Home Phototherapy

Concerns about the dangers of hyperbilirubinemia and the economic and social pressures for early discharge of infants from hospital after delivery have lead to the widespread use of home phototherapy. Because the devices available for home phototherapy do not provide the same degree of irradiance or surface area exposure as those available in the hospital, most home phototherapy, of necessity, is used in the prophylactic rather than in the therapeutic mode. Nevertheless, when used appropriately, home phototherapy poses no obvious hazards to the infant and is certainly much cheaper than hospital treatment.[40,49–52] The use of fiberoptic systems has made it easier to administer phototherapy at home. When compared with other interventions used in the home such as apnea monitors, nasal oxygen or ventilators, phototherapy must certainly rank among the more benign. Home phototherapy does avoid parent–child separation and there is evidence that mothers of infants who receive phototherapy at home are less likely to stop breast-feeding during the period of phototherapy and, if stopped, are more likely to resume breast feeding than women whose infants are treated in the hospital.[53]

Crigler–Najjar syndrome

A rare, but important application of home phototherapy is its use in children with the Crigler–Najjar syndrome. Beyond the neonatal period, the only definitive therapy for these children is a liver transplant, although gene therapy is becoming a distinct possibility. Until this is done, they must rely on phototherapy to prevent extreme hyperbilirubinemia. This has been achieved in most children with type I Crigler–Najjar syndrome by means of specially designed (non commercial) home phototherapy devices that provide adequate phototherapy to the growing child and even the adolescent. As the child gets older, phototherapy becomes less effective, presumably due to thickening of the skin, an increase in skin pigmentation, a decrease in surface area relative to body mass and the need to provide phototherapy only during sleep to allow the normal activities of childhood during the day. To obtain adequate irradiance and sufficient surface area exposure, the most satisfactory systems provide a "tanning bed" configuration. The child lies on a transparent surface directly above special blue fluorescent tubes. Bubble wrap and plastic "lilos" have been used for this purpose but, because of their low porosity, produce patient discomfort.[54-56] Job *et al.* have used a standard mesh or high transmission fabric stretched over an adjustable tension frame.[55] This is similar to a traditional hammock and permits adequate transmission of blue light as well as patient comfort.

Biological Effects and Complications

In spite of the fact that phototherapy has been used in millions of infants for over 30 years, reports of significant toxicity are exceptionally rare.

Toxicity of phototherapy products

Human, animal and *in vitro* studies suggest that the products of photodecomposition have no direct neurotoxic effects.[57,58]

Cell damage

Phototherapy can produce DNA strand breaks in cell cultures and DNA strand breakage increases when cells are irradiated in the presence of 100 µg/ml of bilirubin.[59] Because light penetrates the thin scrotal skin and perhaps even reaches ovaries, it has been suggested that shielding the gonads with diapers may be indicated during phototherapy.[60] However, there is no human or animal evidence to support this practice and limited depth of penetration of light makes this possibility very unlikely.

Skin

Phototherapy bleaches the skin so that skin color cannot be used as a means of assessing serum bilirubin levels in infants receiving phototherapy. Phototherapy lights produce a minimal amount of the ultraviolet portion of light responsible for erythema (below 320 nm). In addition, the interposed Plexiglass^{TM} essentially eliminates the passage of shortwave and middle wave UV light from fluorescent lamps. The light from halogen lamps also contains only traces of ultraviolet. Thus erythema should not normally occur in infants receiving phototherapy. However, bilirubin is a photosensitizer and, in some circumstances, could possibly act as a photodynamic agent in the presence of light and produce damage. Severe blistering and photosensitivity during phototherapy for jaundice have been described in infants with congenital erythropoietic porphyria.[61] The presence of congenital porphyrias should be considered absolute contraindications to the use of phototherapy.

Two recent reports document the development of purpura or bullous eruptions in infants with hemolytic disease and transient porphyrinemia who received phototherapy.[62,63] Mallon et al. describe the development of multiple blisters and erosions on exposed sites in a 32-week gestation male infant who had hydrops fetalis secondary to erythroblastosis.[62] The neonatal course was complicated by severe anemia respiratory distress, thrombocytopenia, hypotension, oliguria, hypoglycemia and electrolyte disturbance. Intensive phototherapy with special blue tubes was administered at an irradiance of $20-25 \mu W/cm^2/nm$. The total bilirubin level peaked at $386 \mu mol/l$ (22.6 mg/dl) and the direct reacting fraction was $254 \mu mol/l$ (14.9 mg/dl). After phototherapy was discontinued on day 8, blisters developed on the infant's trunk and limbs. Total plasma porphyrin levels were markedly elevated.

Paller et al.[63] described 5 infants with erythroblastosis fetalis and a sixth who had profound anemia from twin–twin transfusion. All of these neonates developed purpuric patches at sites of maximal exposure to standard blue light phototherapy 24 hours after initiation of the phototherapy. No eruptions occurred in shielded sites. All infants had significant direct hyperbilirubinemia and plasma proto- or coproporphyrins were elevated in the 2 infants in which they were measured. Skin biopsy showed purpura without significant inflammation or keratinocyte necrosis.

Significant accumulation of coproporphyrins has been well described in infant with the bronze baby syndrome, which occurs exclusively in phototherapy exposed infants who also have cholestasis. This may not explain the elevated erythrocyte porphyrins found in one of Paller's infants. In all of these infants the eruptions cleared spontan-eously. Porphyrins absorb light maximally in the soret band (400–410 nm) with lesser bands occurring in the long visible range (580–650 nm).[63] Erythema has also occurred in occasional neonates treated with tin protoporphyrin and then exposed to daylight fluorescent phototherapy. The rash cleared after discontinuing the phototherapy. An eruption identical to that described in the infants reported by Paller was also described in a single infant who had erythroblastosis fetalis due to anti-E and anti-C blood antigens.[64] Pediatricians should be aware of the possibility of a transient, benign, purpuric eruption occurring in infants who have received transfusions, developed cholestasis and are receiving phototherapy. There appears to be a strong link between elevation in the plasma porphyrin levels and the likelihood of the development of cutaneous lesions in infants exposed to phototherapy.

Other photosensitizors may also be hazardous in infants receiving phototherapy. A 32-week gestation neonate who received intravenous fluorescein for angiography was subsequently exposed to phototherapy. This infant developed a partial thickness burn probably related to the phototoxicity from the fluorescein which has been shown to produce photosensitization by generation of a super oxide anion when exposed to light at a wavelength of 480 nm in the visible light range.[65] Hussain and Sharief[66] described the development of a partial thickness burn of the back in a 25 week gestation, 880 g infant receiving phototherapy with a fiberoptic system (Ohmeda BiliBlanket). This infant required assisted ventilation and inotropic support and died at age 85 hours. There was an extensive, erythematous, denuded area of skin on the back which resembled a partial thickness burn and from which serous fluid oozed. The Ohmeda company issued a medical device safety alert on January 26, 1996 in which they reported that 4 extremely premature infants ($\leq$25 weeks gestation) had developed purplish-red necrotizing lesions during the use of the BiliBlanket phototherapy system. In all of these infants, conditions were present that might reduce skin integrity such as birth trauma, hypotension, poor perfusion of the skin or bacterial contamination of the incubator or bed. Birthweights ranged from 540–800 g. It is difficult to know whether any of these were thermal burns and the company's report stated that "a thermal burn etiology is extremely unlikely." Nevertheless, it is important to note that the skin of these extremely premature infants is remarkably fragile. Finally, 2 neonates have been described who developed erythema (one was blistering) following exposure to daylight fluorescent lamps without Plexiglass™ shielding.[67]

Children with type I Crigler–Najjar syndrome receiving phototherapy for 2–3 years often develop pigmented lesions and tanning as well as skin atrophy.[68]

Bronze baby syndrome

Infants with cholestatic jaundice who are exposed to phototherapy may develop a dark, greyish-brown discoloration of the skin, serum and urine.[69,70] The pathogenesis of this syndrome is unknown, but it occurs exclusively in infants with cholestasis and may be related to an accumulation of porphyrins in the plasma. Jori and colleagues[71] produced an animal model of the bronze baby syndrome by ligating the common bile duct in adult Wistar rats and subjecting them to phototherapy. This syndrome generally has no deleterious consequences although one full term infant with the bronze baby syndrome who died, was shown to have kernicterus at autopsy.[72] The maximal serum bilirubin level in this infant was 308 µmol/l (18 mg/dl) with a direct reacting bilirubin of 70 µmol/l (4.1 mg/dl).

Eye damage

Light can be toxic to the retina. We exposed newborn stump-tail monkeys, lying in standard nursery incubators in the supine position and facing the light source, to daylight phototherapy lights (400 foot candles). No mydriatic drops were used and the monkeys could open and close their eyes as desired. The control eye was sutured closed and covered with a patch. Twelve hours to 7 days of exposure to phototherapy produced severe and progressive damage to the retina.[73] In a subsequent study, investigators exposed monkeys to light for 3–10 days then returned them to normal environments for 10 months before they were sacrificed.[74] If the original exposure was for less than 3 days, there was substantial recovery in retinal cytoarchitecture. The exposed retinas, however, showed some loss of rod and cone cells when compared with controls, a process that is similar to the normal aging process in the mammalian retina. The eyes of infants receiving phototherapy should therefore be protected with appropriate eye patches. If a patch slipped and the infant did suffer some phototoxic retinal damage, it is quite possible that visual acuity, electro-retinography and ophthalmic examination may be normal, despite considerable loss of tissue. Nevertheless, such an eye might later show the effects of premature aging. Displaced eye patches may also obstruct nares and produce apnea. In follow-up studies of infants whose eyes were adequately shielded, clinical assessment of visual function and electroretinography have been normal.[75,76] Shielding eyes, by depriving newborns of visual stimuli might be harmful. The pattern of visual evoked potential responses (PVEP) in preterm infants whose eyes had been shielded until they reached 32 weeks post conceptional age were compared with those in infants with unshielded eyes. At 41 and 51 weeks postconception and at age 3 years, no differences between the groups were found in the PVEP responses.[77]

Patching of eyes

Commercially available eyeshields, if properly applied, prevent more than 98% of light transmission.[78] It should be noted, however, that in addition to the potential risk of irritation or even corneal abrasion from eye patches, there is an increase in bacterial pathogen isolation and purulent conjunctivitis in infants whose eyes are patched (compared with those whose eyes are protected by a head box made of light-proof plastic).[79]

Diarrhea

Infants receiving phototherapy have an increased incidence of diarrhea[80] and stools become darker and have a greenish tinge.[5] The diarrhea is probably not the result of a phototherapy-induced lactase deficiency.[81–83] Diarrhea associated with photo-therapy is most likely a secretory diarrhea related to the increased excretion of unconjugated bilirubin into the gut. Jährig et al. have demonstrated changes in the transepithelial potential difference in the duodenum in newborns undergoing phototherapy suggesting a relation between functional membrane lesions and the local bilirubin concentration.[84]

Insensible water loss, thermoregulation and blood flow

Acute changes in the thermal environment occur directly after the initiation of phototherapy.[85] Infants receiving phototherapy have an increase in peripheral blood flow[86] and this in turn may increase the insensible water loss. Insensible water loss may increase by as much as 80 to 190% in infants nursed in nonservocontrolled incubators.[87] The use of servocontrolled incubators mitigates these effects.

Blood flow

Using Doppler blow flow velocity, Yao *et al.* have demonstrated that phototherapy diminishes the expected postprandial increase in blood flow velocity in the superior mesenteric artery.[88] They suggest that phototherapy-induced peripheral vasodilation diverts blood from the intestines and limits the normal neonatal postprandial response. This may be related to some of the phototherapy-induced intestinal disturbances that have been observed in newborns.

Although Amato *et al.* found that phototherapy produced no changes in cerebral blood flow velocity (CBF) in preterm infants,[89] Benders *et al.* found as much as 20–30% mean increase in CBF in preterm infants of 32 weeks gestation or less.[90] This could be the result of a photochemical reaction to light and might also increase the risk of intraventricular hemorrhage. In the same study, a previously closed ductus arteriosus reopened in 10 of 22 infants.[90]

Growth

Infants receiving phototherapy gained less weight in the first week of life than those not receiving phototherapy but showed catch-up growth in the next 2 weeks. One 2 year follow-up of infants who had received phototherapy suggested that their head growth may be impaired although their neurologic performance did not differ from controls.[91] Other studies that have followed the growth of infants receiving phototherapy for 2 to 6 years have demonstrated no effect on weight, length or head circumference.[80,92]

A 6-year follow-up of children in the NICHHD Cooperative Phototherapy Study showed no differences between the phototherapy or control groups in any aspect of developmental outcome.[93]

Other effects on clinical, chemical and hematologic parameters

Phototherapy does not decrease the bilirubin-binding capacity of albumin. It does appear to lower the oxygen binding capacity of erythrocytes and increase the tendency to spherocyte formation. An increase in lipid peroxidation in the erythrocytic membrane has been observed and studies of osmotic fragility of erythrocytes exposed to phototherapy are conflicting. Changes have been observed in serum gonadotropins during and after phototherapy. Luteinizing hormone (LH) levels decline within 24–48 hours after phototherapy but increase 6–9 days after phototherapy is discontinued.[94] Increases in LH and follicle stimulating hormone (FH) have been observed 3–4 weeks after phototherapy is administered to preterm girls. Phototherapy produced a decline in serum concentration of nonsterified fatty acids and free tryptophan but had no effect on serum enzymes. Serum concentrations of riboflavin and tocopherol decrease during phototherapy and hypocalcemia has been observed in preterm infants and newborn rats.[94] There is no effect on the daily blood sugar profile and a decline in immunoreactive prostaglandin A has been observed. Mild degrees of thrombocytopenia are more common in infants exposed to phototherapy and a slight rise in IgM and a small decrease in IgG have been seen.

Ductus arteriosus

A relationship has been described between the use of phototherapy and the risk of patent ductus arteriosus in very low birthweight infants.[90,95,96] *In vitro*, constricted arteries relax when exposed to light and the normal oxygen-induced constriction of the ductal rings of preterm animals is inhibited if light is present.[97] The possible mechanisms for this *in vivo* effect are not clear, but may be related to a mechanism similar to nitric oxide-induced vasorelaxation.[96]

References

1. Dobbs, R.H. and Cremer, R.J., Phototherapy, *Arch. Dis. Child.* 1975; **50**: 833–836.
2. Cremer, R.J., Perryman, P.W. and Richards, D.H., Influence of light on the hyperbilirubinemia of infants, *Lancet* 1958; **1**: 1094–1097.
3. Obes-Polleri, J. and Hill, W.S., La fototerapia en las ictericas del recien nacido, *Rev. Chile. Ped.* 1964; **25**: 638.
4. Lucey, J.F., Ferreiro, M. and Hewitt J., Prevention of hyperbilirubinemia of prematurity by phototherapy, *Pediatrics* 1968; 1047–1054.
5. Jährig, K., Jährig, D. and Meisel, P., eds., Phototherapy: Treating neonatal jaundice with visible light. München: Quintessenz Verlags-GmbH, 1993.
6. ECRI, Fiberoptic phototherapy systems, *Health Devices* 1995; **24**: 134–150.
7. Agati, G., Fusi, F., Donzelli, G.P. and Pratesi, R., Quantum yield and skin filtering effects on the formation rate of lumirubin, *J. Photochem. Photobiol. B.* 1993; **18**: 197–203.
8. Tan, KL., The pattern of bilirubin response to phototherapy for neonatal hyperbilirubinemia, *Pediatr. Res.* 1982; **16**: 670–674.
9. Haycock, G.B., Schwartz, G.J. and Wisotsky, D.H., Geometric method for measuring body surface area: a height-weight formula validated in infants, children, and adults, *J. Pediatr.* 1978; **93**: 62–66.
10. McDonagh, A.F. and Lightner, D.A., "Like a Shrivelled Blood Orange" – Bilirubin, jaundice and phototherapy, *Pediatrics* 1985; **75**: 443–455.
11. McDonagh, A.F. and Lightner, D.A., Phototherapy and the photobiology of bilirubin, *Sem. Liver Dis.* 1988; **8**: 272–283.
12. Christensen, T. and Kinn, G., Bilirubin bound to cells does not form photoisomers, *Acta. Paediatr.* 1993; **82**: 22–25.
13. Agati, G., Fusi, F. and Pratesi, R., Evaluation of the quantum yield for $E->Z$ isomerization of bilirubin bound to human serum albumin. Evidence of internal conversion processes competing with configurational photoisomerization, *J. Photochem. Photobiol. B.* 1993; **17**: 173–180.
14. Ennever, J.F., Blue light, green light, white light, more light: treatment of neonatal jaundice, *Clin. Perinatol.* 1990; **17**: 467.
15. McDonagh, A.F. and Ramonas, L.M., Jaundice phototherapy: Microflow cell photometry reveals rapid biliary response of Gunn rats to light, *Science* 1978; **20**: 829–829.
16. Ennever, J.F., Knox, I., Denne, S.C. and Speck, W.T., Phototherapy for neonatal jaundice, *in vivo* clearance of bilirubin photoproducts, *Pediatr. Res.* 1985; **19**: 205–208.
17. Costarino, A.T., Ennever, J.F., Baumgart, S., Speck, W.T., Paul, M. and Polin, R.A., Bilirubin photoisomerization in premature neonates under low- and high-dose phototherapy, *Pediatrics* 1985; **75**: 519–522.
18. Knox, I., Ennever, J.F. and Speck, W.T., Urinary excretion of an isomer of bilirubin during phototherapy, *Pediatr. Res.* 1985; **19**: 198–201.
19. McDonagh, A.F. and Maisels, M.J. Photoisomerization of bilirubin in Crigler–Najjar patients. In: Kappas, A., Lucey, J., eds. Treatment of Crigler–Najjar syndrome, conference proceedings. Rockefeller University, New York City, 1996.
20. Lund, H.D. and Jacobsen, J., Influence of phototherapy on the biliary bilirubin excretion pattern in newborn infants with hyperbilirubinemia, *J. Pediatr.* 1974; **85**: 262–267.
21. Lightner, D.A. and McDonagh, A.F., Molecular mechanisms of phototherapy for neonatal jaundice, *Accts. Chem. Res.* 1984; **17**: 417–424.
22. Maisels, M.J., Neonatal Jaundice. In: Sinclair, J.C. and Bracken, M.B., eds. Effective care of the newborn infant. Oxford: Oxford University Press, 1992; 507–561.

23. Maisels, M.J., Is exchange transfusion for hyperbilirubinemia in danger of becoming extinct? *Pediatr. Res.* 1999; **45**: 210A.

24. Jährig, K., Jährig, D. and Meisel, P., Dependence of the efficiency of phototherapy on plasma bilirubin concentration, *Acta. Paediatr. Scand.* 1982; **71**: 293–299.

25. Brown, A.K., Kim, M.H., Wu, P.Y.K. *et al.*, Efficacy of phototherapy in prevention and management of neonatal hyperbilirubinemia, *Pediatrics* 1985; **75** (suppl): 393–400.

26. Tan, K.L., Comparison of the efficacy of fiberoptic and conventional phototherapy for neonatal hyperbilirubinemia, *J. Pediatr.* 1994; **125**: 607–612.

27. Donzelli, G.P., Pratesi, S., Rapisardi, G., Agati. G., Fusi, F. and Pratesi R., 1-day phototherapy of neonatal jaundice with blue-green lamp [letter], *Lancet* 1995; **346**: 184–185.

28. Eggert, P. and Stick, C., The distribution of radiant power in a phototherapy unit equipped with a metal halide lamp, *Eur. J. Pediatr.* 1985; **143**: 224–225.

29. Seidman, D.S., Moise, J., Ergaz, Z. *et al.*, A new blue light emitting phototherapy device vs conventional phototherapy: a prospective randomized controlled application in term newborns, *Pediatr. Res.* 1998; **43**: 193A.

30. Vreman, H.J., Wong, R.J. and Stevenson, D.K., Light-emitting diodes: A novel light source for phototherapy, *Pediatr. Res.* 1998; **44**: 804–809.

31. Maisels, M.J., Bilirubin. On understanding and influencing its metabolism in the newborn infants, *Pediatr. Clin. North Am.* 1972; **19**: 447–447.

32. Maisels, M.J. and Newman, T.B., Kernicterus in otherwise healthy, breast-fed term newborns, *Pediatrics* 1995; **96**: 730–733.

33. Hansen, T.W.R., Acute management of extreme neonatal jaundice – the potential benefits of intensified phototherapy and interruption of enterohepatic bilirubin circulation, *Acta. Paediatr.* 1997; **86**: 843–846.

34. Holtrop, P.C., Ruedisueli, K. and Maisels, M.J., Double versus single phototherapy in low birth weight newborns, *Pediatrics* 1992; **90**: 674–677.

35. Eggert, L.D., Stick, C. and Schroeder, H., On the distribution of irradiation intensity in phototherapy. Measurements of effective irradiance in an incubator, *Eur. J. Pediatr.* 142, 58–61. 1984. (GENERIC). Ref Type: Generic.

36. Tan, K.L., Lim, G.C. and Boey, K.W., Efficacy of "high-intensity" blue-light and "standard" daylight phototherapy for non-haemolytic hyperbilirubinemia, *Acta. Paediatr.* 1992; **81**: 870–874.

37. Garg, A.K., Prasad, R.S. and Hifzi, I.A., A controlled trial of high-intensity double-surface phototherapy on a fluid bed versus conventional phototherapy in neonatal jaundice, *Pediatrics* 1995; **95**: 914–916.

38. Tan, K.L., Phototherapy for neonatal jaundice, *Clin. Perinatol.* 1991; **18**: 423–439.

39. George, P. and Lynch, M., Ohmeda Biliblanket vs Wallaby Phototherapy System for the reduction of bilirubin levels in the home-care setting, *Clin. Pediatr.* (Phila.) 1994; **33**: 178–180.

40. Schuman, A.J. and Karush, G., Fiberoptic vs conventional home phototherapy for neonatal hyperbilirubinemia, *Clin. Pediatr.* (Phila.) 1992; **31**: 345–352.

41. Tan, K.L., Efficacy of bidirectional fiberoptic phototherapy for neonatal hyperbilirbinemia, *Pediatrics* 1997; **99**: 5.

42. Tan, K.L., Efficacy of fluorescent daylight, blue, and green lamps in the management of non-hemolytic hyperbilirubinemia, *J. Pediatr.* 1989; **114**: 132–137.

43. Donzelli, G.P., Moroni, M., Pratesi, S., Rapisardi, G., Agati, G. and Fusi, F., Fibreoptic phototherapy in the management of jaundice in low birthweight neonates, *Acta. Paediatr.* 1996; **85**: 366–370.

44. Costello, S.A., Nyikal, J., Yu, V.Y. and McCloud, P., BiliBlanket phototherapy system versus conventional phototherapy: a randomized controlled trial in preterm infants [see comments], *J. Paediatr. Child Health* 1995; **31**: 11–13.

45. Rubaltelli, F.F., Zanardo, V. and Granati, B., Effect of various phototherapy regimens on bilirubin decrement, *Pediatrics* 1978; **61**: 838–841.

46. Maurer, H.M., Shumway, C.N., Draper, D.A. and Hossaini, A.A., Controlled trial comparing agar, intermittent phototherapy, and continuous phototherapy for reducing neonatal hyperbilirubinemia, *J.Pediatr.* 1973; **82**: 73–76.

47. Lau, S.P. and Fung, K.P., Serum bilirubin kinetics in intermittent phototherapy of physiological jaundice, *Arch. Dis. Child.* 1984; **59**: 892–894.

48. Wu, P.Y., Hodgman, J.E., Kirkpatrick, B.V., White, N.B.J and Bryla, D.A., Metabolic aspects of phototherapy, *Pediatrics* 1985; **75**: 427–433.

49. Slater, L and Brewer, M.F., Home versus hospital phototherapy for term infants with hyperbilirubinemia: A comparative study, *Pediatrics* 1984; **73**: 515–519.

50. Rogerson, A.G., Grossman, E.R., Gruber, H.S. and Boynton, R.C., Cuthbertson JG. 14 years of experience with home phototherapy, *Clin. Pediatr.* Phila. 1986; **25**: 296–299.
51. Meropol, S.B., Luberti, A.A., De Jong, A.R. and Weiss, J.C., Home phototherapy: use and attitudes among community pediatricians, *Pediatrics* 1993; **91**: 97–100.
52. Plastino, R., Buchner, D.M. and Wagner, E.H., Impact of eligibility criteria on phototherapy program size and cost, *Pediatrics* 1990; **85**: 796–800.
53. James, J., Williams, S.D. and Osborn, L.M., Home phototherapy for treatment of exaggerated neonatal jaundice enhances breast-feeding, *Am. J. Dis. Child.* (abstract) 1990; **144**: 431–432.
54. Hughes-Benzie, R., Uttley, D.A. and Heick, H.M., Crigler–Najjar syndrome type I: management with phototherapy crib mattress [letter], *Arch. Dis. Child.* 1993; **69**: 470.
55. Job, H., Hart, G. and Lealman, G., Improvements in long term phototherapy for patients with Crigler–Najjar syndrome type I, *Phys. Med. Biol.* 1996; **41**: 2549–2556.
56. Yohannan, M.D., Terry, H.J. and Littlewood, J.M., Long term phototherapy in Crigler–Najjar syndrome, *Arch. Dis. Child.* 1983; **58**: 460–462.
57. Silberberg, D.H., Johnson, L., Schutta, H. and Ritter L., Effects of photodegradation products of bilirubin on myelinating cerebellum cultures, *J. Pediatr.* 1970; **77**: 613–613.
58. Haddock, J.H. and Nadler, H.L., Bilirubin toxicity in human cultivated fibroblasts and its modification by light treatment, *Proc. Soc. Exp. Biol. Med.* 1970; **134**: 45–48.
59. Rosenstein, B.S. and Ducore, J.M., Enhancement by bilirubin of DNA damage induced in human cells exposed to phototherapy light, *Pediatr. Res.* 1984; **18**: 3–6.
60. Speck, W.T., Effect of phototherapy on fertilization and embryonic development, *Pediatr. Res.* 1979; **13**: 506–506.
61. Tonz. O., Vogt. J., Filippini, L., Simmler, F., Wachsmuth, E.D. and Winterhalter, K.H., Severe light dermatosis following phototherapy in a newborn infant with congenital erythropoietic urophyria, *Helv. Paediatr. Acta.* 1975; **30**: 47–56.
62. Mallon, E., Wojnarowska, F., Hope, P. and Elder, G., Neonatal bullous eruption as a result of transient porphyrinemia in a premature infant with hemolytic disease of the newborn, *J. Am. Acad. Dermatol.* 1995; **33**: 333–336.
63. Paller, A.S., Eramo, L.R., Farrell, E.E., Millard, D.D., Honig, P.J. and Cunningham, B.B., Purpuric phototherapy-induced eruption in transfused neonates: relation to transient porphyrinemia, *Pediatrics* 1997; **100**: 360–364.
64. Crawford, R.I., Lawlor, E.R. and Wadsworth, L.D., Transient erythroporphyria of infancy, *J. Am. Acad. Dermatol.* 1996; **35**: 833–834.
65. Kearns, G.L., Williams, B.J. and Timmons, O.D., Fluorescein phototoxicity in a premature infant, *J. Pediatr.* 1985; **107**: 796–798.
66. Hussain, K. and Sharief, N., Dermal injury following the use of fiberoptic phototherapy in an extremely premature infant, *Clin. Pediatr.* (Phila.) 1996; **35**: 421–422.
67. Siegfried, E.C., Stone, M.S. and Madison, K.C., Ultraviolet light burn: a cutaneous complication of visible light phototherapy of neonatal jaundice, *Pediatr. Dermatol.* 1992; **9**: 278–282.
68. Kappas, A. and Lucey, J., Treatment of Crigler–Najjar syndrome. Conference proceedings. New York: Rockefeller University, New York, 1996.
69. Kopelman, A.E., Brown, R.S. and Odell, G.B., The "bronze" baby syndrome: A complication of phototherapy, *J. Pediatr.* 1972; **81**: 466–466.
70. Rubaltelli, F.F., Jori, G. and Reddi, E., Bronze baby syndrome: A new porphyrin-related disorder, *Pediatr. Res.* 1983; **17**: 327–330.
71. Jori, G., Reddi, E. and Rubaltelli, F.F., Bronze baby syndrome: an animal model, *Pediatr. Res.* 1990; **27**: 22–25.
72. Clark, C.F., Torii, S., Hamamoto, Y. and Kaito, H., The "bronze baby" syndrome: postmortem data, *J. Pediatr.* 1976; **88**: 461–464.
73. Messner, K.H., Maisels, M.J. and Leure-DuPree, A.E., Phototoxicity to the newborn primate retina, *Invest. Ophthalmol. Vis. Sci.* 1978; **17**: 178–182.
74. Messner, K.H., Light toxicity to newborn retina, *Pediatr. Res.* 1978; **12**: 530.
75. Bhupathy, K., Sethupathy, R., Pildes, R.S. *et al.*, Electroretinography in neonates treated with phototherapy, *Pediatrics* 1978; **61**: 189–189.
76. Dobson, V., Coruett, R.M. and Riggs, L.A., Long-term effect of phototherapy on visual function, *J. Pediatr.* 1975; **86**: 555.
77. Roy, M.-S., Caramelli, C., Orquin, J. *et al.* Effects of early reduced light exposure on central visual development in preterm infants, *Acta. Paediatr.* 1999; **88**: 459–461.

78. Robinson, J., Moseley, M.J., Fielder, A. *et al.*, Light transmission measurements in phototherapy eye patches, *Arch. Dis. Child.* 1991; **66**: 59–61.
79. Fok, T.F., Wong, W. and Cheng, A.F., Use of eyepatches in phototherapy: effects on conjunctival bacterial pathogens and conjunctivitis, *Pediatr. Infect. Dis. J.* 1995; **14**: 1091–1094.
80. Drew, J.H., Marriage, K.J., Bayle, V.V., Bajraszewski, E. and McNamara, J.M., Phototherapy – short and long-term complications, *Arch. Dis. Child.* 1976; **54**: 454–454.
81. Ebbesen, F., Edelsten, D. and Hertel, J., Gut transit time and lactose malabsorption during photo-therapy. 2. A study using raw milk from the mothers of infants, *Acta. Paediatr. Scan.* 1980; **69**: 69–71.
82. Ebbesen, F., Edelsten, D. and Hertel, J., Gut transit time and lactose malabsorption during photo-therapy. I. A study using lactose-free human mature milk, *Acta. Paediatr. Scand.* 1980; **69**: 65–68.
83. Bujanover, Y., Schwartz, G., Milbauer, B. and Peled, Y., Lactose malabsorption is not a cause of diarrhea during phototherapy, *J. Pediatr. Gastroenterol. Nutr.* 1985; **4**: 196–198.
84. Jährig, K., Ballke, E.H., Koenig, A. and Meisel, P., Transepithelial electric potential difference in newborns undergoing phototherapy, *Pediatr. Res.* 1987; **21**: 283–284.
85. Dollberg, S., Atherton, H.D. and Hoath, S.B., Effect of different phototherapy lights on incubator characteristics and dynamics under three modes of servocontrol, *Am. J. Perinatol.* 1995; **12**: 55–60.
86. Oh, W. and Karecki, H., Phototherapy and insensible water loss in the newborn infant, *Am. J. Dis. Child.* 1972; **124**: 230–232.
87. Wu, P.Y.K. and Hodgman, J.E., Insensible water loss in preterm infants: Changes with post-natal development and non-ionizing radiant energy, *Pediatrics* 1974; **54**: 704–712.
88. Yao, A.C., Martinussen, M., Johansen, O.J. and Brubakk, A.M., Phototherapy-associated changes in mesenteric blood flow response to feeding in term neonates, *J. Pediatr.* 1994; **124**: 309–312.
89. Amato, M., Donati, F. and Markus, D. Cerebral hemodynamics in low-birth-weight infants treated with phototherapy, *Eur. Neurol.* 1991; **31**: 178–180.
90. Benders, M.J.N.L., van Bel, F. and van de Bor, M., The effect of phototherapy on cerebral blood flow velocity in preterm infants, *Acta. Paediatr.* 1998; **87**: 791.
91. Teberg, A.J., Hodgman, J.E. and Wu P.Y.K., Effect of phototherapy on growth of low birth weight infant – two year follow up, *J. Pediatr.* 1977; **91**: 92–95.
92. Lucey, J.F., Another view of phototherapy, *J. Pediatr.* 1974; **84**: 145–145.
93. Scheidt, P.C., Bryla, D.A., Nelson, K.B., Hirtz, D.G. and Hoffman, H.J., Phototherapy for neonatal hyperbilirubinemia: Six year follow-up of the NICHD clinical trial, *Pediatrics* 1990; **85**: 455–463.
94. Maisels, M.J., Neonatal jaundice, In: Avery, G.B., Fletcher, M.A. and MacDonald, M.G. Neonato-logy: pathophysiology and management of the newborn. 4th ed. Philadelphia: J.B.Lippincott, Co, 1999; 630–725.
95. Rosenfeld, W., Sadhev, S., Brunot, V., Jhavri, R., Zabaleta, I. and Evans, H.E., Phototherapy effect on the incidence of patent ductus arteriosus in premature infants: Prevention with chest shielding, *Pediatrics* 1986; **78**: 10–14.
96. Barefield, E.S., Dwyer, M.D. and Cassady, G., Association of patent ductus arteriosus and photo-therapy in infants weighing less than 1000 grams, *J. Perinatol.* 1993; **13**: 376–380.
97. Clyman, R.I. and Rudolph, A.M., Patent ductus arteriosus: a new light on an old problem, *Pediatr. Res.* 1978; **12**: 92–94.
98. Maisels, M.J., Neonatal jaundice, In: Avery, G.B., Fletcher, M.A. and MacDonald MG. Neonatol-ogy: pathophysiology and management of the newborn. J.B.Lippincott Co., 5th ed. Philadelphia, 1999; 765–820.
99. Maisels, M.J., Why use homeopathic doses of phototherapy? *Pediatrics* 1996; **98**: 283–287.

13 Pharmacological Approaches to the Prevention and Treatment of Neonatal Hyperbilirubinemia

Timos Valaes

Department of Pediatrics, Tufts University School of Medicine, Boston, Massachusetts, USA

Kernicterus – bilirubin encephalopathy – can and has been prevented but cannot be reversed once it has occurred. With prevention, in general, as the ratio of cases prevented to the number treated decreases, the risks and costs of treatment need to be minimized so that the risk-benefit and cost-benefit ratios remain favorable. The management strategies that succeeded in preventing kernicterus – exchange transfusion (ET) and phototherapy (PT) – in terms of simplicity and cost cannot be considered ideal. This is particularly true now that cost containment has led to early (<48 h) post-delivery discharge. In this environment the concern is not only the cost of monitoring neonatal jaundice and of readmission for the treatment of significant hyperbilirubinemia, but also the possibility of kernicterus as a consequence of early discharge and failure to detect and prevent dangerous hyperbilirubinemia in a timely fashion.[1]

Simply stated jaundice is always the result of bilirubin production exceeding bilirubin elimination. In the neonate an active enterohepatic circulation of bilirubin is an additional factor increasing the imbalance. The actual kinetics of these processes are complex but for the purpose of this discussion we will consider their effect on bilirubin balance. The total serum bilirubin concentration (TSB) at any time (t) during the first few days of life is related to the rate of *de novo* bilirubin production (a), the rate of bilirubin enterohepatic circulation (b) and the rate of bilirubin elimination (c) as shown in the following equation:

$$\mathrm{TSB}_t = \mathrm{TSB}_o + \sum (a + b)_t - \sum (c)_t \qquad (13.1)$$

where TSB_o represents cord blood TSB.

This equation indicates that an infinite combination of (a), (b) and (c) can result in the same TSB_t. Moreover the level of TSB and the direction and rate of change at a time point (t) does not depend on the absolute values of (a) or (b) or (c) but on the

---

Address for correspondence: 53 Demetrakopoulou Street, VOULA 166 73 GREECE, Tel/Fax: 301 8991702

level of imbalance between these factors. These factors are in constant flux in the newborn period with (*a*) and (*b*) decreasing and (*c*) increasing with age. The rate of change is related to a host of specific and nonspecific factors making clinical prediction of the course of neonatal hyperbilirubinemia difficult. Pharmacologic or other interventions should moderate the course of neonatal bilirubinemia if either the rate of the *de novo* bilirubin production (*a*) is reduced or the enterohepatic circulation of bilirubin (*b*) is curtailed or if bilirubin elimination (*c*) is promoted. The mechanism of action of a pharmacologic agent and the predominant pathogenetic mechanism of hyperbilirubinemia in a clinical group do not determine the efficacy of the agent in moderating the course of neonatal jaundice in the particular group. This should be obvious from the above Equation (13.1) and has been confirmed in clinical trials of all the agents tested so far. Expressing this fact differently we can state that every case of neonatal hyperbilirubinemia is multifactorial and its course can be modified by favorably shifting the contribution of any of the three factors (*a*, *b*, *c*) that according to Equation (13.1) determine the level of TSB.

In presenting the various pharmacologic agents that have been clinically tested for the prevention or treatment of neonatal jaundice, the chronological order of their clinical introduction will be followed rather than the order of the metabolic steps affected. Drugs used to promote hepatic bilirubin biotransformation will be presented before the recently introduced agents inhibiting bilirubin production. For a detailed account of the earlier efforts the reader is referred to previous reviews.[2,3]

PHARMACOLOGIC INDUCTION OF THE HEPATIC TRANSPORT OF BILIRUBIN

Hepatic enzyme induction has found a useful clinical application in the enhancement of hepatic transport of bilirubin when it is either genetically defective or transiently inadequate as in the newborn infant. Phenobarbital (PB) is known to be a strong inducer of hepatic enzymes while the long history of its use in pregnancy and the newborn period provided some assurance of safety. Patients with genetic defects in bilirubin clearance provided the first successful clinical application of PB. In fact the initial separation of Crigler–Najjar type I from type II (Arias syndrome) is based on the response of the latter to PB.[4] In adults with the type II defect treated with PB at a dose of ≥ 60 mg/day TSB decreased within a few days and a new steady state, at $\sim 50\%$ of the pretreatment level was reached after 2–3 weeks of treatment. On discontinuing treatment TSB increased gradually to return to the original pretreatment level again in 2–3 weeks. Studies in these patients as well as in rodents and primates proved that PB enhanced hepatic bilirubin transport by affecting all four steps (1) uptake from the circulation (2) intrahepatocyte binding or storage (3) conjugation with glucuronic acid (4) biliary excretion. Recently the sequencing of the gene encoding for the family of uridinediphosphoglucuronoside glucuronosyltransferase (UGT) isoforms illuminated important aspects of bilirubin metabolism, related genetic defects, and the effect of PB.[5]

Phenobarbital in Neonatal Bilirubinemia

Antenatal phenobarbital for the prevention of neonatal bilirubinemia

In 1968 Trölle reported a reduced incidence of jaundice in the neonates of epileptic or pre-eclamptic women treated with PB during pregnancy.[6] This observation was followed by a succession of studies[3] that led to the following conclusions: A daily dose of 60 to 100 mg of PB for at least 10 days before delivery reduced the 4th day TSB of term infants with no incompatibility by ~50% and a daily dose of 30 mg, even when treatment was started at 32 weeks of gestation, resulted in a smaller (~30%) reduction in TSB. In a study of 2863 Greek neonates, the administration of 100 mg PB daily for ≥ 10 days reduced the incidence of marked hyperbilirubinemia (TSB ≥ 16.0 mg/dl, 274 µmol/l) from all causes from 6.6% to 1.1% ($p < 0.0001$ OR 6.07, 95% CI 3.5–10.5) and the incidence of exchange transfusion from 1.4% in the controls to 0.23% in the PB treated group ($p = 0.0014$ OR 6.26, 95% CI 1.9–21.0).[7]

Postnatal phenobarbital for the prevention and treatment of neonatal bilirubinemia

PB at a dose of 5 to 10 mg/kg/day po or im for the first 4 to 5 days of life decreased the mean TSB concentration starting from the third day of treatment. The maximum effect was reached on the 5th day or later. Preventive postnatal PB significantly reduced the need for exchange transfusion in Rhesus hemolytic disease and in G6PD deficiency.[8,9] Therapeutic use of postnatal PB after the development of significant hyperbilirubinemia due to ABO incompatibility, G6PD deficiency or undetermined causes also reduced the need for ET.[10]

The combination of PB (10 mg/kg/day po) and diethylnicotinamide-coramine® (100 mg/kg/day po) was used successfully in central and eastern Europe to prevent significant hyperbilirubinemia in preterm infants and in Rhesus hemolytic disease.[3] Finally a combination of antenatal PB (≥ 3 days) and postnatal treatment for 3 to 5 days was found to be as effective in preventing non-specific hyperbilirubinemia as antenatal PB for ≥ 10 days.[11]

Safety of perinatal phenobarbital exposure

Barbiturates have been used frequently in pregnancy and the neonatal period. The most important immediate complication of the antenatal use of PB at a dose used for the prevention of neonatal hyperbilirubinemia is hemorrhagic disease of the newborn due to depression of the vitamin K-dependent clotting factors. Vitamin K_1 administration (1 mg im) at birth rapidly corrects the clotting abnormality.[12] This should be combined with administration of Vitamin K_1 10 mg im at the beginning of labor to protect the fetus from hemorrhage following intra-partum trauma. No sedation, withdrawal or behavioral changes have been documented following perinatal PB at the dose and schedules used for neonatal jaundice.

Because PB – and other enzyme inducing agents – lack specificity, it is difficult to exclude long-term untoward effects with confidence. Together with the hepatic transport of bilirubin, PB also accelerates other metabolic processes in the developing and the mature organism. Due to species-specific differences, animal observations can serve to raise the questions but cannot answer them. Follow up at 5–7 years of the Greek cohort showed either no difference from controls or some advantages for the PB group in physical growth, intelligence, fine motor and visuomotor integration.[7] A second follow up at the age of 15 to 17 years aiming at assessing sexual development and behavioral organization has been completed but a full analysis has not as yet been published.

Other Inducers of Hepatic Transport of Bilirubin

Flumicinol (Zixoryn®) is a non-sedative hepatic enzyme inducer that has been investigated in Europe and in limited clinical studies in the USA. The pharmacologic and clinical evidence so far does not indicate any advantage of Flumicinol over PB in terms of efficacy in ameliorating hyperbilirubinemia and it lacks the extensive animal and clinical work that has been done to establish the safety of PB.

AGENTS INTERCEPTING THE ENTEROHEPATIC CIRCULATION OF BILIRUBIN

After biliary excretion, bilirubin conjugates are hydrolyzed to unconjugated bilirubin which can be reabsorbed from the entire length of the bowel. This process is minimized after the establishment of bacterial flora that reduce bilirubin to urobilinogens.[13] Thus the contribution of the enterohepatic circulation to neonatal jaundice is expected to decrease as postnatal age advances, except when there are conditions that lead to a delay in the establishment of intestinal flora such as the use of broad spectrum antibiotics, exclusive parenteral nutrition and possibly breast feeding. Although there is clearly some contribution of the enterohepatic circulation of bilirubin to neonatal jaundice, the magnitude of this contribution in infants with significant hyperbilirubinemia is unknown. Attempts to interrupt the process with agents sequestering bilirubin in the bowel (charcoal, agar, cholestyramine) have failed to produce clinically significant reductions in TSB.[3] Preliminary data suggest that bilirubin oxidase (BOX) reduces bilirubin products in the stools, but the effect on the course of neonatal bilirubinemia is at best marginal.

DECREASING BILIRUBIN PRODUCTION BY INHIBITING HEME OXYGENASE

Heme oxygenase (HO) is the rate limiting enzyme in the enzymatic degradation of heme (ferroprotoporphyrin) to bilirubin, CO and iron, and certain synthetic metalloporphyrins, in which the central iron atom of heme is replaced by other metals, are capable of inhibiting HO activity and heme metabolism.[14] Tin-protoporphyrin (SnPP) and, more effectively, tin-mesoporphyrin (SnMP) will competitively inhibit HO. Because they have a much higher affinity than heme for the heme-binding site of

HO, these compounds competitively displace heme from its binding to HO. Moreover, in contrast to iron, tin does not activate oxygen and thus the metalloporphyrin is not metabolized and overall the production of bilirubin is decreased. The biliary excretion of heme is increased in equimolar fashion to the decreased excretion of bilirubin.[15] Thus, the inhibition of heme degradation to bilirubin does not lead to an accumulation of heme in the body. This is in agreement with other evidence that the formation of bilirubin is not indispensable for the elimination of the breakdown products of hemoglobin and other hemoproteins.[3]

The liver has the ability to excrete intact heme in the bile whenever the normal pathway for the formation of bilirubin is overwhelmed by an excessive heme load[16] or by inhibition of HO.[17] Nevertheless, in the adult, the contribution of the alternative pathway is normally negligible in contrast to the fetus and, to a lesser degree, the newborn when the alternative pathway is the predominant one in the bile. Reabsorbtion of heme from the bowel (most likely involving formation of bilirubin by intestinal HO) decreases the heme content of meconium relative to bile.[18]

In view of the above, administration of HO inhibitors in the neonatal period is expected to have complex effects on heme and bilirubin metabolism that include: (a) Intensification and prolongation of the alternative pathway – heme excretion in the bile with a commensurate reduction in bilirubin formation; (b) an increased in stool heme elimination both as a result of (a) and inhibition of intestinal HO resulting in reduced heme (and iron) reabsorbtion from the bowel[19] and (c) some degree of heme degradation by bacterial flora.[20] The time course of effects (b) and (c) are expected to be in the opposite direction. After a single systemic administration of a HO inhibitor, effect (b) is likely to be short-lived due to the rapid turnover rate of enterocytes, while effect (c) will be accentuated as more bacterial flora will populate the bowel as the infant ages. The predicted amelioration of hyperbilirubinemia[21] has been confirmed in a series of clinical trials involving all the important clinical groups[22–26] while a negative iron balance has been observed only after prolonged HO inhibitor administration.[27]

Clinical Trials of Heme Oxygenase Inhibitors to Moderate the Course of Neonatal Bilirubinemia

Clinical trials assessing the efficacy and safety initially of SnPP and subsequently of SnMP started in September 1985 and continue to this day. Because of its photophysical properties and stability, SnMP is the preferred HO inhibitor[28] and the only one currently in use in clinical trials. Randomized controlled trials in Coombs positive ABO incompatible term neonates showed that prophylactic administration of small doses of SnPP produced a decrease in the incremental change in TSB values (versus the control infants) that was apparent within 24 hours of administration of the drug.[22] In addition, SnPP reduced the need for phototherapy in the treated infants by 43%.

The issue of dosage and schedule of administration – single or split doses given 24 h apart – was addressed in six randomized, placebo-controlled, fully masked studies in which 517 preterm neonates (gestational age 210 to 251 days and birthweight 1500–2500 g) were enrolled.[23] Tin-mesoporphyrin was administered im within the

Timos Valaes

first 24 hours of life in doses of $1-6\,\mu$mol/kg (preventive use). At the highest dose used (6 μmol/kg) SnMP reduced PT requirements by 76% (vs controls) and at the same time maximum TSB was reduced by 19% and the area under the TSB curve by 43% (Figure 13.1). A dose-dependent shift to the left (lower) of the distribution of maximum TSB values was observed without a change in the age at which maximum TSB values were reached. This indicates that SnMP did not delay the postnatal improvement in bilirubin elimination. With the step-wise dose increase up to 6 μmol/kg there was no indication that the point of diminishing returns had been reached. It is likely that higher doses will result in a further increase in efficacy. There appears to be no advantage of split doses over a single dose of the same total amount but the issue of repeat doses in selected cases was not addressed.

The only short-term untoward effect of SnMP treatment was an increased frequency in PT-associated photosensitivity erythema from 1.6% in the control group to 13% in the SnMP group that were treated with special blue light ($p = 0.0005$ OR 9.5, 95% CI 2.1–42). All five treated infants that accidentally received white light PT developed erythema. The erythema appeared within the first 24 hours after initiation of PT and its frequency was unrelated to dose or time interval between SnMP administration and initiation of PT. The erythema subsided 24–48 h later without blistering, desquamation or discoloration even in the cases where PT was continued. Thus

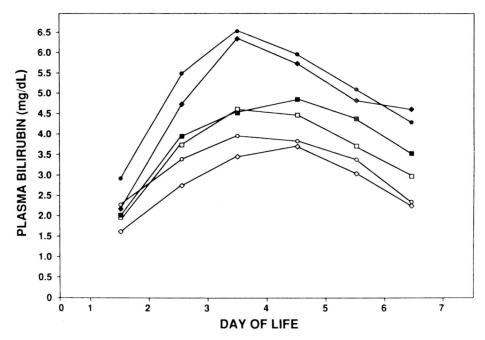

Figure 13.1. Effect of increasing doses of SnMP on the mean increase in plasma bilirubin concentration (actual values – value at enrollment) in the control and tin-mesoporphyrin treated groups Control ●; SnMP₁ ◆; SnMP₂ ☐; SnMP₃ ■; SnMP₄ ○; SnMP₆ ◇; SnMP₁–SnMP₆ refer to doses of SnMP in μmol/kg. From Valaes *et al.*[23]

erythema was an unpredictable, self-limited and clinically insignificant reaction to combined SnMP and PT treatment.

The efficacy of special blue light PT and SnMP (6 μmol/kg/birthweight) to control established hyperbilirubinemia (therapeutic use) has been compared in 2 randomized studies.[24,25] In the first, healthy term and in the second near term (35–37⁶⁄₇ weeks) neonates were enrolled. Direct Coombs positive and G6PD deficient infants were excluded. None of the neonates required ET and switch-over to PT was not required for any treated with SnMP. In both the intrapair and intergroup analyses SnMP proved the superior treatment on the basis of shorter (by ~30) hours length of required observation, fewer bilirubin measurements and shorter hospital stay. Similar results were obtained in another group of term breast fed infants where the use of SnMP entirely eliminated the need for PT to control hyperbilirubinemia.[25]

Finally in a randomized sequentially analyzed trial in a cohort of G6PD deficient neonates the preventive (first day of life) and therapeutic (if and when an age-specific threshold TSB was reached) use of SnMP (6 μmol/kg) were compared. Irrespective of trial arm, none of the 86 enrolled neonates required ET or PT while 20 of 60 G6PD deficient infants in a previous cohort in the same population studied with the same methods required PT and one infant required two ET. In the intrapair analyses preventive use appeared to be superior to therapeutic intervention with SnMP.

Overall, in the trials completed so far 681 neonates have received SnPP or SnMP and, of these, 374 received 6 μmol/kg SnMP. At this dose PT was not required for any of the 312 term or near term infants. Apart from the increased incidence of photosensitivity erythema following PT, comprehensive examinations at 3 and 18 months of corrected age and surveillance at 5 years using a structured telephone interview (completed for about half of the enrolled infants so far) have failed to raise any suspicion of short or long-term untoward effects due to SnPP or SnMP.

DECREASING BILIRUBIN PRODUCTION BY INHIBITING HEMOLYSIS

Controlled trials have confirmed that the administration of IVIG to infants with Rh hemolytic disease will significantly reduce the need for exchange transfusion.[29–31] IVIG will also likely mitigate the course of severe ABO hemolytic disease.[32] The doses have ranged from 500 mg/kg given over 2 hours soon after birth to 800 mg/kg given daily for 3 days. Anti D coated erythrocytes are removed from the circulation through antibody-dependent lysis by cells of the reticuloendothelial system. The mechanism of action of IVIG is unknown, but it is possible that it might alter the course of Rh hemolytic disease by blocking Fc receptors, thus inhibiting hemolysis.

CONCLUSIONS AND RECOMMENDATIONS

With the exception of the Crigler–Najjar syndrome, neonatal jaundice is a self-resolving condition and all methods of management aim at gaining time, while preserving life and neurological integrity, until the problem is resolved. ET replaces vulnerable with normal red cells and is still the management of choice for severe hemolysis due to isoimmunization or G6PD deficiency (see Chapters 5,10,11). In all other cases, the TSB threshold for action should take into consideration the clinical group, the age of the infant (in hours) and the time-frame of action of the available methods of intervention. The effect of ET on TSB is immediate and dramatic and this intervention should be used when kernicterus is imminent. Intensive PT can influence the course of neonatal hyperbilirubinemia fairly rapidly. We suspect that the effect of SnMP is slower in the first few hours but, 24 h after its administration, the effect on hyperbilirubinemia is equal to that of PT. However SnMP is superior to PT as its action is sufficiently long-lasting to cover the critical period with a single dose and the time of necessary observation is shorter. Sick preterm infants and those remaining NPO and on antibiotics are the exception to this statement. For these cases, PT is the intervention of choice. Whether the ultimate solution to neonatal hyperbilirubinemia can be achieved by giving SnMP to all neonates at the time of birth, depends on whether the accumulating experience with SnMP reaches the level of efficacy and safety already achieved by vitamin K prophylaxis for hemorrhagic disease of the newborn.

References

1. Brown, A.K. and Johnson, L., Loss of concern about jaundice and the reemergence of kernicterus in full-term infants in the era of managed care. In: Fanaroff, A.A., Klaus, M. eds. *Yearbook of Neonatal and perinatal Medicine* Mosby, St. Louis MI, 1996, pp. XVII–XXVIII.
2. Vaisman, S.L. and Gartner, L.M., Pharmacologic treatment of neonatal hyperbilirubinemia, *Clin. Perinatol.* 1975; **2**: 37–58.
3. Valaes, T. and Harvey-Wilkes, K., Pharmacologic approaches to the prevention and treatment of neonatal hyperbilirubinemia, *Clin. Perinatol.* 1990; **17**: 245–273.
4. Arias, I.M., Gartner, L.M., Cohen, M., Ben-Ezzer, J. and Levi, A.J., Chronic nonhemolytic unconjugated hyperbilirubinemia with glucuronyl transferase deficiency: clinical biochemical, pharmacological, and genetic evidence for heterogeneity, *Am. J. Med.* 1969; **47**: 395–409.
5. Roy-Chowdhury, J., Roy-Chowdhury, N., Wolkoff, A.W. and Arias, I.M., Heme and bile pigment metabolism. In: Arias, I.M., Boyer, J.L., Fausto, N., Jakoby, W.B., Schachter, D.A. and Shafritz, D.A. eds. *The Liver biology and Pathology.* 3rd ed. Raven Press, New York, N.Y. 1994, pp. 471–504.
6. Trölle D., Phenobarbitone and neonatal icterus, *Lancet* 1968; **1**: 251–252.
7. Valaes, T., Kipouros, K., Petmezaki, S., Solman, M. and Doxiadis, S.A., Effectiveness and safety of prenatal phenobarbital for the prevention of neonatal jaundice, *Pediatr. Res.* 1980; **14**: 947–952.
8. McMullin, G.P., Hayes, M.F. and Arora, S.C., Phenobarbitone in Rhesus hemolytic disease, *Lancet* 1970; **2**: 949–952.
9. Meloni, T., Cagnuzzo, G. and Dove, A., Phenobarbital for prevention of hyperbilirubinemia in glucose-6-phosphate dehydrogenase-deficient newborn infants, *J. Pediatr.* 1973; **82**: 1048–1051.
10. Yeung, C.Y. and Field, E., Phenobarbitone therapy in neonatal hyperbilirubinaemia, *Lancet* 1969; **2**: 135–139.
11. Trölle, D., Decrease of total serum bilirubin concentration in newborn infants after phenobarbitone treatment, *Lancet* 1968; **2**: 705–708.
12. Valaes, T. and Petmezaki, S., Disturbance of coagulation in the newborn following phenobarbital administration in the last part of pregnancy, *Iatriki* 1973; **24**: 325–332 (in Greek).
13. Billing, B.H., Intestinal and renal metabolism of bilirubin including enterohepatic circulation. In: Ostrow, J.D., ed. *Bile pigments and jaundice.* New York and Basel: Marcel Dekker Inc., 1986, pp. 255–269.
14. Drummond, G.S., Valaes, T. and Kappas A., Control of bilirubin production by synthetic heme analogs: Pharmacologic and toxicologic considerations, *J. Perinatol.* 1996; **16**: 572–579.

15. Kappas, A., Simionatto, C.S., Drummond, G.S, Sassa, S. and Anderson, K.E., The liver excretes large amounts of heme into bile when heme oxygenase is inhibited competitively by Sn-protoporphyrin, *Proc. Natl. Acad. Sci. USA* 1985; **82**: 896–900.

16. McCormack, L.R., Liem, H.H., Strum, W.B, Grundy, S.M. and Müller-Eberhart U., Effects of haem infusion on biliary secretion of porphyrins, haem and bilirubin in man, *Eur. J. Clin. Invest.* 1982; **12**: 257–262.

17. Berglund, L., Angelin, B., Blomstrand, R., Drummond, G.S. and Kappas, A., Sn-protoporphyrin lowers serum bilirubin levels decreases biliary bilirubin output, enhances biliary heme excretion and potently inhibits microsomal heme oxygenase activity in normal human subjects, *Hepatology* 1988; **8**: 625–631.

18. Valaes, T., Drummond, G.S. and Louis, F., Variation in heme metabolism and bilirubin production as determinants of neonatal bilirubinemia. In: Xanthou, M. and Bracci, R., eds. *Neonatal Haematology and Immunology* Amsterdam Excerpta Medica 1990, pp. 71–78.

19. Böni, R.E., Huch-Böni, R.A., Galbraith, R.A. *et al.*, Tin-mesoporphyrin inhibits heme oxygenase activity and heme-iron absorption in the intestine, *Pharmacology* 1993; **47**: 318–329.

20. Engel, R.B., Matsen, J.M. and Chapman, S.S. Carbon monoxide production from heme compounds by bacteria, *J. Bacteriol.* 1972; **1120**: 1310–1315.

21. Drummond, G.S. and Kappas, A., Prevention of neonatal hyperbilirubinemia by tin protoporphyrin IX, a potent competitive inhibitor of heme oxidation, *Proc. Natl. Acad. Sci. USA* 1981; **78**: 6466–6470.

22. Kappas, A., Drummond, G.S., Manola, T., Petmezaki, S. and Valaes, T., Sn-protoporphyrin use in the management of hyperbilirubinemia in term newborns with direct Coombs-positive ABO incompatibility, *Pediatrics* 1988; **81**: 485–497.

23. Valaes, T., Petmezaki, S., Henschke, C., Drummond, G.S. and Kappas, A., Control of jaundice in preterm newborns by an inhibitor of bilirubin production: studies with tin-mesoporphyrin, *Pediatrics* 1994; **93**: 1–11.

24. Kappas, A., Drummond, G.S., Henschke, C. and Valaes, T., Direct comparison of Sn-mesoporphyrin, an inhibitor of bilirubin production, and phototherapy in controlling hyperbilirubinemia in term and near-term newborns, *Pediatrics* 1995; **95**: 468–444.

25. Martinez, J.C., Garcia, H.O., Otheguy, L.E. *et al.*, Control of severe hyperbilirubinemia in full-term newborns with the inhibitor of bilirubin production Sn-mesoporphyrin (SnMP), *Pediatrics* 1999; **03**: 1–5.

26. Valaes, T., Drummond, G.S. and Kappas, A., Control of hyperbilirubinemia in glucose-6-phosphate dehydrogenase-deficient newborns using and inhibitor of bilirubin production, Sn-mesoporphyrin, *Pediatrics* 1998; **101**(5): 5URL: http://www.pediatrics.org/cgi/content/full/101/5/el

27. Kappas, A., Drummond, G.S. and Galbraith, R.A., Prolonged clinical use of a heme oxygenase inhibitor: Hematological evidence for an inducible but reversible iron-deficiency state, *Pediatrics* 1993; **91**: 537–539.

28. Delaney, J.K., Manzerall, D., Drummond, G.S. and Kappas, A., Photophysical properties of Sn-protoporphyrins: Potential clinical implications, *Pediatrics* 1988; **81**: 498–504.

29. Dagoglu, T., Ovali, F., Samanci, N. *et al.*, High-dose intravenous immunoglobulin therapy for haemolytic disease, *J. Internat. Med. Res.* 1995; **23**: 264–271.

30. Voto, L.S., Sexer, H., Ferreiro, G. *et al.*, Neonatal adminstration of high-dose intravenous immunoglobulin and rhesus hemolytic disease, *J. Perinat. Med.* 1995; **23**: 443–451.

31. Rubo, J., Albrecht, K., Lasch, P. *et al.*, High-dose intravenous immune globulin therapy for hyperbilirubinemia caused by Rh hemolytic disease, *J. Pediatr.* 1992; **121**: 93–99.

32. Hammerman, C., Kaplan, M., Vreman, H.J. and Stevenson, D.K., Intravenous immune globulin in neonatal ABO isoimmunization: Factors associated with clinical efficacy, *Biol. Neonate.* 1996; **70**: 69–74.

Index